Dementia Care

To Edwin and Eileen Adams,
and to Gary and Elizabeth Witchell

For Baillière Tindall

Publishing manager: Jacqueline Curthoys
Project manager: Ewan Halley
Project development editor: Karen Gilmour
Design direction: Judith Wright
Project controller: Pat Miller
Marketing manager: Hilary Brown

Dementia Care

Developing Partnerships in Practice

Edited by

Trevor Adams MSc RMN RGN CertEd CPNCert
Lecturer, European Institute of Health and Medical Sciences,
University of Surrey, Guildford, UK

Charlotte L. Clarke BA PhD MSc PGCE RN
Research Fellow, University of Northumbria at Newcastle,
Newcastle upon Tyne, UK

Foreword by

Caroline Cantley BSc PhD DipSW
Director, Dementia North,
Newcastle upon Tyne, UK

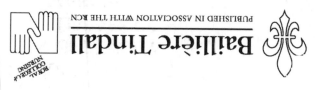

Baillière Tindall

PUBLISHED IN ASSOCIATION WITH THE RCN

LONDON EDINBURGH NEW YORK PHILADELPHIA SYDNEY TOKYO TORONTO

Baillière Tindall
An imprint of Harcourt Publishers Limited

© Harcourt Brace and Company Limited 1999
© Harcourt Publishers Limited 2001

First published 1999
  Reprinted 2001

ISBN 0 7020 2278 0

British Library of Cataloguing in Publication Data
A catalogue record for this book is available from the British Library

Library of Congress Cataloging in Publication Data
A catalog record for this book is available from the Library of Congress

Note
Medical knowledge is constantly changing. As new information becomes
available, changes in treatment, procedures, equipment and the use of
drugs become necessary. The authors and the publishers have, as far as it
is possible, taken care to ensure that the information given in this text is
accurate and up to date. However, readers are strongly advised to
confirm that the information, especially with regard to drug usage,
complies with the latest legislation and standards of practice.

The
publisher's
policy is to use
**paper manufactured
from sustainable forests**

Printed in China

Contents

Contributors

Trevor Adams MSc RMN RGN CertEd CPNCert
Lecturer, European Institute of Health and Medical Sciences, University of Surrey, Guildford, UK

Christine E. Carter BSc RMN
Mental Health Lecturer, St Bartholomew's School of Nursing and Midwifery, City University, London, UK

Charlotte L. Clarke BA PhD MSc PGCE RN
Research Fellow, Faculty of Health, Social Work and Education, University of Northumbria at Newcastle, Newcastle upon Tyne, UK

Jane Crisp BA MA PhD
Senior Lecturer, School of Film, Media and Cultural Studies, Griffith University, Nathan 411, Australia

Jane Gilliard BA CQSW
Director, Dementia Voice, Blackberry Hill Hospital, Bristol, UK

Malcolm Goldsmith BSocSc
Rector of St Cuthbert's Episcopal Church, Edinburgh; formerly Research Fellow, Dementia Services Development Centre, University of Stirling, UK

Mick Hill MA DipNurs RGN RMN RNT CertEd
Senior Lecturer, Faculty of Health, Social Work and Education, University of Northumbria at Newcastle, Newcastle upon Tyne, UK

John Keady DipPP RMN RNT CertEd
Lecturer in Nursing, School of Nursing and Midwifery, University of Wales, Bangor, Fron Heulog, Bangor, Gwynedd, Wales, UK

Ruth Lesser BA BSc PhD FRCSLT
Professor, Department of Speech, University of Newcastle, Newcastle upon Tyne, UK

Liz Matthew MA RMN RN CPNCert
Directorate Manager, Mental Health Services Older People, Community and Priority Services NHS Trust, Tameside General Hospital, UK

Kevin J. McKee BSc PhD Cpsychol
Lecturer, Centre for Aging and Rehabilitation Studies, University of Sheffield, Northern General Hospital, Sheffield, UK

Tracy Packer RGN
Development Nurse (Dementia Services), Blackberry Hill Hospital, Bristol, UK

Lisa Perkins PhD RCSLT
Research Associate, Department of Speech, University of Newcastle, Newcastle upon Tyne, UK

Jan Reed BA PhD RN CertMoralPhil
Professor of Health Care for Older People, Faculty of Health, Social Work and Education, University of Northumbria at Newcastle, Newcastle upon Tyne, UK

Jill Walton BSc MSc RGN
Chorleywood Bottom, Chorleywood, Hertfordshire, UK

Anne Whitworth BappSci MA PhD
Director Clinical Education, University of Newcastle upon Tyne, Newcastle, UK

Foreword

Partnership between professional practitioners and service users is important in much health and welfare provision. Practitioners in many fields have embraced this idea with enthusiasm. However, they have often found that achieving successful partnerships is complicated.

In dementia care, ideas about partnership have been slow to develop. Most efforts to develop partnerships have focused on practitioners and carers. Now ideas about partnerships are being extended to include people with dementia themselves. Their inclusion brings many new considerations and challenges.

In this book, Trevor Adams and Charlotte Clarke provide a timely review of the issues. Everyone involved in working to improve the lives of people with dementia will be concerned with their central questions: how can practitioners, carers and people with dementia work together for better dementia care? How can we ensure that we value and share the knowledge, skills, and experience of all parties?

Trevor Adams and Charlotte Clarke address these issues of partnership from a variety of angles. From a theoretical perspective, the book discusses the knowledge bases and 'discourses' that shape dementia care. From a research perspective, there is discussion of paradigms, methodologies and substantive findings with practice relevance. From a practice perspective, there is a particular focus on how better to engage and communicate with people with dementia. Throughout the book the authors seek to understand the different perspectives of people with dementia, of carers and of health-care practitioners. Approaching the issues from a variety of angles in this way advances our understanding and generates new thinking about the development of care.

There is currently substantial energy and enthusiasm for change. The commitment and values of practitioners are significant factors in bringing about improvements in care. The drive for 'evidence-based' practice means that it is increasingly important for developments to be underpinned by sound theory and research. This book demonstrates the value of linking theory, research and practice in exploring partnerships in dementia care.

Practitioners, students and researchers in the field of dementia care will find this a thought-provoking collection. It will be a valuable resource in stimulating ideas, debate and innovation in practice.

Caroline Cantley BSc, PhD, DipSW

Introduction

A PARTNERSHIP APPROACH TO DEMENTIA CARE

Promoting a partnership approach to health and social care will, at present, raise few eyebrows, supported as it is by policy directives which articulate the benefits of such an approach in both service planning and care delivery (Audit Commission, 1992; Department of Health, 1994). However, the reality of such an apparently well-intentioned idea as 'partnership' is that frustration and confusion may be generated in all parties to the extent that its implementation may be superficial in the extreme. The area of dementia care is particularly complex, and problems become exacerbated so that even the most straightforward of issues are fraught with technical difficulties. Indeed, identifying who it is that could be in partnership is worthy of some explication. Recently the term 'partnership' has been used with reference to interagency and interprofessional collaboration, but we wish to break away from this level of organisational and practice cooperation and devote our attention in the book to a partnership between the person with dementia, family members and professional carers. This interpretation of partnership allows sensitivity to the position of those who are experiencing dementia and who are users of health and social care services.

Dementia care services have been the concern of agencies for some time. The reasons are probably multiple:

- An increase in the proportion of the population that is vulnerable to developing dementia, i.e. older people
- A concern to manage limited health-care resources, in particular for those with chronic illnesses who are heavy users of health and social care
- A recognition that the medical model of health care has limited application in some aspects of dementia management, since 'cure' is not an option
- A challenge to the therapeutic nihilism associated with older people and chronic mental health problems which has perpetuated passivity and pessimism for people with dementia.

Furthermore, the visibility of the role of family carers in Western societies has changed significantly in recent decades, from that of unseen but assumed supporter, to becoming, at times, the primary focus of intervention from health and social care organisations.

One response to these issues has been the development of care models as alternatives, or complements, to the traditional medical model. These alternative models seek to raise the profile of the contribution of psychological and social phenomena in the construction and management of dementia care. These approaches have often been 'closed down' by biomedical research, which seeks to examine the significant physiological and biochemical changes occurring in dementia. However, people possess different ways of knowing about dementia, although they may lack the means to articulate that knowledge in a way which is 'scientifically' credible. These alternative, non-medical, ways of understanding dementia are possessed by nurses and therapists who have sustained contact with someone with dementia, and by family carers. Moreover, there is a knowledge of dementia that belongs to individuals themselves. All these people therefore possess forms of knowledge which are at times marginalised within a biomedical framework, but which are derived from the lived experiences of being, or being with, someone with dementia.

This book is intended to highlight these differing forms of knowledge of dementia and dementia care, and to make them visible. There is an arrogance in assuming that one's own knowledge is the only one that is relevant to a situation, and that knowledge is complete. Exposing the myth of such a stance is the intention of this book. The features of these differing knowledges can be located in three areas: philosophy, practice and policy.

• Philosophy

There has been a substantial shift towards the recognition of psychosocial aspects of dementia care, promoted through the work of writers such as Gubrium (1986), Fox (1989) and Hanson (1989, 1997). However, the approach is particularly indebted to the work of Tom Kitwood (1997) and his associates at the University of Bradford. Kitwood has put forward a view of dementia care that has brought about a radical shift in the thinking of health-care professionals and family carers about the nature of dementia and the ways in which the care of people with dementia should be provided and evaluated. Above all, he has brought into the discussion the people with dementia themselves, who were previously lost in a welter of neuronal and neurochemical deficits. This shift towards recognising the person despite their dementia is a central feature of alternative ways of knowing of dementia.

● Practice

The move towards developing psychosocial interventions for people with dementia probably began in the late 1970s and the early 1980s with the work of Pattie and Gilleard (1979) who developed rating scales, for example the Clifton Assessment Procedures for the Elderly (CAPE) scale, to measure the effectiveness of psychosocial interventions for people with dementia. The 1980s heralded the development of reality orientation and later validation therapy, which provided therapeutic intervention to help people with dementia, and therefore challenged the prevailing idea of 'therapeutic nihilism'. More recently, Kitwood's work on personhood has supported the development of dementia care mapping (a person-centred approach to dementia care) and the development of 'a new culture of dementia' (Fox, 1995; Kitwood and Benson, 1995). Through work such as that of Cheston (1996), Sutton (1997) and Meisen and Jones (1997), it is hoped that the momentum towards psychosocial approaches to dementia care will be maintained, and practice will continue to develop.

● Policy

The social orientation to dementia and dementia care has taken place at a time when the main health and social policy thrust has been towards the provision of care in the community. This is one reason why dementia care has had to take account of the individual within the context of the family as well as wider social contexts. Dementia care also accommodates many professional groups, and whilst seeking to remain distant from biomedical knowledge of dementia, it must be recognised that the medical profession have made a considerable contribution to the establishment of multidisciplinary teams of practitioners. In support of these policy changes, there has been a growth in infrastructure to promote changes in dementia care practice. For example, in Britain a major contribution has been made by the Dementia Services Development Centre at Stirling University since its inception in the 1980s. More recently, there has been a move to establish a network of centres throughout Britain, with centres being located in Bristol, Newcastle upon Tyne and elsewhere. We look forward to the work that these newly established centres will undertake in the future development of dementia care.

It is not the intention of this book to provide answers to any of the multitude of questions about dementia and dementia care, nor is it our belief that this is possible. This book will perhaps raise only more questions about working in partnership in dementia care, but we hope it will initiate debates among the practitioners who read it. These debates can only be initiated here; they must be brought alive by practitioners and researchers in the area. The only answers will be found as the debates are addressed to each and every person with dementia and their families, for each situation is different, possessing as it does its own personal and historical context which is richer and denser than any tapestry of care that can be depicted here. This is a task for all of us who aspire to develop care for people with dementia.

Trevor Adams
Charlotte Clarke

REFERENCES

Audit Commission (1992) *The Community Revolution: Personal Social Services and Community Care*. London: HMSO.

Cheston, R. (1996) Stories and metaphors: talking about the past in a psychotherapy group for people with dementia. *Ageing and Society* **16**, 579–602.

Department of Health (1994) *Working in Partnership: A Collaborative Approach to Care*. London: HMSO.

Fox, L. (1995) Mapping the advance of the new culture in dementia care. In: Kitwood, T. & Benson, S. (eds) *The New Culture of Dementia Care*. London: Hawker.

Fox, P. (1989) From senility to Alzheimer's disease: the rise of Alzheimer's disease movement. *Millbank Quarterly* **67**, 58–103.

Gubrium, J. (1986) *Old Timers and Alzheimer's: the Descriptive Organisation of Senility*. Greenwich: JAI Press.

Hanson, B. (1989) Definitional deficit: a model of senile dementia in context. *Family Process* **28**, 281–298.

Hanson, B. (1997) Who's seeing whom? General systems theory and constructivist implications for senile dementia intervention. *Journal of Aging Studies* **11** (1), 15–25.

Kitwood, T. (1997) *Dementia Reconsidered*. Buckingham: Open University Press.

Kitwood, T. & Benson, S. (1995) *The New Culture of Dementia Care*. London: Hawker.

Meisen, B. & Jones, G.M.M. (1997) *Care-giving in Dementia: Research and Applications*, Vol. 2. London: Routledge.

Pattie, A.H. & Gilleard, C. (1979) *Manual of the Clifton Assessment Procedures for the Elderly (CAPE)*. Kent, Hodder & Stoughton.

Sutton, L. (1997) *Whose memory is it anyway?* PhD dissertation, University of Southampton.

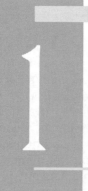

Dementia care partnerships: knowledge, ownership and exchange

Charlotte L. Clarke

KEY ISSUES

- There are differing knowledges of dementia, dementia care and the person with dementia

- It is a myth that any single knowledge base represents an entire and relevant knowledge

- Sharing of knowledge may result in effective interventions but is fraught with moral, ethical and practical problems

- Partnerships in care move beyond consensus and collaboration to a mutual appreciation of each other's knowledge

INTRODUCTION

In seeking a partnership in care between people with dementia, family carers and professional carers, there is a need to articulate some of the tensions that have dogged development in this area. Years have been spent, for example, in seeking the best ways to ensure compliance with a professional knowledge base. Lip-service has been paid to user involvement in collaborative developments, and consensus has been sought where there can be none if the full mosaic of diversity of knowledge is acknowledged.

Control, and power, in health and social care has been vested in those whose knowledge has been most prized. From this arises a continuum, ranging from a single, highly prized knowledge base which seeks compliance (people with dementia being profoundly powerless), to multiple, equally prized knowledge bases which provide the foundation for a partnership in care. At intermediate points along this continuum are consensus and collaboration, which have the potential for partnership but which risk superficiality in their implementation.

Powell-Cope (1994) argues that a partnership in health-care relationships exceeds the undirectionality of 'caring'. It is an interactive process in which all parties expect their knowledge to be received with 'respect and regard', and each works towards a relationship in which such knowledges can be therapeutically exchanged. The difficult issues which have obstructed the development of meaningful partnerships between professionals, people with dementia and their family carers centre around the varying domains of knowing of dementia and dementia care. The implications for dementia care of each domain of knowledge is presented in Table 1.1, but it is acknowledged that to portray such information in tabular form makes the divisions in knowledge too fixed and absolute, and belies the more probable situation of fluid exchange between knowledge domains. In brief, a pathophysiological domain emphasises the inevitable decline of individuals and their relationships such that the professional view is held as dominant. A psychosocial domain emphasises the socially constructed view of dementia and family caring as a burden such that the view of the person with dementia may be marginalised. An interactional (and also constructivist) domain emphasises the importance of the relationships held by the person with dementia such that an emphasis is placed on working alongside them. A socio-critical domain emphasises the need to emancipate people with dementia from care activities that underline dependency and loss of self, such that care partnerships can be actively negotiated.

This chapter presents a broad picture of the contemporary knowledge of dementia care, family caregiving and partnership. Drawing on a wide professional and theoretical literature base, various positions of knowledge are put forward and their implications for working in partnership explored. In seeking to span the areas of knowledge held as well as to open debates about the complexities of sharing knowledge, it has to be hoped that each individual issue is not swept past without due attention. The intention is only to initiate thoughts. It is the purpose of subsequent chapters to add depth and explore issues in all their richness.

KNOWING ABOUT DEMENTIA AND DEMENTIA CARE
Dementia: physical, social and political aspects

'Dementia' is an evolving concept whose definition has changed over time. For example, in the eighteenth century dementia was not defined specifically as a cognitive deficit nor associated with a particular age group (Berrios, 1987). In contemporary Western society there are two ways in which the term 'dementia' is used (Lishman, 1987): first, as a general term indicative of a single clinical entity; second, as a specific term indicative of one of a variety of pathological disorders. As a specific term, dementia

Table 1.1 Differential knowledge domains of dementia care

Domain	Pathophysiological	Psychosociological	Interactional	Sociocritical
Causality and diagnosis of dementia	Physical cause. Early identification sought as an essential precursor to treatment	Physical cause with social and psychological influences. Socially 'different' and cognitively incompetent	Emphasis on the social creation of dementia. Diagnosis may undermine self and relationships	Dementia socially and culturally constructed. Diagnosis may be empowering
Trajectory of future	Dementia medicalised. Emphasis on inevitable decline	Although no 'cure', symptoms and behaviours can be managed	Positive future through continuance of relationships	Continuance of 'person'
Role of person with dementia	Objectified. Views not sought. Denied part in decisions about care. No recognition of 'self'	Stigmatised. Limited choice offered. 'Self' severely affected	Some involvement in decision-making. 'Self' defined through relationship with others	Views fully sought. Given real opportunity to participate in decisions. 'Self' acknowledged
Role of family carer	Caring seen as a chore. Regarded as a semiprofessional	Caring seen as a necessary burden. Regarded as a co-client or resource	Caring seen as part of family relationship. Reciprocity important	May become a 'superseded' carer. Carer is an inappropriate term
Role of health and social care professional	Care focus on needs of family carer. Interventions emphasise 'geriatric routine', containment, pharmaceutical management, carer education and search for a cure	Aim to 'bring back' person with dementia. Interventions emphasise the 'real' world, e.g. reality orientation	Individualized care sought within family context. Interventions emphasise self-validation and life history work	Able to appreciate and work with 'other' realities. Interventions may seek to work with the individuals as active members of social framework, e.g. family therapy
Degree of partnership	Professional view dominant. Patient compliance sought	Professional and family carer views dominant. Collaboration/consensus sought	Some voice afforded to person with dementia. Consensus and partnership sought	Equality of each party. Partnership actively negotiated

includes those distinct diseases that have received recognition to date, for example\Alzheimer's diseasè, Pick's disease, diffuse Lewy body disease, vascular dementia and Huntington's chorea.

Neuropathologically, dementia is viewed as a progressively deteriorating condition, its diagnosis depending on an arbitrary dividing line drawn at some point in a continuum of disability. Consequently, prevalence depends upon where that line is drawn to demarcate normal ageing from dementia (Clarke, 1995), and is subject to the line being 'redrawn' as assessment techniques become more sophisticated, earlier diagnosis becomes increasingly sought, and society adjusts its definitions of 'normal' and 'abnormal'.

Identifying the prevalence of dementia is complicated by both the difficulty of defining dementia and methodological issues such as the cultural transferability of assessment tools (Ineichen, 1996). However, one widely acknowledged feature of dementia is that its incidence rises markedly with age. Hofman et al (1991) reviewed 23 European epidemiological studies of dementia and concluded that the prevalence rises from 1.0% in those aged 60–64 years to 32.3% in those aged 90–94 years, the figures nearly doubling with every 5 years of increase in age. In the UK in 1993 there were estimated to be 635 735 people with dementia (Alzheimer's Disease Society, 1993).

The dementias are associated with specific vascular, neurological and neurochemical changes. For example, Alzheimer's disease may be characterised by excessive neuron loss, amyloid deposition, neuritic plaques, neurofibrillary tangles and neurochemical changes; diffuse Lewy body dementia may be characterised by the presence of senile plaques and Lewy bodies; and vascular dementia may be characterised by vascular damage to cerebral tissue. A more detailed description of the biomedical pathology of dementia is presented in Chapter 12 by Jill Walton. Typically, people with dementia present with disturbances of memory, orientation, intellect, behaviour and mood (Adams, 1997).

Kitwood (1989), Hanson (1989) and Harding and Palfrey (1997) challenge the assumption of a linear relationship between neuropathology and the presenting problems of dementia. Kitwood suggests that the dementing process should be viewed as the outcome of the interplay between two factors: the first is neurological impairment, and the second is the individual psychology of the person together with the social psychology with which the person is surrounded (Kitwood and Bredin, 1992).

However, the experience of dementia has been rarely linked with wider historical and social forces. This may be a consequence of the medicalisation of dementia where the problem of dementia is located with the diagnosis bearer, a perspective promulgated by the individualistic focus of dementia care practice and research. The experiences of dementia may also be influenced by the life course as well as the political economy of old age (Townsend, 1981), the medicalisation of old age (Riley et al, 1988), ageism (Blytheway, 1995), assumptions about the limited abilities of older people (Banks and Blair, 1997) and therapeutic pessimism (Butler et al, 1991). Kitwood (1990) argues that wider social phenomena such as the decline of Western capitalism and rising unemployment, as experienced by many older people, are likely to contribute to a person's experiences of dementia.

Hanson (1989) adopts an interpersonal approach to dementia and proposes that the symptoms of dementia are created within a family context, emphasising the role of the family in giving meaning to, reacting to and acting upon indicators of dementia. Hanson (1997) presents a model of dementia in which 'the social construction of senile dementia begins at home and is driven by families who construct and maintain problems and are thus at the core of treatment seeking, compliance and effectiveness' (p. 17). In support of such an approach she draws attention to the observed influence of the family on the individual, the mediation of dementia by race and gender, and the debates about the medicalisation of normal ageing.

Hall (1996) moves beyond the position of the family as constructors of dementia in examining the processes by which society continually redefines what is acceptable within it through the 'cultural and self-defined meanings or ingrained patterns of oppression and discrimination that underpin establishing diagnostic categories' (p. 17). Harding and Palfrey (1997) further extend the debate, asserting that the biomedical model of dementia leads not to an objective diagnosis but to a position of 'moral rectitude'. Value judgments are placed on diagnostic indicators – short-term memory is rated as more worthy than long-term memory, strict compliance with social inhibitions is assumed to be more normal than less compliance, and the inability to communicate coherently is depicted as the fault of the individual rather than the more rational observer.

At a sociopolitical level, Fox (1989) has argued that the construction of Alzheimer's disease in Western society is related to political manoeuvres between various research agencies in their pursuit of research funding. A similar case could perhaps be made in relation to services seeking to shift the financial liability of dementia care (Badger et al, 1989). The 'location' of dementia as an illness is also a concern of social policy, Hopton and Glenister (1996) being critical of the 1994 review of mental health nursing, *Working in Partnership* (DoH, 1994) for failing to clarify whether people with dementia are best served by being cared for within mental health services or within general medical services.

Thus, the problems facing someone with dementia may not be directly linked to the extent of physiological change. As with so many illnesses, the knowledge about dementia, its presentation and significance depend on a variety of physical, social and psychological factors as well as on the professions' and society's interpretation and management of it.

Responding to dementia: policy and practice

Throughout the world, societies have established a model of mental health care that emphasises the containment and isolation of people with mental health problems from the rest of society, for example in Russia (Sosnovsky and Valentine, 1995) and in Britain (Prior, 1993). Rural areas became home to glorious architecture which signified the benevolent but excluding nature of care until recent times (Prior, 1993). The colloquial expression for such institutions as 'bins' typifies this approach to care: somewhere neat and tidy in which unwanted things could be put.

People with dementia have been faced with a triple problem. Firstly, their care was located in places isolated from the rest of society; secondly, their illness was perceived as having no resolution other than decline and eventual death; thirdly, people with dementia are usually elderly and therefore subject to ageism in care resourcing. Often, having dementia meant being cared for on the 'back wards' of the mental health institution – the bottom of the bin.

The staff who have worked with people with dementia have been faced with similar societal attitudes, discouraging and devaluing their professional practice (Means and Smith, 1994), as discussed by Tracy Packer in Chapter 15. The difficulties faced by professional carers in 'dealing' with people with dementia have been extensively researched. For example, in Scandinavia, Kuremyr et al (1994) found that a close staff–patient relationship caused emotional strain, whilst more task-oriented practices caused guilt at the apparent lack of a close relationship. Astrom et al (1990, 1991) found that staff 'burn-out' correlated with reduced empathy and less positive attitudes, and was therefore a crucial concept in caring for older people with dementia.

More recently, social policies have responded to pressure from professional and lay groups. Institutional exposés (e.g., Goffman, 1961; Martin, 1984) have swung public opinion against the containment of older people with dementia. However, the general population remains nervous about the integration of people with mental health problems in the community, and such people continue to lack opportunities to participate as active members of society (Prior, 1993), thus potentially merely creating a dispersion of deviance and a lack of acceptance by society, rather than integration within that society. In Britain, policy now emphasises a shift from service-led to needs-led assessment and care provision (DoH, 1989), but Richards (1994) warns that the pressures on limited service resources and the fear of legal challenge if identified needs are not fulfilled may simply result in a shift from 'service eligibility criteria' to the service's definition of 'eligible need'. In this way 'need' becomes socially constructed and reflects, in large part, the ability of services and professional workers to deliver care both strategically (Caldock, 1996) and interpersonally, a point also alluded to by McWalter et al (1994).

A professional knowledge base of dementia care has gradually evolved and there is now a plethora of publications and guidelines – for example, the guidelines of the Royal College of Nursing (1994). For practitioners, this knowledge arises from past experiences and education of caring for people with dementia. In particular, Clarke and Heyman (1998) argue that professionals have a knowledge of the pathology of dementia, with its implications of inevitable decline, which is applied to individual people. This may assume that each individual will comply with this aggregated knowledge of dementia. Individual variation has limited acceptance, and the values and meanings associated with the family carer's personal domain of caring may lack acknowledgment (Clarke and Heyman, 1998).

From this baseline of knowledge, professional carers must seek a knowledge of each individual who has dementia in order to contextualise their care. However, this is not always an easy step. In Chapter 14, Trevor Adams explores the work of community psychiatric nurses with older people with dementia, whilst Chapter 13, discusses the inappropriate care that may be offered to people with dementia and their families if care fails to be contextualised for each individual situation. For professional carers, clinical decision-making in dementia care is inextricably embedded in an ethical framework (Hurley et al, 1995), an issue explicated in Chapter 4 by Malcolm Goldsmith.

The dominant construction of old age and mental illness as a biomedical problem affects the nature of professional care (see Chapter 3 by Michael Hill). In a study of older people in a large hospital in the UK, Koch and Webb (1996) found that older people were contained on age-specific wards, felt treated as objects as a result of the 'geriatric routine' from which there was little daily deviation, and their care needs were 'reduced' to nursing practices such as hygiene and medication. These deprivations in care were complied with stoically, patients aware of the disapproval which would greet them if they complained. Koch and Webb (1996) argue that nursing care is greatly influenced by the medical model of care which interprets old age as a time of physiological decay. Such a pathological construction of age (Benner and Wrubel, 1989):

> … *puts helpers in a superior position and those they help in an inferior position. To be helped or be in need of help means that one is incompetent, wrong, hapless, helpless, or stupid. (p. 187)*

Reed and Watson (1994) found limitations in the use of a medical model of care by nurses in long-term care environments, and Davis (1980) reported that chronically ill patients were cared for on the 'narrowly conceived acute disease modality of care'. In dementia care, interventions have been developed which are minimally therapeutic for the individual and which emphasise their safe containment, for example most traditional forms of respite care; whilst health in older age or with a chronic illness has frequently been regarded as unattainable and therefore health promotion activities are considered irrelevant (McWilliam et al, 1996).

In parallel with, and in reaction to, the developing knowledge of the pathophysiology of dementia, discussed earlier, there has been a striving for a psychosocial model of dementia care. This has resulted in the growth of therapeutic interventions with people with dementia that seek to promote social and psychological wellbeing, for example through reality orientation and validation therapy – see Phair and Good (1995) for some detail of such interventions. Adams (1997) identifies a number of reasons for this quiet but resolute revolution in professional care against the dominant pathophysiological model. These are:

- A powerful critique of the 'biomedicalisation of dementia'
- The move from institutional to community care, demanding a professional response to family carers
- The development of multidisciplinary professional practice, providing opportunity for a variety of perspectives to be considered.

Beyond the emergence of the psychosocial aspect of dementia care has been a recent acknowledgement of the interpersonal and interactional aspects both of the experience of dementia and of dementia care. From the interactionist standpoint, that people exist in their relationship with others and their surroundings, Kitwood and Bredin (1992) argue that as cognitive ability changes, so interrelationships become increasingly essential if a sense of self is to be maintained, a view also advanced by Orona (1990) and Sabat and Harré (1992). Particularly effective within this knowledge domain are interventions such as family nursing (Freidemann, 1993) which is increasingly popular in the USA, and family therapy (e.g. Richardson et al, 1994).

Kitwood and Bredin (1992) and Kitwood (1993) argue for a sense of relative wellbeing to be the goal of professional care for people with dementia. They identify four 'global sentient states' which must be protected if wellbeing is to be maintained: a sense of personal worth, a sense of agency (control of personal life or self-determination), social confidence and hope. The medicalisation of dementia strips the individual of these rights. Perceived to be cognitively incompetent, people with dementia risk being denied a sense of self-determination, their personal worth is rendered valueless, and any social confidence and hope is consequently shattered. The implications of a medicalised, pathophysiological approach for all forms of chronic illness and for older people are increasingly debated. Defining health and wellbeing so narrowly results in dissatisfaction for all involved when there is a failure to be 'cured', or even 'managed' effectively such that physiological decline is reversed or halted. Hall (1996) argues that the processes of care within a psychiatric medical model, for example the diagnostic process, result in 'a contrived and sanctioned dehumanisation of the person', a point also made by Kevin McKee in Chapter 7 in relation to research with people with dementia. Similarly, Richards (1994) argues that professional assessment may be disempowering for the client. This is far from the equality required for an effective partnership.

A 'vicious circle' is entered on seeking diagnosis. Once the diagnosis of dementia is established the pathophysiological model offers little hope for the future. The diagnostic label influences expectations, which in turn creates a self-fulfilling prophecy for the individual and the family (Hall, 1996). Brown (1995) argues that the diagnosis is central to subsequent social constructions of the illness experience. The diagnosis of dementia, perhaps like that of any chronic mental health illness, can have a devastating impact on the individual's identity, from exposure to the disempowering and dehumanising attitudes of society (Handyside and Heyman, 1995; Hall, 1996).

Clarke and Keady (1996) challenge the wisdom of pursuing this approach for people with dementia, since diagnosis may, at times, be inappropriate to an individual's experiences and emphasise the pathology (Lewis, 1995). It may serve merely to expose features of the condition that people with dementia are working to keep hidden and private (Robinson et al, 1997); for example, Keady and Nolan (1994a) found 'covering up' to be a key stage in the experience of dementia.

The social consequences of diagnosis may, however, be welcome. Broom and Woodward (1996) identify diagnosis as the key to obtaining medical insurance for services in the USA. Further, symptoms are validated and can be negotiated as 'the illness not the person' within family relationships, thus serving to protect the position of the person with dementia within the family context (Clarke and Heyman, 1998). Adams (1997) urges that assessment be seen as a therapeutic intervention and the commencement of an effective care relationship between the professional, the individual and the family. In this way, argue Patterson and Whitehouse (1990), assessment ceases to be disabling but, rather, increases awareness within a family of their own strengths and abilities. Harding and Palfrey (1997) argue that the label of dementia 'appears to be required of all save the sufferers themselves' (p. 125).

In dementia care, individual care and family care are often addressed concurrently as the care focus shifts from the 'untreatable' dementia to the 'manageable' impact of caring on the family carer. Hurley et al (1995) found that nursing staff made no distinction between their assessments of the person with dementia and their assessment of the family. Such a concurrency of care may be a somewhat naïve approach, however. Clarke and Heyman (1998) found that there was at times an inherent tension between the care needs of the individual and those of the family, such that professional carers had to make a distinction between caring for the person with dementia and caring for the family. Haug (1994) also identifies potential conflict between the older person as health-care consumer, and the family carers as seekers of support.

Very often professional carers are caught in a web of ethical dilemmas from which no solution is entirely satisfactory. Take, for example, the potential (and frequent) dilemma faced when a minibus arrives to take a person with dementia to the local day centre, to find that the person firmly refuses to go; the family carer is fraught, has had little sleep and despairs at the possible lack of a break that day. To what extent is it acceptable to cajole, not to say coerce or bribe, the person with dementia into the minibus? Accept the biomedical model and the answer becomes relatively easy. Even working within a psychosocial model, it can be argued that day care provides necessary stimulation and social contact for the person with dementia and relieves the stress of the family. However, working within an interactional model creates unresolvable dilemmas, as cajoling is seen to destroy just a little more of the individual's self-determination and rights.

In a challenging editorial, Chinn (1996) asks why, in the face of clear inability to 'cure' a disease, do nurses and other medical care providers continue to move within a frame of reference oriented towards cure? Why, indeed! She proposes one starting point: 'the development of viable frameworks that keep the interests, the experience, and the voice of the person with chronic illness in the centre'. Let us keep this goal in mind in seeking to develop health and social care for people with dementia.

Articulating the voice of dementia

Buried beneath all these issues is the actual person with dementia. These people have remained largely invisible to researchers, planners and practitioners. Research and practice in dementia care do not have a very proud history in this respect. Very often, the views of people with dementia are made known only through the selective screen of their families, upon whom the responsibility for this is devolved. Cotterell and Schulz (1993) suggest that 'the person with dementia is often relegated to the status of an object rather than a legitimate contributor to the research process' (p. 205).

There are undoubtedly pragmatic methodological challenges in facilitating the perspective of the person with dementia in social critical and participatory research (Henderson, 1995) and as service users in policy and practice development. However, various ways in which this may be achieved are outlined by Goldsmith (1996) and Winner (1996). The problems are no more insurmountable than with other groups with challenging communication and cognitive processes, for example people with learning disabilities (Heyman and Huckle, 1995; Booth and Booth, 1996).

Primarily, there needs to be a belief that people with dementia have something to say that merits the intention of others to listen. As Goldsmith (1996) describes, this was not always the case at the outset of his study:

> It was as though there were three set positions. The first was that people with dementia cannot be understood, and they need to have decisions made for them – the 'we know best, poor things' approach. The second was that although in theory it was a good idea to hear their views, it really is not practical, but it is good that we hold on to the concept. The third view was a sort of gut reaction that it must be possible somehow, and that we need to keep working away at it until we find a way through. (p. 18)

Several of the chapters in this book are concerned with the ways in which people with dementia can be heard more effectively in research and practice. For example, in Chapter 4, Malcolm Goldsmith explores the particular problems that emerge when people are not able to speak for themselves. In Chapter 5, Jane Crisp encourages a positive construction of people with dementia which allows others to more fully appreciate their language and communication. In Chapter 6, Anne Whitworth, Lisa Perkins and Ruth Lesser write of the potentially unique interaction between people with dementia, their family carers and speech and language therapists, in which everyone's distinct knowledge and skills are utilised to create more effective communication for the people with dementia and their carers.

An important consideration in seeking to 'hear' people with dementia, is the extent to which they, as people, have changed (Goldsmith, 1996). Within the biomedical framework, the impact of dementia is seen as so pervasive that the person is substantially and irreversibly changed. Such a position permits people to be treated as 'socially dead' before their physical death (Sweeting and Gilhooly, 1997). Within a social constructivist framework, the experience of dementia is largely influenced by the way the person with dementia is regarded by others. This approach has advantages for those who do not have dementia: it allows them to distance themselves from those with dementia, and reinforces their definition of themselves as 'normal' and 'sane' (Hall, 1996). This is the 'them' and 'us' situation criticised by Kitwood (1993) and in Chapter 3 by Michael Hill. This point is explored in Chapter 8 by Jan Reed in respect of older people in nursing homes who protect an image of themselves by emphasising their difference from other residents with dementia.

In using social constructivist theory to illuminate the destructive pattern of social interactions with people with dementia which undermines any sense of 'self', Sabat and Harré (1992) note the lack of cooperation of other people in maintaining and developing the public self (rather than the impact of the disease itself). This issue is explored further in Chapter 5 by Jane Crisp.

Within a more interactional and social critical framework, people continue unchanged despite their dementia, either through their relationships with others or as wholly 'themselves'. However, Kelly and Field (1996) argue that whilst a core sense of self and identity persists, the consequences of chronic illness have to be 'incorporated permanently into conceptions of self and are likely to become a basis for the imputation of identity by others'. Kitwood and Bredin (1992) propose that people with dementia should be cared for within a framework that preserves their 'personhood', that social part of existence in which human beings relate to others. Little exploration has been undertaken of the implications of someone with dementia potentially retaining some insight, or self-knowledge (Fairbairn, 1997).

In emphasising the importance of functioning within the domains known to those without dementia, there is a failure to acknowledge any other form of reality. Shomaker (1989), Frank (1995) and Crisp (1995), however, illustrate the reality and rationality of someone with dementia which exists without constraints of, for example, notions of the present time (temporality). This may perhaps be accessed if there is a commitment to developing a partnership of care with people with dementia.

Some forms of intervention seek to work within the realities of the person with dementia. Life history work, for example, seeks to contextualise older people within their evolving, and continually redefined, life to create meaning within it (Hargrave, 1994; Murphy and Moyes, 1997). Bleathman and Morton (1992) remark on the communication abilities of people with dementia within validation therapy. Killick (1997) describes working with people with dementia as a writer in residence, stating that:

> I am confident that it is possible to communicate with a person with dementia. I am confident that I will be able to write down what they have to say. I am confident that what they have to say will be coherent and illuminating. (p. 32)

KNOWING ABOUT FAMILY CARING
Identification and kinship

Family carers are involved in an increasing amount of health-care activity and there are an estimated 1.7 million co-resident family carers in Britain (Redding, 1991). However, there has been a considerable amount of conflict about just who does the caring within the home setting. The traditional view has been that middle-aged women shoulder the greatest part of family caring. Indeed, a major contention of British feminist research in this area in the 1980s was that home-based care can be defined as the unpaid work of female relatives within the private domain of the family – see, for example, Graham (1991).

The emphasis on female caring has, however, obscured other dimensions of caring such as the involvement of male carers (Arber and Ginn, 1990; Matthew et al, 1990), age, race and class. Chapter 10 by Liz Matthew seeks to address this deficit in knowledge about dementia care, but there remains a lack of knowledge about spouse carers, and in this area Chapter 9 by Christine Carter makes an important contribution. Keith (1995) also challenges the traditional view of a single primary carer as a possible artefact of research and clinical approaches which fall short of considering the perspectives of other family members.

Kinship plays a crucial part in maintaining dependent people in the community, despite the social changes of recent decades which include kin dispersal and smaller local extended families (Willmott, 1986). Qureshi and Simons (1987) and Ungerson (1987) found there to be a hierarchy of kinship obligations, held by both informal networks and by professionals, in which women are exposed to 'considerable ideological and material pressure' to care, irrespective of their personal wishes and circumstances. In contrast, the work of Finch and Mason (1993), examining intergenerational family responsibilities, emphasised that responsibility is developed and created over time rather than being inherent in a specific relationship. The traditional view of the care receiver as passive and the caregiver as active is therefore challenged as the two-directional nature of family caring situations is realised (Horwitz et al, 1996).

Affection, power and work

The reasons for caring for a dependent relative have been explored at length since the 1970s. Various reasons have been postulated, for example: kinship (Abrams and Bulmer, 1985), reciprocity (Hirschefeld, 1981; Abrams and Bulmer, 1985), religion or altruism (Abrams and Bulmer, 1985; Wade, 1991), obligation (Pratt et al, 1987), affection (Cicirelli, 1983; Motenko, 1989) and mutuality (Hirschefeld, 1981; Qureshi and Walker, 1989). Gilleard (1984) wrote of the complex reasons for being a family carer: 'concepts of mutuality, affection, closeness and reciprocity are interlinked, but seem to entail differing elements in the supporter–dependant relationship' (p. 82). The work of Arber and Gilbert (1989) serves as a reminder that many family carers do not make a conscious decision about caring, but 'drift' into the situation as the person with dementia gradually deteriorates.

In particular, reciprocity (Abrams and Bulmer, 1985) and the centrality of the role played by the person with dementia in the carer's life (Colerick and George, 1986) have been cited as central to family caring. However, this approach to understanding family care may be perhaps somewhat idealistic. Reciprocity in caring is not necessarily a direct, equal and concurrent exchange but rather is an exchange of symbolism which is equated over a life course (Horwitz et al, 1996) and it is ensured that no-one over-receives or over-reciprocates (Finch and Mason, 1993). Komter (1996), studying reciprocity in the Netherlands, argues that consequently those who can give least over their life course receive the least in return. This is particularly pertinent for people who are chronically ill (Horwitz et al, 1996) or older (Komter, 1996). For example, unless older people with dementia have anticipated their need to receive care they may not have previously 'over provided' within their family in recompense. Reciprocity can be seen, therefore, not always as a neat mechanism for family exchange, but as a form of power which reinforces the inequalities within each society.

Importantly, family caring extends beyond the domain of the family home into care environments such as hospitals (Laitinen and Isola, 1996; Nolan et al, 1996) and entails a great deal more than the negotiation of family roles and responsibilities. Whilst the act of caring may incorporate management of the 'physical aspects of living such as eating, bathing or going to the toilet' (Kelly and Field, 1996), such intimate physical care transforming family relationships, caring activities may be far more pervasive in the family's activities.

Bowers (1987), interviewing 27 older people and at least one of their children, identified five categories of caring. The traditional 'hands on' form of caring is categorised as *instrumental* caring. Other categories of caring were *anticipatory* (behaviour or decisions based on possible need), *preventive* (an active monitoring role), *supervisory* (a 'checking on' function), and *protective*. This last category, the most difficult and important type of care provided, includes the important notion of protecting the older person's self-image rather than simply the person's physical wellbeing, an issue debated earlier in this chapter. Recently these categories have been reconsidered by Nolan et al (1995) and have been extended to include preservative, (re)constructive and reciprocal components of care which are considered to have a temporal relationship, each replacing the preceding component as it becomes functionally redundant because of the changing needs of the person with dementia.

Caring – drudgery or pleasure?

Family members have themselves been seen as victims of dementia, Zarit et al (1985) writing that there is probably no other disease that involves families so much or has such devastating effects. The standard view of family caring has made the assumption that caring for someone with dementia is, and will always be, a drudgery. Negative imagery of dementia and dementia care have long been a feature within professional and lay domains, for example Coates (1995), and in academic papers; for example McCarty (1996) identifies the core category of the 'living death' of a parent with Alzheimer's disease.

The 1980s was a period of fruition for numerous studies, particularly in the USA, about the problems associated with caring; for example, being unable to leave the dependant (Baines, 1984), disruptive behaviour (Poulshock and Deimling, 1984) and the detrimental effect of caring on the carers' health, particularly their emotional health (for example, Chenoweth and Spencer, 1986; Haley et al, 1987). Many of these earlier studies relied on either carer complaints or measures of burden, although these may present only a selective view of the problems faced by family carers, and Vitaliano et al (1991) question the validity of some of the measures used. Studies have also been restrictive in their selection of samples of family carers. For example, retrospective data are a common feature, collected after the cessation of caring (e.g. Bloomfield, 1986), and carers may have already been known to carer associations (e.g. Jackson et al, 1986) or identified professional groups (e.g. Adams, 1987).

The factors that family carers find stressful are evidently complex. In an extensive literature review, Parker (1990) suggests that it is unreliable and contradictory to link the amount of carer stress experienced to factors such as the degree of dementia present because of the multiplicity of influential factors. Indeed, Opie (1992), in a study of community care and family caring in New Zealand, states that 'stress is embedded in caring and not an outcome of it'. Similarly, Kahana and Kinney (1991) write that:

> Some critics argue that stress researchers probably are more responsible for the creation of caregiving stress than are either caregivers or the recipients of their care. (p. 138)

Contrary to the findings of the substantial number of studies highlighting the negative effects of caring on carer health, some studies have been more positive. Motenko (1989), interviewing 50 women caring for their husbands with dementia, and Grant and Nolan (1993), using a postal questionnaire, emphasise the rewards and gratifications, rather than problems and difficulties, which influence the burden experienced.

Increasingly, carer burden has been conceptualised within a transactional model of stress in which an individual's perceptions of events are important and factors mediate the relationship between the stressor and the response (Nolan et al, 1990; Schulz et al, 1990). Factors mediating the degree of subjective burden experienced by carers of people who are cognitively impaired have been identified as including seeking social support (Neundorfer, 1991); positive reappraisal of the situation (Neundorfer, 1991); self-efficacy (Mowat and Laschinger, 1994); and powerlessness (Davidhizar, 1994).

The impact that dementia has upon the relationship between the individual and family carers is also of crucial importance: this includes experiences of loss (Barnes et al, 1981; Gabow, 1989); confusion over uncharacteristic behaviour of the person with dementia (Chenoweth and

Spencer, 1986); and the adoption of altered roles within the relationship (Barnes et al, 1981; Cantor, 1983) which may involve modifying a complex set of generationally linked rights, responsibilities, obligations and awareness of self and others (Steinmetz and Amsden, 1983). However, these alterations in relationships and roles are not necessarily perceived as negative by carers. Fitting et al (1986) interviewed 54 carers of spouses with dementia and found that 25% of the husbands reported having an improved relationship with their spouse since caring began. Ungerson (1987) comments that there were those 'for whom [giving care] seemed to bestow a certain satisfaction, even, in one or two cases, an extraordinary kind of joy'. Farren et al (1991), Clarke (1995) and Askham (1995) argue that an important factor is the family carer's ability to find meaning in the caring situation.

In addition, family carers are frequently placed in situations where they carry the responsibility for decision-making. This may be in situations of urgency, for example discharge from hospital (Nolan et al, 1996), and may sometimes be on behalf of the person with dementia when family carers act as 'surrogate' or 'proxy' decision-makers (Hurley et al, 1995).

That the person with dementia and the family carer are in a relationship that contributes to the perceptions of self for both of them is easily forgotten in the search to maintain the identify of the person with dementia. Orona (1990) writes:

> As the Alzheimer's persons changed to the point of being unrecognisable, the caregiving relatives lost remnants of their own identity as the impaired partners were no longer able to reciprocally participate in the relationship. (p. 1255)

From the late 1980s a number of qualitative studies, often using grounded theory, have examined the experiences of caring from this more interactionist perspective. Often the studies have acknowledged the processes developed over a caring 'career' or trajectory. These studies are founded on the acknowledgment that caring occurs in the context of a maze of relationships and social support networks. Lewis and Meredith (1988) constructed 'caring biographies' with 41 daughters who had ceased caring for their mothers. A caring matrix was developed for each caring situation to express the unique mix of relationships, circumstances and attitudes.

A number of temporal models have been explored, identifying the stages of going through the caring process. Wilson's illuminative study articulated the experiences of 20 carers of people with dementia (Wilson, 1989a,b). A basic sociopsychological problem was identified, termed 'coping with negative choices'. Management of negative choices was by 'surviving on the brink', a process of three stages ('taking it on', 'going through it' and 'turning it over'), each with a number of associated strategies. Similarly, Willoughby and Keating (1991) identify the taking on and relinquishing of control as central to caring for someone with dementia. In Canada, research by Wuest et al (1994) has illuminated the experiences of 15 family carers looking after people with Alzheimer's disease. A basic social process of 'becoming strangers' was found, identifying the stages of 'dawning' (a gradual awareness of changes), to 'holding on' (strategies being used to sustain the relationship) through finally to 'letting go' (the estranged carer relinquishing care).

Clarke (1997) explored the interrelationships between family carers, people with dementia and professional carers. The centrality of the continuing relationship between the person with dementia and the carer was identified, and this affected the three basic social processes of normalising, a defining and redefining of the relationship as normal for them (Clarke, 1995); interfacing, a negotiation of professional carer involvement (Clarke and Heyman, 1998); and interacting, the process of family and professional carers working to care for the person with dementia (described in some detail in Chapter 13).

Family carers – delivering or receiving care?

Family carers have an ambiguous relationship with health and social care professionals (Twigg, 1989a), being variously described as either a social problem or a solution to the increased demands on services (Robinson, 1988), and as anything from a resource to a victim of exploitation (Nolan and Grant, 1989). Pitkeathley (1989) identifies three common attitudes that professionals hold towards carers: ignoring them, feeling guilty about them or being impatient with them. Only recently have family carers and their needs been acknowledged as a political health and social care issue. For example, in Britain the Carers (Recognition and Services) Act (1995) requires carer need to be assessed.

However, there has not been an easy transition to the consideration of family carers. Three possible models for working with family carers were identified by Twigg (1989a): as resource, co-worker or co-client. Twigg and Atkin (1994) describe a fourth model of family carer, the superseded carer. In the latter model, which has had limited application to older people, the service aim is to 'free disabled people from relationships of dependence' and to dispense with the need for a family carer.

As a resource, family carers represent the assumed, but not acknowledged, group who provide the majority of care in the community. Their needs are not identified or addressed. Family caring assumes a position of subservience to the professional dominance and decision-making of the health and social services. Services have been developed to provide occasional breaks from such resource provision, for example day and respite care, although the benefits of such interventions for family carers have been regularly questioned (Twigg, 1989b; Nolan and Grant,

1992). Skills training and support is often offered to enhance their ability to care (Glosser and Wexler, 1985; Russell et al, 1989).

As co-workers, family carers work in nominal collaboration with services, their needs met so that they may continue to care. However, the relationship between the family carer and the person with dementia is undermined and the latter becomes the 'cared for'. Questions remain about whether adoption of this model has resulted in the traditional inequality of service distribution; female carers, for example, being seen as 'natural' carers (Graham, 1991), and therefore offered fewer resources than male carers (Badger et al, 1990). This issue is discussed further in Chapter 9 by Christine Carter in relation to women caring for their husbands, and in Chapter 10 by Liz Mathew in relation to male carers' management of caregiving.

As co-clients, the model promoted in current public policy in Britain – for example, the Carers (Recognition and Services) Act (1995) – the needs of the carer are seen to take precedence over those of the dependant at times, and the family carer is rendered pathological. However, Clarke (1997) argues that emphasising the needs of carers simply creates another patient who must be cared for; the paternalism with which health and social care envelops patients threatens to engulf the family carers as well. In the same way that the person who has dementia is rendered irrelevant by the medicalisation of dementia care (Kitwood, 1990), so the knowledge base on which family caring is founded is rendered irrelevant. The knowledge base of professional carers is assumed to be the correct and dominant one, as discussed by Robinson (1994) in relation to chronic illness. Various professional interventions have evolved to help family carers cope with the pressures which render them a co-client, for example pre-bereavement counselling – detailed in Adams (1997) and discussed in Chapter 10 by Liz Matthew.

In a thought-provoking paper, Robinson (1994) suggests a move towards a professional's focus on the relationships between families and the individual with a chronic illness, such a perspective inviting health and social care professionals to 'open space for, and be curious about, the beliefs, ideas and experiences of families'. Professional interventions are not directed towards the person with dementia and/or the family carer, but are directed towards the family's functioning. Similarly, Davis (1996) calls for interventions that 'enable families to function as a caregiving unit', whilst Jenkins and Price (1996) propose assisting family carers to find meaning in their experiences and preserve the personhood of the individual with dementia. Ultimately, perhaps, use of the word 'carer' and in particular 'caregiver' is inappropriate in that it emphasises a disorder in a family member and consequently a disorder in family functioning. It is notable that several family carers do not recognise themselves as such, regarding their activity as an inherent part of family exchange (Bell et al, 1987).

Directly in contrast to the medicalising effects of a biopathological model is the emerging model of normalisation (Clarke, 1997). This offers a way of understanding dementia care and family caring which, as Robinson (1993) describes, is 'clearly contradictory to the story of deviance, difficulty, and despair'. In adopting this model, family carers are seen as consumers of services, and their own knowledge base of the individual with dementia is seen as equal to the dementia knowledge base of professional carers. There are, indeed, early indications of the family carer's knowledge base being accessed in practice to inform service interventions (Keady and Nolan, 1994b).

COMPLIANCE, CONSENSUS, COLLABORATION AND PARTNERSHIP

It is pertinent to restate Powell-Cope's (1994) argument that a partnership in health-care relationships exceeds the unidirectionality of 'caring' and demands a mutual exchange. In moving beyond the search for compliance and consensus with a dominant single knowledge base, there needs to be an emphasis on respecting diverse knowledge bases to develop therapeutic health-care relationships. Coates and Boore (1995), in relation to chronic illness, emphasise that participation in care does not mean compliance or acquiescence to ready-made decisions but requires active involvement throughout the process. However, there are a number of issues which have obstructed the development of meaningful partnerships between professionals, people with dementia and their family carers:

- Power through the status of knowledge, some knowledge bases being more highly valued and therefore dominant over other less valued (usually lay) perspectives of health and illness.
- Power through the ability to effect action, there being structural constraints on the ability of individuals outside of health and social care organisations to influence the development of those services. For example, services users are a dispersed group who lack a 'critical mass' in identifying and responding to common problems. Further, the dialogue of the white middle classes is most audible to professionals, and so responding to the service user's perspective may therefore perpetuate social inequalities.
- Professional – client relationships, which have been dominated by attention to interpersonal communication models for many years, emphasising the exchange of information between parties. However, this work has failed to recognise the context of that communication as being within a health-care relationship, to the detriment of its therapeutic potential.
- The superficiality of consensus and collaboration, which can be thought of as 'pseudo-partnership' models in which the need to have agreement is recognised but the agenda is established by only one party.

Professional dominance

Accepting a pathophysiological knowledge of dementia as dominant, with scant recognition of the psychosocial and interactional knowledges of dementia care, results in an emphasis on the abnormal, the pathological and the prognosis of relentless deterioration. A participatory approach to care planning and decision-making is undermined. It does, however, offer structure and some meaning to events and allows planning to be made for future problems (Broom and Woodward, 1996) although arguably contributing to their creation (Clarke and Keady, 1996). Medical sociologists, for example Bond (1992), perceive such a professionally dominant model of care as objectifying the individual who has dementia and medicalising the experience of dementia. Bond (1992) identifies four implications of medicalisation:

- Expert (professional) control, resulting in the professional knowledge base being highly regarded, as professionals are seen to have a monopoly of knowledge about anything relating to disease and illness: the 'doctor knows best' approach (Haug, 1994).
- Social control, in which health and social care professionals act as agents for social values through care and are able to legitimise social status through diagnosis.
- Individualisation of 'deviant' behaviours, denying the social context of illness and distancing the person with dementia from the family caring relationship. Consequently services have evolved that seek to remove the person with dementia from the environment (to day care and respite care for example), rather as though such an individual is a rotten tooth which needs to be extracted from an otherwise healthy mouth.
- Depoliticisation of behaviour from the social environment, resulting in a lack of acknowledgment of the impact of social and environmental factors on the presentation of dementia, and marginalising the perspective of the person with dementia.

The sociological and professional literature on health-care relationships traditionally portrays the dominance of health-care ideologies at the expense of the patient (e.g. Freidson, 1970; Brooking, 1989; Rundle, 1992). Although there has now been recognition of the need to avoid professional dominance (Rundle, 1992; Haug, 1994), even those approaches to health care that emphasise a partnership have been criticised; for example, Glenister (1994) writes that:

> In reality patient participation often proceeds on the basis of conflicting ideologies, for example the psychiatric and the lay perspectives, and the dominance of the former is maintained by inequalities of power and status. (p. 803)

Webb (1994), in relation to partnership in child care in social work, argues that moving towards the values of shared care, empowerment and self-advocacy is constrained by the everyday power relations and forms of exchange between professionals and clients, and by the professional and institutional contexts that structure those exchanges. Hewison (1995) discusses how control is exerted by nurses through their use of language, which creates barriers to effective nurse–patient interactions and so constrains the development of more open, collaborative relationships. That often-experienced frustration 'functional fudge' (Biehal, 1993) is used to avoid confrontation of the routine responses to service users which further deny their individuality and hamper their participation. Power is therefore held and exercised by both individuals and by institutional structures (Pappas, 1990).

Webb (1994) portrays social work as a system of patronage which is inherently caught in its conflicting but complementary aspects of hierarchical relationships of power (resulting in a sense of fear and gratitude in its recipients) and forms of social exchange and reciprocity (resulting in a sense of bond and exchange). Clients, therefore, oscillate between compliance and praise for services they are offered, and resentment at the interfering nature of care interventions (with varying degrees of non-compliance).

At the level of policy, although the 1994 review of mental health nursing in the UK (DoH, 1994) called for many changes in mental health-care practice, it is criticised by Hopton and Glenister (1996) for failing to address the issue of power relations between staff and patients. The law is always there as the often unstated threat of the ultimate power vested in professionals. Indeed, Coyne et al (1996) argue that knowledge that the law can be enforced contributes to an adversarial relationship rather than one of cooperation and partnership. They cite the mandatory reporting in the USA of suspected cases of abuse of people with dementia to punitive agencies, as potentially jeopardising the relationship of trust between the client and the professional.

Service user dominance

Power, as exercised by patients or clients, may be an overt refusal to comply with professional directives, but is perhaps most likely to be exercised subtly. In a study of the medicalisation of menstruation, Bransen (1992) found that women retained control over when they allowed the intervention of health care. Power was not considered to be inevitably undesirable if it was the result of processes of interacting forces rather than the traditional 'top-down' model. Such a contention is supported by Clarke and Heyman (1998), health and social care being 'let in' to people's lives rather than being imposed solely by professionals. Not only did family carers control the entry of professional carers into their lives, they then modified and adapted professional carer proposals to meet their own purposes, a phenomenon referred to by Hasselkus (1988). Calnan (1984) also writes of the lack of evidence from interactionist studies of:

> ...the patient naturally deferring to superior medical competence, being duped into accepting medical authority through medical ideology or through bourgeois ideology and being mystified by scientific knowledge. (p. 83)

Further, family carers may also release information to professional carers in ways which support their own view (Clarke and Heyman, 1998). This selective disclosure occurs in a variety of ways, for example before diagnosis when the family carer 'covers' for the person with dementia (Keady and Nolan, 1994a), and in the control of information according to perceptions of professional carer intervention. For example, information about the severity of dementia may be withheld because of the perceived consequences of professional carers knowing it, such as unwanted admission into permanent residential care.

May (1992a, b) draws on Foucault's concepts of 'clinical gaze', in which health-care professionals exercise an assumed right to 'know' patients. He discusses the patient's power in relation to the extended clinical gaze of nursing, beyond the physical body and into the psychosocial sphere. This extended clinical gaze, May argues, can be resisted by remaining silent, by not allowing access to 'private domains'. This right to silence is upheld by people with dementia and their family carers as another way in which they exert power over health and social care agencies. The knowledge of professionals is therefore limited to that deemed appropriate by their profession. They do not have knowledge that is relevant to the social and emotional constituents of the individual patient's care (Henderson, 1994).

Similarly, individuals who are ill do not necessarily simply react to their illness, passively complying with the demands of care interventions. Rather, they are likely to become active managers who balance the intrusion of illness, health and social care with their own lifestyle. Much work in this area has focused on chronic illness, for example Coates and Boore (1995) in relation to diabetes care, and Chapter 11 by John Keady and Jane Gilliard illuminates this area of active management in relation to the early experiences of dementia.

Professionals and service users in partnership

It is evident that the issues of consensus, collaboration and partnership are complex. Partnership does not 'just happen' because it is written into a policy document somewhere, but rather it strikes to the heart of professional practice: the relationship which professionals have with their clients in the context of their respective backgrounds. A seminal study by

Robinson and Thorne (1984) argued for the relationship between professionals and the families of those with chronic illness to be regarded as a process. The relationship was seen to evolve through three stages: first, naïve trusting, in which family and professionals do not share the same perspective because they belong to conceptually distinct but interdependent cultural systems; second, disenchantment, in which, realising the discrepancy in their perspectives, the professionals and family become adversaries; third, guarded alliance, in which trust in each other's competencies is gained and mutually satisfying care can be negotiated. So often, though, it appears that the relationship with professionals becomes entrenched in the phase of disenchantment, with the family seen as demanding or overanxious; so infrequently is that stage resolved, and the potential for collaboration realised.

In a study examining the process of reaching a consensus between staff and family members over end-of-life decisions for people with dementia, Hurley et al (1995) are explicit about the amount and nature of work needed to achieve a relationship in which consensus can be negotiated. The work required to achieve a state of readiness (in both staff and family) for consensus is identified as 'interactive preparation' requiring adjustment, caring and knowing, and the catalysts of timing and trust. Without such work, issues of collaboration, consensus and partnership in care are hollow, with neat paperwork but ingenuous in practice – a case of 'we agree because I say we agree'! Indeed, Webb (1994) states that written contracts may be used as a device to help the professional ensure that the individual does not renege from the receipt of care. Further, Biehal (1993), using findings from the Social Work in Partnership project which aimed to develop a model of practice that encouraged greater user participation, found that whilst shared records were developed, professionals gave a low priority to (or reframed) the problems and goals defined by the service user. Price (1996) describes the shift in professional practice to an understanding of the patient's own goals as requiring a change in the relationship from that of patient and teacher, to that of client and facilitator.

Increasingly, policies are emphasising the importance of user involvement in service planning (e.g. DoH 1994). Despite recognition of the divergence between lay and professional perspectives on health and health care (e.g. Heyman, 1995), little attempt is made to ensure that users have a full contribution in decision-making, Glenister (1994) arguing that professional carers prefer to work with passive recipients of their care. Indeed, Richards (1994) argues that the purchaser–provider split in many health and social care reforms undermines such an opportunity for participation and emphasises the potential power of providers. Beihal (1993) comments that the short notice for, say, discharge, precludes user participation in decision-making. Hopton and Glenister (1996) note the 'tokenist' approach to user participation on policy committees. However, these papers all fall short of considering how people with dementia may be allowed to participate and be involved in either service planning or their own care delivery. It would appear to be hard enough for any user to become truly involved, even without dementia being an added reason for discrimination and isolation from planning. Further, not all services recognise family carers as users and so their involvement in service planning may not be encouraged (Twigg and Atkin, 1991).

Winner (1996) articulates some of the common assumptions made about partnership with people with dementia: 'that they may have difficulty in articulating needs and preferences; that judgment about potentially complex issues may be impaired; that understanding about new ideas and information may be difficult; that they are unlikely to have insight into their own situations and therefore require protection' (p. 72). In considering the part that people with dementia may play in their care as service users, Winner emphasises the need for ongoing assessment, early establishment of communication, continuity of information, valuing of relationships and, perhaps most importantly, for self-determination to be seen as appropriate.

In seeking to find an effective model of working with both family carers and people with dementia it is necessary to move beyond the traditional dyads of health and social care relationships, and consider each individual as one of a number of partners involved in identifying and meeting care needs for the whole situation. There are, as highlighted throughout this chapter, many alliances, coalitions, role differences and ideological variations within and between families and various professional groups (Silliman, 1989; Clarke, 1995). Silliman (1989) highlights the inherent instability of triadic relationships which 'easily decay into coalitions of two against one'. The problems of such a situation are outlined in the earlier discussion about models of working with family carers.

A number of studies, however, focus on the extended patient–doctor exchange without embedding that encounter in a longer-term health-care relationship. For example, Adelman et al (1987) identify three ways in which the third person may act in a triadic relationship: as an advocate, actively engaged in the interaction; as a passive recipient, disengaged from the interaction; or as an antagonist, either ignoring the patient's agenda or opportunistically using the situation to address their own concerns.

Powell-Cope (1994), studying the interactions between family carers, professional carers and people with acquired immune deficiency syndrome (AIDS), found that negotiating partnerships was a fundamental process. This process included the dimensions of conveying information, knowing, being accessible and maintaining belief. Hanson (1997) calls for 'a fluid participatory experience of analysis, diagnosis, and intervention which sees all parts, clinicians and families included, contributing to the whole process' when working with people with dementia. To achieve this requires a commitment to appreciating and valuing other knowledge bases and to equipping ourselves to be able to access such knowledge when working with people with dementia and their families.

A partnership requires the dynamics of isolated exchanges to be understood within the context of longer-term health and social care relationships. Neither, by itself, can constitute a partnership. Further, in moving away from an emphasis on the individual to developing partnerships in care, there is a need to focus attention on the dynamics of both the interactions and the relationships between each individual. These spaces between people are not vacant; they are filled with the very factors that appear to confound partnerships in health care and which have been articulated throughout this chapter. It is in this nebulous and fluid space that the search for effective partnerships may be fruitfully located.

CONCLUSION

A tremendous breadth of knowledge about dementia, dementia care, family caring and professional responses exists. This chapter has, perhaps necessarily sweepingly, highlighted just some of these areas of knowledge. In particular, it has sought to articulate some of the tensions inherent in the work in this area. Meaningful triadic relationships are about the mutual appreciation of each other's knowledge and a willingness to regard each other's knowledge as of equal worth. However, not all domains of knowing about dementia and dementia care promote such an approach, as summarised in Table 1.1. No-one, least of all people with dementia, can benefit from health and social care that is built on the arrogance of dominant knowledge. Partnerships in care are about sharing knowledge in a symbiotic fashion to enhance patient care and professional knowledge. Indeed, Hasselkus (1988) argues that there is a need for professional and family carers to recognise the context of meaning in which their expertise is embedded, and challenges both types of carer to make these meanings accessible to each other. The remainder of this book sets out to explore some of the many ways in which this process can be obstructed, and seeks to identify ways in which these beliefs about working with people with dementia and their family carers can be taken forward in practice.

REFERENCES

Abrams, P. & Bulmer, M. (1985) Policies to promote informal social care: some reflections on voluntary action, neighbourhood involvement, and neighbourhood care. *Ageing and Society* 5, 1–18.

Adams, T. (1987) How does it feel to be a caregiver? *Community Psychiatric Nursing Journal* 7, 11–17.

Adams, T. (1997) Dementia. In: Norman I. & Redfern S. (eds) *Mental Health in Elderly People*. Edinburgh: Churchill Livingstone.

Adelman R.D., Greene M. & Charon R. (1987) The physician – elderly patient – companion triad in the medical encounter: the development of a conceptual agenda. *Gerontologist* **27**, 729–734.

Alzheimer's Disease Society (1993) *Deprivation and Dementia*. London: Alzheimer's Disease Society.

Arber, S. & Gilbert, N. (1989) Men: the forgotten carers. *Sociology* **23**, 111–118.

Arber, S. & Ginn, J. (1990) The meaning of informal care: gender and the contribution of elderly people. *Ageing and Society* **10**, 429–454.

Askham, J. (1995) Making sense of dementia: carers' perceptions. *Ageing and Society* **15**, 103–114.

Astrom, S., Nilsson, M., Norberg, A. & Winblad, B. (1990) Empathy, experience of burnout and attitudes towards demented patients among staff in geriatric care. *Journal of Advanced Nursing* **15**, 1236–1244.

Astrom, S., Nilsson, M., Norberg, A., Sandman, P. & Winblad, B. (1991) Staff burnout in dementia care – relations to empathy and attitudes. *International Journal of Nursing Studies* **28**, 65–75.

Badger, F., Evers, H. & Cameron, E. (1989) *The Community Care Project: Community Service Provision and Clients with Dementia*. Report No. 29. Department of Social Medicine, University of Birmingham.

Badger, F., Cameron E. & Evers, H. (1990) Waiting to be served. *Health Service Journal* **100**, 54–55.

Baines, E. (1984) Caregiver stress in the older adult. *Journal of Community Health Nursing* **1**, 257–263.

Banks, E.J. & Blair, S.E.E. (1997) The contribution of occupational therapy within the context of the psychodynamic approach for older clients who have mental health problems. *Health Care in Later Life* **2**, 85–92.

Barnes, R.F., Raskind, M.A., Scott, M. & Murphy, C. (1981) Problems of families caring for Alzheimer patients: use of a support group. *Journal of the American Geriatrics Society* **554**, 80–85.

Bell, R., Gibbons, S. & Pinchen, I. (1987) *Action Research with Informal Carers of Elderly People*. Cambridge: Health Education Services.

Benner, P. & Wrubel, J. (1989) *The Primacy of Caring, Stress and Coping in Health and Illness*. Menlo Park: Addison-Wesley.

Berrios, G.E. (1987) Dementia during the seventeenth and eighteenth centuries: a conceptual history. *Psychological Medicine* **17**, 829–837.

Biehal, N. (1993) Changing practice: participation rights and community care. *British Journal of Social Work* **23**, 443–458.

Bleathman, C. & Morton, I. (1992) Validation therapy: extracts from 20 groups with dementia sufferers. *Journal of Advanced Nursing* **17**, 658–666.

Bloomfield, K. (1986) Ask the family. *Nursing Times* **82**, 28–30.

Blytheway, B. (1995) *Ageism*. Buckingham: Open University Press.

Bond, J. (1992) The politics of caregiving: the professionalisation of informal care. *Ageing and Society* **12**, 5–21.

Booth, T. & Booth, W. (1996) Sounds of silence: narrative research with inarticulate subjects. *Disability and Society* **11**, 55–69.

Bowers, B.J. (1987) Intergenerational caregiving: adult caregivers and their aging parents. *Advanced Nursing Science* **9**, 20–31.

Bransen, E. (1992) Has menstruation been medicalised? Or will it never happen? *Sociology of Health and Illness* **14**, 98–110.

Brooking, J.J. (1989) A survey of current practices and opinions concerning patient and family participation in hospital care. In: Wilson-Barnett, J. & Robinson, S. (eds) *Directions in Nursing Research*. London: Scutari Press.

Broom, D.H. & Woodward, R.V. (1996) Medicalisation reconsidered: towards a collaborative approach to care. *Sociology of Health and Illness* **18**, 357–378.

Brown, P. (1995) Naming and framing: the social construction of diagnosis and illness. *Journal of Health and Social Behaviour* (extra Issue) 34–52.

Butler, R.N., Lewis, M. & Sunderland, T. (1991) *Ageing and Mental Health: Positive Psychological and Biomedical Approaches*, 4th edn. New York: MacMillan.

Caldock, K. (1996) Multidisciplinary assessment and care management. In: Phillips, J. & Penhale, B. (eds) *Reviewing Care Management for Older People*. London: Jessica Kingsley.

Calnan, M. (1984) Clinical uncertainty: is it a problem in the doctor-patient relationship? *Sociology of Health and Illness* **6**, 74–85.

Cantor, M.H. (1983) Strain among caregivers: a study of experience in the United States. *Gerontologist* **23**, 597–604.

Carers (Recognition and Services) Act (1995) London: HMSO.

Chenoweth, B. & Spencer, B. (1986) Dementia: the experience of family caregivers. *Gerontologist* **26**, 267–272.

Chinn, P.L. (1996) Living with chronic illness (editorial). *Advances in Nursing Science* **18**, vi.

Cicirelli, V.G. (1983) Adult children and their elderly parents. In: Brubaker, T. (ed.) *Family Relationships in Later Life*. London: Sage.

Clarke, C.L. (1995) Care of elderly people suffering from dementia and their co-resident informal carers. In: Heyman, B. (ed). *Researching User Perspectives On Community Health Care*. London: Chapman & Hall.

Clarke, C.L. (1997) In sickness and in health: remembering the relationship in family caregiving for people with dementia. In: Marshall, M. (ed.) *The State of the Art in Dementia Care*. London: Centre for Policy on Ageing.

Clarke, C.L. & Heyman, B. (1998) Risk management for people with dementia. In: Heyman, B. (ed.) *Risk, Health and Health Care: A Qualitative Approach*. London: Chapman & Hall.

Clarke, C.L. & Keady, J. (1996) Researching dementia care and family caregiving-extending ethical responsibilities. *Health Care in Later Life* **1**, 85–95.

Coates, D. (1995) The portrayal of family carers in dementia: some critical observation. *Health and Social Care in the Community* **3**, 267–270.

Coates, V.E. & Boore, J.R.P. (1995) Self-management of chronic illness: implications for nursing. *International Journal of Nursing Studies* **32**, 628–640.

Colerick, E.J. & George, L.K. (1986) Predictors of institutionalisation among caregivers of patients with Alzheimer's disease. *Journal of the American Geriatrics Society* **34**, 493–498.

Cotterell, V. & Schulz, R. (1993) The perspective of the patient with Alzheimer's disease: a neglected dimension of dementia research. *Gerontologist* **33**, 205–211.

Coyne, A.C., Potenza M. & Berbig, L.J. (1996) Abuse in families coping with dementia. *Aging* **367**, 93–95.

Crisp J. (1995) Making sense of the stories that people with Alzheimer's tell: a journey with my mother. *Nursing Inquiry* **2**, 133–140.

Davidhizar, R. (1994) Powerlessness of caregivers in home care. *Journal of Clinical Nursing* **3**, 155–158.

Davis, M.Z. (1980) The organisational, interactional and care-orientated conditions for patient participation in continuity of care: a framework for staff intervention. *Social Science and Medicine* **14A**, 39–47.

Davis, L.L. (1996) Dementia caregiving studies: a typology for family interventions. *Journal of Family Nursing* **2**, 30–55.

[DoH] Department of Health (1989) *Caring for People: Community Care in the Next Decade and Beyond*. London: HMSO.

[DoH] Department of Health (1994) *Working in Partnership: A Collaborative Approach to Care*. London: HMSO.

Fairbairn, A. (1997) Insight and dementia. In: Marshall, M. (ed.) *The State of the Art in Dementia Care*. London: Centre for Policy on Ageing.

Farren, C., Keane-Hagerty, E., Salloway, E., Kupferer, S. & Wilken, C. (1991) Finding meaning: an alternative paradigm for Alzheimer's disease family caregivers. *Gerontologist* **31**, 438–489.

Finch, J. & Mason, J. (1993) *Negotiating Family Responsibilities*, London: Routledge.

Fitting, M., Rabins, P., Lucas, M.J. & Eastham, J. (1986) Caregivers for dementia patients: a comparison of husbands and wives. *Gerontologist* **26**, 248–252.

Fox, P. (1989) From senility to Alzheimer's disease: The rise of Alzheimer's disease movement. *Milbank Quarterly* **67**, 58–103.

Frank, B.A. (1995) People with dementia can communicate – if we are able to hear, In: Kitwood, T. & Benson, S. (eds) *The New Culture of Dementia Care*. London: Hawker.

Freidson, E. (1970) *Professional Dominance: The Social Structure of Medical Care*. Chicago: Aldine.

Friedemann, M. (1993) The concept of family nursing. In: Wegner, G.D. & Alexander, R.J. (eds) *Readings in Family Nursing*. Philadelphia: Lippincott.

Gabow, C. (1989) The impact of Alzheimer's disease on family caregivers. *Home Healthcare Nurse* **7**, 19–21.

Gilleard, C.J. (1984) *Living With Dementia – Community Care of the Elderly Mentally Infirm*. London: Croom Helm.

Glenister, D. (1994) Patient participation in psychiatric services: a literature review and proposal for a research strategy. *Journal of Advanced Nursing* **19**, 802–811.

Glosser, G. & Wexler, D. (1985) Participants' evaluation of educational support groups for families with Alzheimer's disease or other dementias. *Gerontologist* **25**, 232–236.

Goffman, E. (1961) *Asylums: Essays on the Social Situations of Mental Patients and Other Patients*, New York: Anchor.

Goldsmith, M. (1996) *Hearing the Voice of People with Dementia – Opportunities and Obstacles*. London: Jessica Kingsley.

Graham, H. (1991) The concept of caring in feminist research: the case of domestic service. *Sociology* **25**, 61–78.

Grant, G. & Nolan, M. (1993) Informal carers: sources and concomitants of satisfaction. *Health and Social Care* **1**, 147–159.

Haley, W.E., Brown, E.G., Brown, S.L., Berry, J.W. & Hughes, G.H. (1987) Psychological, social and health consequences of caring for a relative with senile dementia. *Journal of the American Geriatrics Society* **35**, 405–411.

Hall, B.A. (1996) The psychiatric model: a critical analysis of its undermining effects on nursing in chronic mental illness. *Advances in Nursing Science* **18**, 16–26.

Handyside, E. & Heyman, B (1995) Mental illness in the community: the role of voluntary and state agencies. In: Heyman, B. (eds) *Researching User Perspectives on Community Health Care*. London: Chapman & Hall.

Hanson, B.G. (1989) Definitional deficit: a model of senile dementia in context. *Family Process* **28**, 281–289.

Hanson, B. (1997) Who's seeing whom? General systems theory and constructivist implications for senile dementia intervention. *Journal of Aging Studies* **11**, 15–25.

Harding, N. & Palfrey, C. (1997) *The Social Construction of Dementia – Confused Professionals?* London: Jessica Kingsley.

Hargrave, T.D. (1994) Using video life reviews with older adults. *Journal of Family Therapy* **16**, 259–267.

Hasselkus, B.R. (1988) Meaning in family caregiving: perspectives on caregiver/professional relationships. *Gerontologist* **28**, 686–691.

Haug, M.R. (1994) Elderly patients, caregivers, and physicians: theory and research on health care triads. *Journal of Health and Social Behaviour* **35**, 1–12.

Henderson, A. (1994) Power and knowledge in nursing practice: the contribution of Foucault. *Journal of Advanced Nursing* **20**, 935–939.

Henderson, D.J. (1995) Consciousness raising in participatory research: method and methodology for emancipatory nursing inquiry. *Advances in Nursing Science* **17**, 58–69.

Hewison A. (1995) Nurses' power in interactions with patients. *Journal of Advanced Nursing* **21**, 75–82.

Heyman, B. & Huckle, S. (1995) How adults with learning difficulties and their carers see 'the community'. In: Heyman, B. (ed.) *Researching User Perspectives On Community Health Care*. London: Chapman & Hall.

Heyman, B. (1995) Introduction. In: Heyman, B. (ed.) *Researching User Perspectives on Community Health Care*. London: Chapman & Hall.

Hirschefeld, M.J. (1981) Families living and coping with the cognitively impaired, In: Copp, L.A. (ed.) *Recent Advances In Nursing: Care of the Aging*. New York: Churchill Livingstone.

Hofman, A., Rocca, W.A., Brayne, C. et al (1991) The prevalence of dementia in Europe: a collaborative study of 1980–1990 findings. *International Journal of Epidemiology* **20**, 736–748.

Hopton, J. & Glenister, D. (1996) Working in partnership: vision or pipe dream? *Critical Social Policy* **16**, 111–119.

Horwitz, A.V., Reinhard, S.C. & Howell-White, S. (1996) Caregiving as reciprocal exchange in families with seriously mentally ill members. *Journal of Health and Social Behaviour* **37**, 149–162.

Hurley, A.C., Volicer, L., Rempusheski, V.F. & Fry, S.T. (1995) Reaching consensus: the process of recommending treatment decisions for Alzheimer's patients. *Advances in Nursing Science* **18**, 33–43.

Ineichen, B. (1996) The prevalence of dementia and cognitive impairment in China. *International Journal of Geriatric Psychiatry* **11**, 695–697.

Jackson, J., Cambridge, P. & Anderson, D. (1986) The experiences and needs of carers of the elderly mentally infirm. *Social Services Research* **14**, 95–127.

Jenkins, D. & Price, B. (1996) Dementia and personhood: a focus for care? *Journal of Advanced Nursing* **24**, 84–90.

Kahana, E. & Kinney, J. (1991) Understanding caregiving interventions in the context of the stress mode. In: Young, R.F. & Olsen, E.A. (eds) *Health Illness and Disability in Later Life – Practice, Issues and Interventions*. Newbury Park: Sage.

Keady, J. & Nolan, M. (1994a) Younger onset dementia: developing a longitudinal model as the basis for a research agenda and as a guide to interventions with sufferers and carers. *Journal of Advanced Nursing* **19**, 659–669.

Keady, J. & Nolan, M. (1994b) The Carer-Led Assessment Process (CLASP): a framework for the assessment of need in dementia caregivers. *Journal of Clinical Nursing* **3**, 103–108.

Keith, C. (1995) Family caregiving systems: models, resources and values. *Journal of Marriage and the Family* **57**, 179–189.

Kelly, M.P. & Field, D. (1996) Medical sociology, chronic illness and the body. *Sociology of Health and Illness* **18**, 241–257.

Killick, J. (1997) Confidences: the experience of writing with people with dementia. In: Marshall, M. (ed.) *The State of the Art in Dementia Care*. London: Centre for Policy on Ageing.

Kitwood, T. (1989) Brain, mind and dementia: with particular reference to Alzheimer's disease. *Ageing and Society* **9**, 1–15.

Kitwood, T. (1990) The dialectics of dementia with particular reference to Alzheimer's disease. *Ageing and Society* **10**, 177–196.

Kitwood, T. (1993) Towards a theory of dementia care: the interpersonal process. *Ageing and Society* **13**, 51–67.

Kitwood, T. & Bredin, K. (1992) Towards a theory of dementia care: personhood and well-being. *Ageing and Society* **12**, 269–287.

Koch, T. & Webb, C. (1996) The biomedical construction of ageing: implications for nursing care of older people. *Journal of Advanced Nursing* **23**, 954–959.

Komter, A.E. (1996) Reciprocity as a principle of exclusion: gift giving in the Netherlands. *Sociology* **30**, 299–316.

Kuremyr, D., Kihlgren, M., Norberg, A., Astrom, S. & Karlsson, I. (1994) Emotional experiences, empathy and burnout among staff caring for demented patients at a collective living unit and a nursing home. *Journal of Advanced Nursing* **19**, 670–679.

Laitinen, P. & Isola, A. (1996) Promoting participation of informal caregivers in the hospital care of the elderly patient: informal caregivers' perceptions. *Journal of Advanced Nursing* **23**, 942–947.

Lewis, J. & Meredith, B. (1988) *Daughters Who Care – Daughters Caring for Mothers at Home*. London: Routledge.

Lewis, S.E. (1995) A search for meaning: making sense of depression. *Journal of Mental Health* **4**, 369–382.

Lishman, W.A. (1987) *Organic Psychiatry*, (2nd edn.) Oxford: Blackwell.

Martin, J.P. (1984) *Hospitals in Trouble*. Oxford: Basil Blackwell.

Mathew, L., Mattocks, K. & Slatt, L.M. (1990) Exploring the roles of men: caring for demented relatives. *Journal of Gerontological Nursing* **16**, (10), 20–25.

May, C. (1992a) Individual care? Power and subjectivity in therapeutic relationships. *Sociology* **26**, 589–602.

May, C. (1992b) Nursing work, nurses' knowledge, and the subjectification of the patient. *Sociology of Health and Illness* **14**, 472–487.

McCarty, E.F. (1996) Caring for a parent with Alzheimer's disease: process of daughter caregiver stress. *Journal of Advanced Nursing* **23**, 792–803.

McWalter, G., Toner, H., Corser, A., Eastwood, J., Marshall, M. & Turvey, T. (1994) Needs and need assessment: their components and definitions with reference to dementia. *Health and Social Care* **2**, 213–219.

McWilliam, C.L., Stewart, M., Brown, J.B., Desai, K. & Coderre, P. (1996) Creating health with chronic illness. *Advances in Nursing Science* **18**, 1–15.

Means, R. & Smith, R. (1994) *Community Care, Policy and Practice*. London: Macmillan.

Motenko, A.K. (1989) The frustrations, gratifications, and well-being of dementia caregivers. *Gerontologist* **29**, 166–172.

Mowat, J. & Laschinger, H.K.S. (1994) Self-efficacy in caregivers of cognitively impaired elderly people: a concept analysis. *Journal of Advanced Nursing* **19**, 1105–1113.

Murphy, C. & Moyes, M. (1997) Life story work. In: Marshall, M. (ed.) *State of the Art in Dementia Care*. London: Centre for Policy on Ageing.

Neundorfer, M. (1991) Coping and health outcomes in spouse caregivers of persons with dementia. *Nursing Research* **40**, 260–265.

Nolan, M. & Grant, G. (1989) Addressing the needs of informal carers: a neglected area of nursing practice. *Journal of Advanced Nursing* **14**, 950–962.

Nolan, M. & Grant, G. (1992) Respite care: challenging tradition. *British Journal of Nursing* **1**, 129–131.

Nolan, M., Grant, G. & Ellis, N. (1990) Stress is in the eye of the beholder: reconceptualising the measurement of carer burden. *Journal of Advanced Nursing* **15**, 544–555.

Nolan, M., Keady, J. & Grant, G. (1995) Developing a typology of family care: implications for nurses and other service providers. *Journal of Advanced Nursing* **21**, 256–265.

Nolan, M., Walker, G., Nolan, J. et al (1996) Entry to care: positive choice or *fait accompli*? Developing a more proactive nursing response to the needs of older people and their carers. *Journal of Advanced Nursing* **24**, 265–274.

Opie, A. (1992) *There's Nobody There: Community Care of Confused Older People*. Oxford University Press.

Orona, C.J. (1990) Temporality and identity loss due to Alzheimer's disease. *Social Science in Medicine* **30**, 1247–1256.

Pappas, G. (1990) Some implications for the study of the doctor-patient interaction: power, structure and agency in the work of Howard Waitzkin and Arthur Kleinman. *Social Science in Medicine* **30**, 199–204.

Parker, G. (1990) *With Due Care and Attention*. London: Family Policies Studies Centre.

Patterson, M. & Whitehouse, P. (1990) The diagnostic assessment of patients with dementia. In: Mace, N. (ed.) *Dementia Care: Patient, Family and Community*. Baltimore: Johns Hopkins University Press.

Phair, L. & Good, V. (1995) *Dementia: A Positive Approach*. London: Scutari Press.

Pitkeathley, J. (1989) *It's My Duty, Isn't It? The Plight of Carers in Our Society*. London: Souvenir Press.

Poulshock, S.W. & Deimling, G.T. (1984) Families caring for elders in residence: issues in the measurement of burden. *Journal of Gerontology* **39**, 230–239.

Powel-Cope, G.M. (1994) Family caregivers of people with AIDS: negotiating partnerships with professional health care providers. *Nursing Research* **43**, 324–330.

Pratt, C., Schmall, V. & Wright, S. (1987) Ethical concerns of family caregivers to dementia patients. *Gerontologist* **27**, 632–638.

Price, B. (1996) Illness careers: the chronic illness experience. *Journal of Advanced Nursing* **24**, 275–279.

Prior, L. (1993) *The Social Organisation of Mental Illness*. London: Sage.

Qureshi, H. & Simons, K. (1987) Resources Within Families: Caring for Elderly People. In: Brannen, J. & Wilson, G. (eds) *Give and Take in Families: Studies in Resource Distribution*. London: Allen & Unwin.

Qureshi, H. & Walker, A. (1989) *The Caring Relationship: Elderly People and their Families*. London: Macmillan Educational.

Redding, D. (1991) Exploding the myth. *Community Care* **893**, 18–20.

Reed, J. & Watson, D. (1994) The impact of the medical model on nursing practice and assessment. *International Journal of Nursing Studies* **31**, 57–66.

Richards, S. (1994) Making sense of needs assessment. *Research Policy and Planning* **12**, 5–9.

Richardson, C.A., Gilleard, C.J., Lieberman, S. & Peeler, R. (1994) Working with older adults and their families – a review. *Journal of Family Therapy* **16**, 225–240.

Riley, M., Foner, A. & Waring, J. (1988) Sociology of old age. In: Smelser, N.J. (ed.) *Handbook of Sociology*. London: Sage.

Robinson, C.A. (1993) Managing life with a chronic condition: the story of normalisation.

Qualitative Health Research **3**, 6–28.

Robinson, C.A. (1994) Nursing interventions with families: a demand or an invitation to change? *Journal of Advanced Nursing* **19**, 897–904.

Robinson, J. (1988) Support systems. *Nursing Times* **84**, 30–31.

Robinson, C.A. & Thorne, S. (1984) Strengthening family 'interference'. *Journal of Advanced Nursing* **9**, 597–602.

Robinson, P., Ekman, S.-L., Meleis, A.I., Winbald, B. & Wahlund, L.-O. (1997) Suffering in silence: the experience of early memory loss. *Health Care in Later Life* **2**, 107–120.

Royal College of Nursing (1994) *Guidelines for Assessing Mental Health Needs in Old Age.* London: RCN.

Rundle, R. (1992) Parsons revisited: a reappraisal of the community nurse role. In: Jolley, M. & Brykczynska, G. (eds) *Nursing Care: The Challenge To Change.* London: Edward Arnold.

Russell, V., Proctor, L. & Moniz, E. (1989) The influence of a relative support group on carers' emotional distress. *Journal of Advanced Nursing* **14**, 863–867.

Sabat, S.R. & Harré, R. (1992) The construction and deconstruction of self in Alzheimer's disease. *Ageing and Society* **12**, 443–461.

Schulz, R., Beigel, D., Morycz, R. & Visintainer, P. (1990) Psychological paradigms for understanding caregiving. In: Light, E. & Lebowitz, B.D. (eds) *Alzheimer's Disease Treatment and Family Stress, Directions for Research.* New York: Hemisphere.

Shomaker, D.J. (1989) Age disorientation, liminality and reality: the case of the Alzheimer's patient. *Medical Anthropology* **12**, 91–101.

Silliman, R.A. (1989) Caring for the frail older patient: the doctor-patient-family caregiver relationship. *Journal of General Internal Medicine* **4**, 237–241.

Sosnovsky, A. & Valentine, K. (1995) Patients' opinions of mental health services in Russia. In: Boykin, A. (ed.) *Power, Politics and Public Policy – A Matter of Caring.* New York: National League for Nursing Press.

Steinmetz, S.K. & Amsden, D.J. (1983) Dependent elders family stress, and abuse. In: Brubaker, T. (ed.) *Family Relationships in Later Life.* London: Sage.

Sweeting, H. & Gilhooly, M. (1997) Dementia and the phenomenon of social death. *Sociology of Health and Illness* **19**, 93–117.

Townsend, P. (1981) The structured dependency of the elderly: a creation of social policy in the twentieth century. *Ageing and Society* **1**, 5–28.

Twigg, J. (1989a) Models of carers: how do social care agencies conceptualise their relationship with informal carers? *Journal of Social Policy* **18**, 53–66.

Twigg, J. (1989b) Not taking the strain. *Community Care* **77**, 16–19.

Twigg, J. & Atkin, K. (1991) *Evaluating Support to Informal Carers – Summary Report.* Social Policy Research Unit, University of York.

Twigg, J. & Atkin, K. (1994) *Carers Perceived – Policy and Practice in Informal Care.* Buckingham: Open University Press.

Ungerson, C. (1987) *Policy Is Personal – Sex, Gender and Informal Care.* London: Tavistock.

Vitaliano, P.P., Young, H.M. & Russo, J. (1991) Burden: a review of measures used among caregivers of individuals with dementia. *Gerontologist* **31**, 67–75.

Wade, S. (1991) Support for carers. *Journal of District Nursing* **10**, 13–19.

Webb, S.A. (1994) 'My client is subversive!' Partnership and patronage in social work. *Social Work and Social Sciences Review* **5**, 5–23.

Willmott, P. (1986) *Social Networks, Informal Care and Public Policy.* London: Policy Studies Institute.

Willoughby, J. & Keating, N. (1991) Being in control: the process of caring for a relative with Alzheimer's disease. *Qualitative Health Research* **1**, 27–50.

Wilson, H.S. (1989a) Family caregivers: the experience of Alzheimer's disease. *Applied Nursing Research* **2**, 40–45.

Wilson, H.S. (1989b) Family caregiving for a relative with Alzheimer's dementia: coping with negative choices. *Nursing Research* **38**, 94–98.

Winner, M. (1996) User choice, care management and people with dementia. In: Phillips, J. & Penhale, B. (eds) *Reviewing Care Management for Older People.* London: Jessica Kingsley.

Wuest, J., Ericson, P.K. & Stern, P.N. (1994) Becoming strangers: the changing family caregiving relationship in Alzheimer's disease. *Journal of Advanced Nursing* **20**, 437–443.

Zarit, S.H., Orr, N.K. & Zarit, J.M. (1985) *The Hidden Victims of Alzheimer's Disease: Families Under Stress.* New York University Press.

2

Developing partnership in dementia care: a discursive model of practice

Trevor Adams

KEY ISSUES

- 'Partnership' and 'social construction of dementia' are important issues in the contemporary provision of dementia care

- The use of language by family carers, health professionals and the media contributes to the experience of people with dementia

- The way in which language about dementia has been used highlights primary family carers and has disadvantaged other family members including the people with dementia themselves

- Various approaches that focus on narrative and discourse can be used to help people with dementia and their families

INTRODUCTION

There are two major themes running through this book. The first is that of 'partnership'. This theme has been emphasised in recent UK health and social care policy documents such as *Working in Partnership* and *A New Partnership for Care in Old Age* (DoH, 1994, 1996). This theme is important in that it counters the excessive individualisation of dementia care that has resulted from the influence of the medical profession (Lyman, 1989). In this dominant model of dementia the main concern is the diagnosis bearer, whereas little attention is given to family, friends, neighbours and the wider aspects of society in the development of dementia and dementia care.

The second theme is that of the social construction of dementia. As Clarke and Adams point out in the introduction to this book, there are various degrees to which a belief in social construction may be held; nonetheless, each of the contributors to this book affirms that to a greater or lesser extent social factors construct the experience of dementia care for people with dementia and their families. Each chapter supports and adds substance to the groundswell of critique that has been directed at the medical model of dementia (Lyman, 1989). Indeed, it is recognised that the idea of partnership is important, as it is a major objective of community care policy to support those families, friends and neighbours who care for dependent older people, including those with dementia, seeing their carers in terms of partnership (DHSS, 1981).

Two distinct research and practice traditions have developed within dementia care. The first tradition focuses on the person with dementia, for example through the development of assessment tools and interventions. The other tradition focuses upon the family and understands it as the main source of support for people with dementia. Knapman and Waite (1995) sum the situation up succinctly, commenting that: 'There is a tension between the rights of and wellbeing of the person being cared for, and those of the primary carer and other family members'. This raises the important question: who is the client? Is it the person with dementia, or is it the family?

In addition to the theme of partnership, a further theme within this book is that the person with dementia has been marginalised in the delivery of dementia care. This approach has been influenced by various sources including feminist writers such as Gilligan (1982); the disability movement who conceptualise people with disabilities as being subject to the discourses of 'the powers that be' in society (Gwilliam and Gilliard, 1996); and post-structuralist writers such as Foucault (1967) who argue that psychiatric discourses determine the practice of psychiatry and are used as a means of exercising power and control in society. This raises further questions about whose voice we are hearing in dementia care: is it the voice of the professional, the family carer or the person with dementia?

This chapter provides a theoretical framework within which these questions may be answered. The main concern, however, is that a socially just form of partnership should exist. Various writers have suggested that the concept of 'partnership' has very little to say about the contribution that each party within the partnership should make to the provision of community care to people with dementia. Opie (1992) comments that in dementia care, partnership 'tends to obscure the power differentials between informal caregivers and service providers' (p. 197). This point is supported by Goss and Miller (1995), who in a wider mental health perspective argue that 'the partnership between carers/users and workers must be equal in power but unequal in effort'.

A PARTNERSHIP APPROACH TO DEMENTIA CARE

The theoretical framework outlined in this chapter sets out the relationship between the person with dementia, the family, health and social care

providers, and the wider society. The framework draws
various writers, notably Silliman (1989). The framework
importance of language in the construction of dementia and

The person with dementia

People with dementia have largely gone unnoticed in studies on dementia
(Cotrell and Schulz, 1993). Whilst there has been much interest in the
neurological and biochemical aspects of dementia, there has been little
interest in the person as a whole (Lyman, 1989). However, the recent
increase in interest in the experience of people with dementia has provided
a welcome new focus to dementia care (Keady, 1996). Various factors have
contributed to the rediscovery of the person with dementia, including the
publication of a number of first-hand accounts of the experience of having
dementia; the continued development of reminiscence work; and the
recognition that people with dementia can possess insight about their
condition – something that by definition was denied in medical
formulations of dementia (McGowin, 1993; Bonat, 1997; Fairbairn, 1997).

Credit should also be given to the work of Tom Kitwood for the rediscovery of the person with dementia. This rediscovery can be seen in
Kitwood's development of a 'psychobiography' of Rose. In this
'psychobiography', Kitwood uses the recollections of members of her family
to write a history of Rose's psychological development within the context of
particular life events (Kitwood, 1990). For example, Kitwood tells the story
of Rose's relationship with her husband, daughter and siblings, including
one for whom she provided particular care. By caring for these people
without caring for herself, Kitwood reveals how Rose had little opportunity
to develop her experiential self, that is, the sense of self resulting from being
accepted, named and validated by other people. Rose's failure to develop
her experiential self was characterised generally by a lack of affect and
difficulty in creating bonds with other people. In its place, Kitwood argues
that Rose began to develop an adapted self, after the death of her husband,
which continued to develop as she responded to subsequent events in her
life. Kitwood (1990) sums up Rose's situation accordingly:

> In her case the experiential self, which might have sustained her sense of
> ontological security, her sense of agency, and her capacity for relatedness
> despite some degree of brain failure, was only poorly developed; and her
> adapted self ... underwent progressive decline; in her case, to vanishing point.
> Psychologically, it would seem that dementia was the inevitable consequence.
> (p. 72)

Moreover, Kitwood understands what happened to Rose in the wider
context of ideological and sociopolitical factors such as economic decline
and the social construction of women.

There are, however, various problems with the work of Kitwood, particularly his development of psychobiography (Adams, 1996; Harding and Palfrey, 1997). Firstly, Kitwood is far too optimistic about the ability of Rose's family to give an accurate account of Rose's life, particularly the times when they were not around such as before they were born. Secondly, Kitwood fails to include Rose's own account of her life, privileging the discourse of her family. Furthermore, little consideration is given to the strategic use of language by Rose's relatives and their choice – unconscious or otherwise – of what should or should not be included in their account. While Kitwood's approach has greatly contributed to the rediscovery of the person with dementia, his failure to acknowledge the weaknesses and limitations of his method raises doubts regarding its credibility as presented.

More recently, however, Kitwood has moved away from using accounts of relatives to develop a fuller psychological history of the person with dementia. Kitwood (1997a,b) has identified seven 'access routes' by which people may 'gain insight into the subjective world of dementia' (Kitwood, 1997a, p. 15):

- Through accounts that have been written by people who have dementia
- By careful listening to what people with dementia say, in some kind of interview or group context
- Attending carefully to what people with dementia say and do in the course of their ordinary life
- Learning through the behaviour of people with dementia
- Consulting people who have undergone an illness with dementia-like features
- Through the use of our own poetic imagination
- Through the use of role play, that is actually taking on the part of someone who has dementia, and living it out in a simulated care environment.

Whilst it is noticeable that Kitwood emphasises the account of the person with dementia more fully, nonetheless Kitwood's work lacks any acknowledgment that the use of language is problematical and socially situated. However, there has been a reversal in this trend, and various 'post-Kitwoodian' writers have emerged. Whilst in many ways these writers are fellow travellers with Kitwood, their work is based on empirical data gained from the people with dementia themselves. This is an important step forward methodologically, though it has to be noted that problems of collecting valid and reliable data still remain and should be properly addressed. In Chapter 11, John Keady and Jane Gilliard provide an example of the trend towards using empirical findings as an access to the person with dementia.

The family

Until recently, the dominant approach in dementia care emphasised the burden incurred by the primary family carer as a result of caring for the person with dementia (Zarit and Edwards, 1996). In this approach, the burden was understood to be physical and emotional, even to the point of contributing to the development of illness in the family carer (Donaldson et al, 1997). However, this focus on the primary family carer is conceptually inadequate, because when a person develops dementia it is not just one member of the family who suffers but the whole family (Garwick et al, 1994). Commonly, when other family members are included in discussions about dementia care, it is only in terms of the support they can provide or the extent to which conflict exists between themselves and the primary carer, rather than their own difficulties (Malonbeach and Zarit, 1991; Semple, 1992; Zarit et al, 1980).

Reconceptualising dementia care in terms of the whole family, rather than just one family carer, is an important shift in thinking and has considerable implications for practice. Firstly, it takes full account of what is happening to all family members. Perry and Olshansky (1996) in a study of families containing people with dementia found that there were differences in how each family member defined and made sense of the situation and that this had consequences for the whole family. In particular, each family member experienced a similar process of coming to terms with changes in the person who had dementia. This process was found to consist of three stages: identifying how the person with dementia was the same as before the disease onset, as well as the differences; redefining the identity of the person with dementia; and rewriting one's relationship with the person with dementia. Perry and Olshansky's paper does much to dispel 'the myth of the solitary family carer' and suggests the development of a family systemic approach to dementia care (Perry and Olshansky, 1996). Moreover, the study also dispels the notion of the family as having a shared meaning as suggested by Patterson (1993), and reveals the family as having multiple perspectives about what is happening to that family. As Wright and Leahey (1994) point out, 'each individual has a role to play in understanding, describing and dealing with the problem' (p. 155).

Reconceptualising the family as containing multiple perspectives also acknowledges the possibility that conflict may occur between the family members and the person with dementia which may contribute to the physical and emotional abuse of the older person with dementia. It also highlights the conflict that may exist amongst the family members themselves as a result of their relative having dementia, for example conflict may develop between brothers and sisters, or between husbands and wives (Zarit and Edwards, 1996; Parker, 1997).

Another benefit of reconceptualising dementia in terms of the family is that one family member is less likely to be singled out as 'the carer'. Often when one person is seen to take on the responsibility of providing care, for a relative with dementia, the rest of the family are happy to acquiesce. Reconceptualising the dementia in terms of the family acknowledges that there are various configurations that families may adopt in providing care for one of their members. This is highlighted by Keith (1995) whose study of caregiving families identifies three ways in which families configure themselves as they care for an older family member. The first configuration relates to the 'primary caregiver', in which one person carries all or most of the responsibility for providing care. The second is characterised by partnership in which 'two offspring contribute relatively equitably to the caregiving work, and more importantly, are equal in authority and responsibility, in making and implementing decisions' (p. 183). Other siblings may also be involved in the caregiving, but their roles are more limited. Partnership is understood by Keith (1995) in qualitative terms as 'sharing the undertaking, consulting with each other, arriving at decisions together, carrying the responsibility jointly, and commiserating about the failings of their siblings' (p. 184), rather than in terms of how many hours each carer puts in. The last caregiving system is characterised by the 'team' approach, in which family members perceive their roles as team members, rather than considering how the work is appropriated.

The health and social care agencies

Health and social agencies contribute to the wellbeing or otherwise of people with dementia and their families. The discourses that constitute professional education and practice by which they categorise and address the problems of people with dementia will affect the lives of people with dementia and their families. However, as Kitwood argues, not all professional practice promotes the 'personhood' of the person with dementia and he argues for the development of a 'new culture of dementia care' (Kitwood, 1997b).

The way in which health and social care professionals manage their caseloads by finding new cases, responding to people with dementia and their family carers, working with other health or social care professionals, and referring cases to other health and social care agencies, will contribute to the experience of people with dementia and the care that they receive. This raises the issue of the organisation of dementia care services, the models of service provision and the amount of money spent on the care of people with dementia and by whom. It also raises issues about the quality assurance of interagency and interprofessional working and the provision of education for professionals and family carers. At the moment there is a considerable amount of rhetoric about the need to work together and the development of partnership. In the UK this has been set into a neo-liberal framework for health and social policy developed in the 1980s by the Thatcher administration and there seems little prospect of change under the Blair administration of the 1990s (Goodwin, 1997). An important part of this framework is 'the mixed economy of care', which was a key concept of the NHS and Community Care Act 1990 (DoH, 1990). The implication was that services should not just be supplied by the state but rather should come from a variety of sources: the private sector, the voluntary sector, and family, friends and neighbours. Indeed, government policy has accepted that the family is the first port of call when an old person needs help, at least since the publication of *Growing Older* in 1981 (DHSS, 1981). However, this raises the question: at what point should formal agencies of support start to support people with dementia, most of whom are elderly, and how should these formal sources of support make contact with the family?

The provision of informal care often places considerable strain upon family carers, as they struggle their way through the first few months (or more) of their relative's dementia (Parker, 1997). Also, considerable difficulties for the family often arise in obtaining help from the health and social services. Not only do families take a long time to realise that one of their members has developed dementia, but they also have difficulty in obtaining help from their general practitioners, who often fail to make an appropriate diagnosis or take appropriate action. Illiffe (1997) argues that within general practice four issues appear important in improving the management of people with dementia: a population perspective that includes assessing the population over the age of 75 years; enhanced diagnostic skills; the recognition by family doctors that a range of supportive responses exist; and the development of good networks between health and social care workers – or in terms of this book, 'good partnership'.

Another increasingly important area of service provision is the voluntary sector. Within this sector of the mixed economy of care, various agencies make a significant contribution to the care of people with dementia and their families. A particularly important organisation in the UK is the Alzheimer's Disease Society (ADS). At a national level this organisation lobbies government agencies through the publication of reports, and provides funding for medical and social research. The ADS was influential along with the Carers National Association in helping to usher in the Carer's (Recognition and Services) Act 1995 (DoH, 1995) which gives carers a statutory right to have their needs assessed by their local authority. At a local level, the ADS organises groups of family carers who meet on a regular basis to provide much-needed mutual support. Clearly, through consultation and partnership with government agencies, the general public, family carers for people with dementia and ultimately the people with dementia themselves will be affected by the work of voluntary agencies such as the ADS.

Societal variables

In addition to the partnership that exists between the person with dementia, the family carers and the health and social care providers, it should also be acknowledged that other, more general, agencies contribute to the development of partnership in dementia care. Whilst these agencies possibly do not have a direct impact upon the construction of dementia care, they are nonetheless important as they mediate the experience of people with dementia, their families, and health and social care agencies. These societal variables include social support networks, the media, the political context and the use of discourse.

Social support networks

Wenger (1994a,b) has undertaken a considerable amount of work on the social networks within which people with dementia are situated. Other work compares the experience of people with dementia and their carers in cities and towns with those living in rural areas. The physical distance between family carers and their relatives with dementia will affect their ability to offer care, and if the family carers live some distance away it is likely to make the carers more tired and exhausted than they would be if they lived nearer, and may even make it impossible for them to continue providing care. Moreover, the nature of the relationships that a person with dementia had with family and friends before the onset of dementia will affect the subsequent support network, as too will the support network of the primary family carer.

The media

Another contributory social factor is the influence of the media upon the experience of dementia, both for sufferers and for carers. This area has generally been neglected, but a number of studies relating to the role of the media in other mental health problems have been undertaken by the Glasgow Media Group (Philo, 1996). Philo (1996) found that the media can exert great influence over audiences, but people are able either to accept or to reject the message. He argues that the media exploit key elements of social cultures which they have in part created – for example, they can exploit people's fear of mental illness, and can also create images that help people feel concern for people who are mentally ill. This supports the use of the media by agencies such as the Alzheimer's Disease Society to raise people's awareness of dementia in a constructive way. An example of this is the ADS annual Awareness Week. For example, part of the 1997 Awareness Week was the publication of a report entitled *No Accounting for Health*, which sought to highlight deficiencies in the provision of care for older people with dementia in the UK (ADS, 1997). Also, the ADS has been active in criticising a television comedy called *Keeping Mum*, which purported to portray the experience of a woman in the early stages of dementia in a comical way. Activity such as this will help challenge dominant notions of dementia as amusing, and properly represent dementia as a tragic event in a person's life.

The public's awareness of dementia will affect the lives of people with dementia and their carers. In another study, Philo (1996) found that media images can have a damaging effect on people with mental illness and their carers and on their immediate social-relationships. Empirical work relating to the representation of dementia in the media would be welcome, particularly relating to the effectiveness of awareness campaigns such as those undertaken by the ADS.

Political contexts

Recent social policy in the UK has been the replacement of large-scale institutionalisation of people with mental illness by a policy of community care within 'a mixed economy of care' (DoH, 1990). This policy reflects the general mood of suspicion about the standards of care in mental hospitals in the 1960s and 1970s fostered by the work of Barton (1959), and Goffman (1961), as well as by government reports, written at a time when the abuses occurring in mental hospitals were revealed through reports in newspapers and television documentaries such as *World in Action* (Martin, 1984; Goodwin, 1997).

The policy of community care has many shortcomings, not least the inappropriate discharge of people with mental illness into community settings (Goodwin, 1997). However, since the problems associated with the care of people with dementia are rather different from those of younger people with mental health problems, the problems that families experience are not so much related to discharge from hospital but to maintaining people in community settings until they have to enter residential accommodation. Nevertheless, the problem of transferring frail older people with dementia has become an issue of recent concern (Trieman and Wills, 1997).

Another political issue that needs to be addressed is the nature of the 'mixed economy of care'. The policy argues that care should be provided by both the informal and formal sectors, that is the statutory, independent and voluntary agencies. This raises the issue of whether people can afford residential care if they need it, and whether the state is retreating from the commitment of an earlier time to provide welfare 'from the cradle to the grave'. This raises two further points: firstly, there is a need for closer partnership in the form of interagency collaboration between all sections of the 'mixed economy of care' in the provision of care to older people with dementia; secondly, there is a need to address criticism regarding the provision of care to people with dementia at a political level, as it is the government through the Department of Health that determines and is responsible for the development of good community care.

An additional point about politics arises in the context of developments in health and social policy aimed at people with mental illness. It has been a concern of government agencies to address the problems of people with 'severe and enduring mental health problems' (DoH, 1997); however, it is not clear whether this term is intended to include people with dementia. In various government documents people with dementia *are* included, but often only in parenthesis. This misses the opportunity to stress that dementia is indeed a severe and enduring mental health problem. The term tends to be applied only to younger people with functional psychoses such as schizophrenia and mania, not to people with organic psychoses such as dementia. The result of this tendency to exclude dementia has been that funds made available to address the problems encountered by the mentally ill have not been shared with people with dementia.

There are signs, however, that there is a move to refocus this policy to include people with dementia within research and practice initiatives directed towards people with severe and enduring mental health problems. This is in line with a paper published by Powell and Slade (1996), who set out five distinct dimensions to the idea of severe mental illness: these are safety; informal and formal support; diagnosis; disability; and duration (SIDDD). As can be seen from Box 2.1, dementia fits readily into each of these dimensions.

The use of discourse

There are many discourses – that is ways of speaking and practice about social phenomena – that construct the experience of people with dementia and their family carers. Glenister and Tilley (1996) outline six discourses they suggest have a bearing on mental health practice:

1. medical discourse
2. social disablement discourse
3. discourse relating to 'communality between the mass and the excluded minority'
4. human rights discourse
5. social integration discourse
6. consumerism.

Other discourses also contribute to the experience of people with dementia, for example community care discourse, ageist discourse and gender-related discourse (Potter and Collie, 1989; Bytheway, 1995). These

Box 2.1 The 'SIDDD' dimensions relating to severe mental illness

- **Safety** has four components:
  unintentional self-harm, self-neglect
  intentional self-harm
  safety of others
  abuse by others, e.g. physical, sexual, emotional, financial.

- **Informal and formal support** has two components:
  help from informal carers including friends and relatives
  help from formal services such as day care centres, paid staff, voluntary services, hospital admissions, medication and detention under the Mental Health Act.

- **Diagnosis** may include:
  psychotic illness
  dementia
  severe neurotic disorders
  personality disorder
  developmental disorder.

- **Disability** with impaired ability to function effectively in the community, which may include problems with:
  employment and recreation
  personal care
  domestic skills
  interpersonal skills.

- **Duration** of any of the above for a minimum period.

From Powell and Slade (1996).

discourses are perpetuated by powerful agencies in society such as the church and professions who communicate their interests through newspapers, books, magazines, academic journals and television.

Clearly there is an interconnection between social support, politics, the media and discourse. They are to some extent overlapping and have an effect on each other. For example, government use of the phrase 'severe and enduring mental health problems' arises in part from a concern in the media about the possibility of violence to the public from people receiving inadequate social support in the community. However, through the proactive use of the media, agencies such as ADS are introducing a new discourse directed at changing government policy and enhancing the support of older people with dementia. In this way the interconnection between the social support, politics, the media and discourse may be used to the advantage of older people with dementia and their family carers. Health and social care professionals too need to be more aware of the discourse they have been brought into, through education and training.

THE INTERDEPENDENT CAREER: PEOPLE WITH DEMENTIA AND THEIR FAMILIES

As a result of the progressive nature of dementia, people with this condition and their families are affected in different ways, at different times. Donaldson et al (1997), in a review of empirical studies relating to the impact of symptoms of dementia upon family carers, found that various recognisable impairments in people with dementia, particularly non-cognitive features of the illness, are an important cause of negative outcomes in family carers. Some writers have suggested that the impairments associated with dementia follow various stages. However, this approach has met with some opposition, notably from Bell and McGregor (1995), who argue that some of the dangers of a staged theory of dementia include a predetermined course of a person's future development; it ties each person into a 'syndrome' and it offers a hopeless and inevitable future of decline. Everyone is different and has a different response to dementia, and so a rigorous staging approach to dementia is inappropriate and unhelpful.

Nevertheless, it is reasonable to suggest that a person with dementia does possess a career in much the same way as a person with any other chronic condition (Bury, 1982). To a certain extent this career will be affected by the onset and type of dementia: for example, Alzheimer's disease has an insidious onset, whereas in multi-infarct dementia the onset is sudden. Whilst every situation is different, nevertheless a clear progression in the development of dementia may be identified. Moreover, there appears to be a progression not only in the development of the dementia but also in the nature and character of family care. Various models have been put forward; although focusing mainly on the primary family carer rather than the whole family, they provide some indication of the various psychosocial stages passed through by families looking after a person with dementia (Wilson, 1989; Willoughby and Keating, 1991; McCarty, 1996).

One particularly worthwhile model is that of Aneshensel et al (1995), which proposes three stages – role acquisition, role enhancement and role disengagement. Throughout the career, the primary carer takes on and relinquishes new roles and activities. Some of these role changes are the result of changes in the location of the person with dementia; for example, initially the person with dementia will be at home, but later on may receive various forms of day care and respite care. Later still, the carer may have to adjust to the person with dementia being admitted to full-time residential or hospital care, and finally, to the person's death. Other changes during the career relate to the sufferer's changing mental, physical and emotional state. Initially, the family carer will have to adjust to a period when the person with dementia is beginning to show signs of forgetfulness. During this period the carer will not be sure whether the person is just going through a bad patch, is being awkward, or has a serious mental illness such as dementia. Ironically, the management of the person with dementia is often most difficult at the early stage of the disorder at a time when health and social care agencies are not involved with the case (Wenger, 1994b). As the dementia progresses, the carer may need to adjust to the increasing inability of the sufferer to cope with previously easy tasks such as collecting pension money or dressing, and so the carer has to take over these tasks. These changes in location and in the ability to undertake tasks will challenge the family carer and require adjustment to these new demands.

Whilst this model has much to recommend it, two points of difference may be suggested. Firstly, there is not just one carer involved in looking after the person with dementia, but potentially the whole family. Secondly, this model focuses primarily on the concept of stress and coping as an underlying theoretical approach, whereas a more social constructionist approach may be valuable.

To summarise, the relationship between the person with dementia and other family members is an interdependent one. What happens to a person with dementia will affect the family, and what happens to the family will have consequences upon the person with dementia.

THE LINGUISTIC CONSTRUCTION OF DEMENTIA CARE

The construction of the person with dementia

A number of writers have examined the importance of language in the construction of social phenomena in general and in dementia in particular (Gergen, 1985; Shotter, 1993; Hyden, 1997). The way in which language provides a descriptive organisation of dementia was the central theme of Gubrium's important book *Old Timers and Alzheimer's* (Gubrium, 1986). More recently, Sabat and Harré (1992) have identified ways in which the personal and social selves are produced in people with dementia through their interaction with other people. They argue that any threatened disappearance of self is not directly linked to the progress of the disease but results from people not understanding what demented people are saying, and positioning people with dementia as helpless and confused. A similar case is made by Kitwood (1997b) who lists various ways of talking to Alzheimer's sufferers that can undermine their personhood, such as treating them as if they are a child (infantilisation) and unnecessarily doing things for them (disempowerment).

Cheston (1996) describes the way in which people with Alzheimer's disease use stories of past events to describe their present experiences.

Cheston (1996) understands stories as having two related functions. Firstly, they enable people to explore their experiences and thus, he argues, stories act as metaphors for the personal experience of having dementia. Secondly, they act as a means of creating a series of social identities. Golander and Raz (1996) similarly see stories as constructive of the identity of people with dementia. For example, they describe a hospital patient, Pinhas, who had 'advanced dementia' and had 'a famous past identity, life achievements'. Although his present behaviour was distasteful, nonetheless the staff on the ward would interpret his presence on the ward favourably in line with his past identity.

Ramanathan-Abbott (1994) describes how the way in which people with dementia are spoken to affects their ability to participate in interviews, and raises the possibility that the ability of people with dementia to recall events and their meaning is grounded in and constructed through interaction, suggesting that the mental health nurses may help to 'create' people's presentation of their dementia. As with any other chronic disability, people with dementia have a biography or story about their life, and it is this story that is the subject of what is said to them but also that out of which they construct meaning to events that are happening in their life (Bury, 1982).

The construction of family care

Various studies demonstrate how linguistic devices contribute to the construction of family care in dementia. Globerman (1995) in a study of caregiving and non-caregiving children of parents with dementia found that stories about themselves as children were important in the family's decision over who should take on the role of the primary family carer. When stories identified a particular child as different, for example that they were 'spoilt' or 'intellectual', they were found not to be given caregiving responsibilities as adults. Moreover, while these unencumbered children were not given caregiving responsibilities, they were still affected by their parent becoming demented, and were found to describe their loss and suffering in terms of identity and selfhood, further undermining the idea that the 'primary carer is the only carer'.

Crisp (1995) applies existing theories about the nature of narrative to the confabulations made by her mother with dementia. She argues that in people with dementia, 'confabulatory story telling becomes a valuable means of social interaction and of maintaining a sense of identity and worth against the inroads of increasing infirmity and dependence' (p. 136).

The construction of professional care

In addition to the way in which people with dementia and their family carers develop meaning in their lives through the use of stories, numerous studies have revealed the importance of language in the construction of people's work. Hunter (1991) argues that doctors use narratives to reason out issues they meet in their practice; so that 'in medicine the case is the basic unit of thought and discourse, for clinical knowledge, however scientific it may be, it is narratively organised and communicated' (p. 51). Other health-care professionals have also been found to use narrative in their work. A study by Mattingly and Fleming (1994) of occupational therapists identified the use of narratives in their reasoning about their clients. These authors make the distinction between 'telling stories', which is a retrospective process, and 'story making', which concerns the way in which therapists work to structure therapy as a coherent plot, not just a series of treatment activities, thus creating dramatic therapeutic events that connect therapy to a patient's life.

Within nursing too, narratives have been found to play a significant role in the patient's reasoning, for example Benner (1982) and Saanddiski (1996) describe the use of narratives in nursing. Häggström and Norberg (1996) found that nurses use maternal language to talk about the people with dementia for whom they care. More specifically, Tilley (1995) argues that psychiatric nurses employ narratives in their work and describes the form and grammar employed in psychiatric nursing narratives. This notion of narrative together with his work on discourse (Glenister and Tilley 1996) is continued in the more recent study by Tilley (1997) of the psychiatric nurse as a 'rhetorician'. Kitwood (1993) notes that in dementia care nurses are often placed in a conflict between two different discourses – the dominant medical discourse to which they are expected to adhere, and what they 'know through experience'. The work of Hunter (1991), Atkinson (1995) and Mattingly and Fleming (1994) suggests that the use of narratives is not just a feature of how nurses undertake their work but is an important characteristic of various health-care professionals, particularly in terms of their ability to make clinical judgments and decisions.

HEARING THE VOICES OF DEMENTIA CARE

An important consideration in the construction of dementia and dementia care is the use of language. Since the publication of Malcolm Goldsmith's book *Hearing the Voice of People with Dementia* (Goldsmith, 1996), recognition is growing that often the contribution and participation of people with dementia has been neglected in favour of that of the primary family carer. However, now that the initial shock produced by the book has been absorbed, it is appropriate to develop a more considered position that sets the voice of the person with dementia within the context of other voices within dementia care such as those of the primary family carer, the other family members and the health-care professionals themselves.

There are various ways in which health practitioners may understand the accounts that are given to them. Firstly, accounts may be understood as windows through which reality is accurately represented. This, however, is a rather simplistic view, since whenever two people see the same event, particularly complex events that occur over prolonged periods, there will be differences between their accounts. It also depends on a realist model of language in which word and meaning are perfectly joined, without ambiguity.

Secondly, accounts may be understood as the means by which people come to their understanding of reality. Therefore a carer may develop a mental explanation of why she is providing care for her husband when she could be doing other things. For example, she may say, '[my husband] would have done the same to me if it was me who had dementia'. In this way, a carer's understanding of what has happened provides a story through which the carer comes to terms with difficult and tragic events. Indeed, this approach may be developed into a means of enabling family carers to transform their feelings of depression and burden by therapeutic work associated with amending their narrative of what has happened. This approach is based on the work of White and Epson (1990) and has usefully been applied to family carers by Clark and Standard (1997).

Thirdly, the telling of the account itself may be understood as 'performative' and situated within the social context. For example, a female carer may spend some time telling a female health practitioner about the difficulties she has experienced with a husband who had been difficult and awkward throughout their marriage, in the hope, (albeit unconscious) that this particular account will elicit a favourable response from the health-care professional and the opportunity to gain a better share of health-care resources.

There are not only various ways in which an account may be understood within dementia care, there are also various accounts that are available and may be drawn upon to describe a particular case. These accounts may come from:

- The person with dementia
- The primary, family carer
- Every family member
- The health-care professional.

The accounts of the carer and of other family members may draw upon the individual's own story and also on the 'family story', the story that the family has developed collectively over the years. The importance of the family story in relationship to health and illness has been elaborated by Bell (1997) and by Mules and Streitberger (1997). The family story includes the way in which the family has collectively understood and interpreted what has happened to them. For example, it may include religious and political elements, feuds, and stories about illness and previous experiences with the health-care provision. Indeed, there may be an intimate relationship between the individual and the family story. Finally, all health-care professionals possess their own story which they can tell in many different ways. These stories are developed from the expert narrative that constitutes their professionalisation as a health-care practitioner, and also from their personal story. For example, health-care professionals who are themselves the daughter or son of a parent with dementia will be able to give a different account from professionals with no experience of dementia in their personal life.

IMPLICATIONS FOR PRACTICE

Firstly, health-care professionals should listen to all the voices associated with the care of a person with dementia. This will include a critical and reflective understanding of their own understanding of the situation, with a particular sensitivity to their own prejudices and blockages to thinking. Within this context clinical supervision may be helpful as a means of helping practitioners in dementia care to reflect and think through the issues involved in casework.

Secondly, health-care practitioners should elicit all the various accounts of the situation that are available. These accounts will show some similarities but also differences of understanding. It is important that the health-care professional takes an agnostic position to these accounts rather than accepting one particular account of the situation, which might compromise the professional's neutrality.

Thirdly, health-care professionals should develop an understanding of the situation based upon all the accounts that have been given. Whilst it is desirable that health-care professionals should develop an objective view of what has happened, their understanding can only be *their* interpretation of the situation. Nonetheless, it is this understanding that has to underpin their health-care professional practice.

Fourthly, health-care professionals should address these accounts in appropriate setting. This will be accomplished either individually, as with the accounts of people with dementia, family carers and other health-care professionals, or in a group setting such as a family meeting or a multidisciplinary team meeting. A non-directive approach should be adopted in which it is not the responsibility of the health-care professional to attempt to 'convert' the other people involved in the care of the person with dementia to a particular view of a situation, but rather to help them come to an understanding that will facilitate the care of the person with dementia within the wellbeing of the family.

To summarise, therefore, this chapter has argued that partnership in dementia care is constructed through the use of language, and that it is through language that the person with dementia, the family carers and health and social care professionals are constructed. This is an important area of interest since the primary way in which government agencies and the professions organise themselves, and organisations such as the ADS operate, is through the use of language. It is hoped that this chapter will encourage other practitioners, researchers and academics to develop an increased understanding of the importance of language in the construction of partnership in dementia care.

REFERENCES

Adams, T. (1996) Kitwood's approach to dementia and dementia care: a critical but appreciative review. *Journal of Advanced Nursing* **23**, 948–952.
Adams, T. (1997) Kitwood's approach to dementia and dementia care: a critical but appreciative review. *Journal of Advanced Nursing* **23**, 948–953.
Adams, T. (1998) A discursive approach to dementia care – implications for mental health nursing. *Journal of Advanced Nursing* (in press).
[ADS] Alzheimer's Disease Society (1997) *No Accounting for Health: Health Commissioning for Dementia*. London: ADS.
Aneshensel, C.S., Pearlin, L., Mullan, J., Zarit, S. & Whittlatch, C. (1995) *Profiles in Caregiving: The Unexpected Career*. San Diego: Academic Press.
Atkinson, P. (1995) *Medical Talk and Medical Work*. London: Sage.
Barton, R. (1959) *Institutional Neurosis*. Bristol: Wright.
Bell, J. & McGregor, I. (1995) A challenge to stage theories of dementia. In: Kitwood, T. & Benson, S. (eds) *The New Culture of Dementia*. London: Hawker.
Bell, J.M. (1997) Illness stories and family nursing. *Journal of Family Nursing* **3** (4), 315–317.
Benner, P. (1982) *From Novice to Expert*. Menlo Park: Addison-Wesley.
Bonat, J. (1997) Approaches to reminiscence. In: Norman, I. & Redfern, S. (eds) *Mental Health Care for Elderly People*. Edinburgh: Churchill Livingstone.
Bury, M. (1982) Chronic illness as a biographical disruption. *Sociology of Health and Illness* **4**, 167–182.
Bytheway, B. (1995) *Ageism*. Buckingham: Open University Press.
Cheston, R. (1996) Stories and metaphors: talking about the past in a psychotherapy group for people with dementia. *Ageing and Society* **16**, 579–602.
Clarke, M.C. & Standard, P.L. (1997) The caregiving story: how the narrative approach informs caregiving burden. *Issues in Mental Health Nursing* **18**, 87–97.
Cotrell, V. & Schulz, R. (1993) The perspective of the patient with Alzheimer's disease: a neglected dimension of dementia research. *Gerontologist* **33** (2), 205–211.
Crisp, J. (1995) Making sense of the stories that people with Alzheimer's tell: a journey with my mother. *Nursing Inquiry* **2**, 133–140.
DeLongis, A. & O'Brien, T. (1990) An interpersonal framework for stress and coping: an application to the families of Alzheimer's disease. In: Stephen, J. Crowther, S., Hobpoll, S. & Tennenhaum, I. (eds) *Stress and Coping in Later-Life Families*. New York: Hemisphere.
[DHSS] Department of Health and Social Security (1981) *Growing Older*. London: HMSO.
[DOH] Department of Health (1990) *NHS and Community Care Act 1990*. London: HMSO.
[DOH] Department of Health (1994) *Working in Partnership*. London: HMSO.
[DOH] Department of Health (1995) Carers (Recognition and Services) Act. London: HMSO.
[DOH] Department of Health (1996) *A New Partnership for Care in Old Age*. Cm 3242. London: HMSO.
[DOH] Department of Health (1997) *Voices in Partnership: Involving Users and Carers in Commissioning and Delivering Mental Health Services*. London: HMSO.
Donaldson, C., Tarrier, N. & Burns, A. (1997) The impact of the symptoms of dementia on caregivers. *British Journal of Psychiatry* **170**, 62–68.
Fairbairn, A. (1997) Insight and dementia. In: Marshall, M. (ed.) *State of the Art in Dementia Care*. London: Centre for Policy on Ageing.

Foucault, M. (1967) *Madness and Civilisation*. London: Tavistock.

Garwick, A., Detzer, D. & Boss, P. (1994) Family perceptions of living with Alzheimer's disease. *Family Process* **33**, 327–340.

Gergen, K. (1985) The social constructionist movement in modern psychology. *American Psychologist* **40**, 266–275.

Gilligan, C. (1982) *In a Different Voice: Psychological Theory and Women's Development*. Cambridge: Harvard University Press.

Glenister, D. & Tilley, S. (1996) Discourse, social exclusion and empowerment. *Journal of Psychiatric and Mental Health Nursing* **3**, 3–5.

Globerman, J. (1995) The unencumbered child: family reputations and responsibilities in the care of relatives with Alzheimer's disease. *Family Process* **34**, 87–99.

Goffman E. (1961) *Asylums*. Harmondsworth. Penguin.

Golander, H.A. & Raz, A.E. (1996) The mask of dementia: images of 'Demented Residents' in a nursing ward. *Ageing and Society* **16**, 269–285.

Goldsmith, M. (1996) *Hearing the Voice of People with Dementia*. London: Jessica Kingsley.

Goodwin, S. (1997) *Comparative Mental Health Policy: From Institutional to Community Care*. London: Sage.

Goss, S. & Millar, C. (1995) *From Margin to Mainstream: Developing User and Carer Centred Community Care*. Community Care / Joseph Rowntree Foundation.

Gubrium, J. (1986) *Old Timers and Alzheimer's: The Descriptive Organisation of Senility*. Greenwich: JAI Press.

Gwilliam, C. & Gilliard, J. (1996) Dementia and the social model of disability. *Journal of Dementia Care* January / February,

Häggström, T. & Norberg, A. (1996) Maternal thinking in dementia care. *Journal of Advanced Nursing* **24**(3), 431–438.

Harding, N. & Palfrey, C. (1997) *The Social Construction of Dementia: Confused Professionals?* London: Jessica Kingsley.

Hunter, K.M. (1991) *Doctors' Stories: The Narrative Structure of Medical Knowledge*. Princeton University Press.

Hyden, L.-C. (1997) Illness and narrative. *Sociology of Health and Illness* **19** (1), 48–69.

Illife, S. (1997) Problems in recognising dementia in general practice: how can they be overcome? In: Marshall, M.M. (ed.) *State of the Art in Dementia Care*. London: Centre for Policy on Ageing.

Keady, J. (1996) The experience of dementia: a review of the literature and the implications for clinical practice. *Journal of Clinical Nursing* **5**, 275–288.

Keith, C. (1995) Family caregiving systems: models, resources, and values. *Journal of Marriage and the Family* **57**, 179–189.

Kitwood, T. (1990) Understanding senile dementia: a psychobiographical approach. *Free Associations* **19**, 60–76.

Kitwood, T. (1993) Towards a theory of dementia care: the interpersonal process. *Ageing and Society* **13**, 51–67.

Kitwood, T. (1997a) The experience of dementia. *Aging and Mental Health* **1** (1), 13–22.

Kitwood, T. (1997b) *Dementia Reconsidered*. Buckingham: Open University Press.

Knapman, C. & Waite, H. (1995) Dementia care: time to ask new questions. *Social Alternatives* **14** (2), 41–43.

Lyman, K. (1989) Bringing the social back in: a critique of the biomedicalization of dementia. *Gerontologist* **29** (5), 597–605.

Malonbeach, E.E. & Zarit, S.H. (1991) Current issues in caregiving to the elderly. *International Journal of Ageing and Human Development* **32** (2), 103–114.

Mattingly, C. & Fleming, M. (1994) *Clinical Reasoning: Forms of Inquiry in a Therapeutic Practice*. Philadelphia: FA Davis.

McCarty, E.F. (1996) Caring for a parent with Alzheimer's disease: process of daughter caregiver stress. *Journal of Advanced Nursing* **23**, 792–803.

McGowin, D. (1993) *Living in The Labyrinth: A Personal Journey Through the Maze of Alzheimer's*. San Francisco: Elder Books.

Moules, N.J. & Streitberger, S. (1997) Stories of suffering, stories of strength: narrative influences in family nursing. *Journal of Family Nursing* **3** (4), 365–377.

Opie, A. (1992) *There's Nobody There*. Oxford University Press.

Parker, I. (1997) *Representing Reality*. London: Sage.

Patterson, J.M. (1993) The role of family meanings in adaption to chronic illness and disability. In: Turnbull, J., Patterson, S.K., Behr, D., Murphy, Marquis, J. Blue-banning (eds) *Cognitive Coping, Families, and Disabilities*, pp. 221–238. Baltimore: Paul H. Brookes.

Perry, J. & Olshansky, E.F. (1996) A family coming to terms with Alzheimer's disease. *Western Journal of Nursing Research* **18** (1), 12–28.

Philo, G., ed. (1996) *Media and Mental Distress*. London: Longman.

Potter, J. & Collie, F. (1989) 'Community Care' as persuasive rhetoric; a study of discourse. *Disability, Handicap and Society* **4** (1), 57–64.

Powell, R. & Slade, M. (1996) Defining severe mental illness. In: Thornicroft, G. & Strathdee, G. (eds) *Commissioning Mental Health Services*. London: HMSO.

Ramanathan-Abbott, V. (1994) Interactional differences in Alzheimer's disease: an examination of AD speech across two audiences. *Language in Society* **23**, 31–58.

Saanddiski, M.J. (1996) Truth/storytelling in Nursing Inquiry. In: Kikuchi, J.F., Simmons, H. & Romyn, D. (eds) *Truth in Nursing Inquiry*. London: Sage.

Sabat, S.R. & Harré, R. (1992) The construction and deconstruction of self in Alzheimer's disease. *Ageing and Society* **12** (4), 443–461.

Semple, S. (1992) Conflict in Alzheimer's caregiving families: its dimensions and consequences. *Gerontologist* **32** (5), 648–655.

Shotter, J. (1993) *Conversational Realities*. London: Sage.

Silliman, R. (1989) Caring for the frail older patient: the doctor-patient-caregiver relationship. *Journal of General Internal Medicine* **4**, 237–241.

Tilley, S. (1995) Notes on narrative knowledge in psychiatric nursing. *Journal of Psychiatric and Mental Health Nursing* **2**, 217–226.

Tilley, S. (1997) The mental health nurse as rhetorician. In: Tilley, S. (ed.) *The Mental Health Nurse: Views of Practice and Education*. Oxford: Blackwell.

Trieman, N. & Wills, W. (1997) The psycho-geriatric population: in transition from hospital to community-based services. In: Leff, J. (ed.) *Care in the Community: Illusion or Reality?* Chichester: Wiley.

Wenger, G.C. (1994a) Social support networks and dementia. *International Journal of Geriatric Psychiatry* **9**, 181–194.

Wenger, G.C. (1994b) Dementia sufferers at home. *International Journal of Geriatric Psychiatry* **9**, 721–733.

White, M. & Epston, D. (1990) *Narrative Means to Therapeutic Ends*. New York: WW Norton.

Willoughby, J. & Keating, N. (1991) Being in control: the process of caring for a relative with Alzheimer's disease. *Qualitative Health Research* **1** (1), 27–50.

Wilson, H.S. (1989) Family caregiving for a relative with Alzheimer's dementia: coping with negative choices. *Nursing Research* **38** (2), 94–98.

Wright, L.M. & Leahey, M. (1994) *Nurse and Families: A Guide to Family Assessment and Intervention*, 2nd edn. Philadelphia: FA Davis.

Zarit, S.H. & Edwards, A.B. (1996) Family caregiving: research and clinical intervention. In: Woods, R.T. (ed.) *Handbook of the Psychology of Ageing*. Chichester: Wiley.

Zarit, S.H., Reever, K. & Bach-Patterson, J. (1980) Relatives of the impaired elderly: correlates of feelings of burden. *Gerontologist* **20** (6), 649–655.

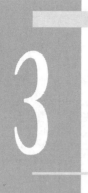

Western medicine and dementia: a deconstruction

T. Michael Hill

KEY ISSUES

- Scientific medicine (traditionally viewed as a superior way of understanding health and illness issues in Western societies) has dominated our understanding of dementia

- Scientific medicine appears to have had limited success in both addressing the needs of people with dementia, and fostering cooperative approaches to care involving other carers

- A more theoretically open-minded approach would consider scientific medicine as offering only one frame of interpretation of dementia amongst many that are possible

- Detailed scrutiny of key medical texts on dementia reveals contradictions around the issues of causation, personhood and dependency, which can be further explored by deconstructive analysis

- Possible avenues of future investigation must transcend traditional debates between the natural and social sciences in order to enhance future possibilities for those with dementia, as well as those involved in care provision

INTRODUCTION

I wish to outline the scope of this chapter in terms of what it does *not* intend to do. Firstly, I do not deny the obvious human misery experienced by individuals and families living with the day-to-day realities of dementia. Nor do I wish in any way to undermine the well-intentioned (and sometimes heroic) efforts of those providing care to people with dementia. I do not even intend to provide a 'critique' (in the traditional sense of the word) of medical thinking in relation to dementia. As I hope will become apparent during the course of this chapter, 'deconstructing' (Derrida, 1978, 1981) medical discourse does not mean denying its legitimacy as a position. However, what I hope to achieve is an account of how medical theories relating to dementia only represent one position amongst the many that are possible. At first sight, it may appear that this aim is rather modest, until we step back and remind ourselves that medical theories have assumed prominence to such an extent that they have almost 'drowned out' other possible understandings of dementia, and have subsequently dominated the context of care provision for the people with dementia. What is intended here is an attempt to put medical accounts of dementia into some sort of proper context, and demonstrate that they do not represent a panacea, or are superior to other valuable sources of knowledge in this arena. In short, I am seeking to 'deprivilege' medical accounts of dementia: in order to do so, it is essential to explore contradictions within medical claims in relation to the issue of dementia. Berrios (1994) argues that:

> *Behavioural states related to what is now called 'dementia' have existed –*
> *and been named differently – since classical times and it is safe to assume that*
> *psychosocial incompetence has been the only feature they all have in common.*
> *(p. 15)*

Following a reading of Berrios' history of the concept of dementia, it is clear that the idea that *cognitive failure* represents the essence of dementia originated in the late nineteenth century. Some of the most prominent contradictions within medical theory addressed below are by no means new. For instance, it has been open to debate since the nineteenth century as to whether the cognitive and behavioural changes associated with dementia represent a distinct disease category, as opposed to being a variant of 'normal' ageing. Berrios (1994) has documented a history of disputes about causation, conceptual shifts and the emergence of the idea that dementia could be accounted for in terms of a discrete lesion, as suggested by the early works of Fuller and of Alzheimer. Perhaps predictably, the variety of ways in which dementia has been understood over time closely mirrors changes in medical thought more generally.

WESTERN MEDICINE AND DEMENTIA

Foucault (1973) argued that the emergence of a scientific world view facilitated major changes in medical knowledge. Specifically the dissection of bodies resulted in a new way of thinking about the body and disease closely allied to the 'hard' physical sciences. Many aspects of medical theory remain deeply rooted in the 'hard scientific' view of the world. However, it would be simplifying matters to assume a simple one-to-one correspondence between medicine and 'hard science'. Medicine has, it seems, changed with the times. Since the 1970s modifications to the traditional 'hard science' approach have been attempted. Of particular note is the emergence of what Engel (1977) has termed 'biopsychosocial medicine'. Armstrong (1987) has suggested that the model was developed in order to rescue psychiatrists who were (and largely still are) torn between pursuing a 'hard science' model of mental illness, and various emerging theories largely drawn from the social sciences. However, the 'new' model of medicine has arguably gained a wider currency than psychiatry, and perhaps is nowadays considered as more or less coterminous with ideas of humanistic medical practice.

Armstrong (1987) identifies that the theoretical foundation of the 'new' model is that of systems theory, which, Engel claims, provides a basis for the 'integration' of biological, psychological and social domains of health and illness. Engel's argument on this point is contentious. He suggests various human 'subsystems' – biological, psychological and social – and claims that whilst each possesses its own particular language and way of understanding the world, they can be integrated on common ground as a means of explaining health and illness. The apparent advantage of this 'integration' is that in attempting to pin down a particular cause of illness, medical theory can now draw upon psychology and sociology, without disturbing the 'hard science' view that physical lesions cause disease in the last instance. This recognition, Engels argues, provides a comprehensive framework that can accommodate the 'hard scientific' *as well as* the holistic elements of medicine. In outlining medical theory, I have been conscious of these broader theoretical changes. In characterising the medical position in relation to dementia, I have restricted my attentions to three principal sources, which I contend are 'ideal typical', rather than indicative in any absolute sense. These sources are:

- The American Psychiatric Association's *Diagnostic and Statistical Manual of Mental Disorders* (DSM-IV) (American Psychiatric Association, 1994)
- The World Health Organization's ICD-10 classification of mental and behavioural disorders, (WHO, 1992)
- The *Oxford Textbook of Psychiatry* (Gelder et al, 1996).

The significance of the first two works lies in the fact that they articulate diagnostic criteria, with the broad aim of achieving reliability of diagnosis in the clinical situation. The third source is included because of its wide readership amongst medical students and general practitioners, as well as those 'new' to the field of psychiatric medicine. This work can thus be seen as significant in disseminating (or perpetuating) medical ideas about dementia.

I wish to make five key claims about the discipline of medicine as it is currently practised:

1. Human beings are seen essentially as machines. Illness is understood in terms of the physical malfunction of parts. The determinants of health and illness are viewed primarily as physical.
2. Medicine aspires to retain a 'hard scientific' approach to issues of health and illness, insofar as medicine claims that health and illness states (as well as the causes of disease) can be objectively measured and differentiated; medicine remains concerned to establish simple causal links between 'pathological agents' and specific disease outcomes.
3. Scientific medicine is inherently reductionist in its approach to health and illness. It is generally argued that in order to understand disease, it is necessary to understand the body in smaller and smaller constituent units. Furthermore, the way in which scientific medicine views the issue of 'cause' places physical causes ahead of psychological and social factors in explaining health and illness. Inherently, this invites the treatment of the mind and body as separate entities, and neglects the role of social and environmental issues in the causation of disease.
4. Scientific medicine remains dominated by the search for 'cures', which can be given 'to' patients in order to rid them of disease regardless of patient participation. Healing activities – involving some form of active participation or partnership between carer and patient – are therefore seen as of secondary importance.
5. Scientific medicine has expansionist tendencies. Medicine has traditionally responded to conflict and challenge in at least two ways: by marginalising the alternative (i.e. denouncing it as secondary or bogus), and by incorporating the potential threat (Armstrong, 1987).

Armstrong (1995) suggests that the emergence of a 'new medicine' is founded upon the idea that the causes of modern-day illnesses are located in the wider social and cultural environment. The form of medical practice that logically follows from this idea is based upon surveillance of the 'normal' state, as normal forms of human life are now seen as problematic. Whilst scientific hospital medicine is concerned with the ill, 'surveillance medicine' focuses upon the total population, by undoing the conceptual distinction between 'healthy' and 'ill'. Areas of life to come under the focus of the 'new' clinical gaze are hygiene, reproduction and childbirth, child-rearing and old age. The medicalisation of old age has specific relevance in relation to medical views of dementia. As well as its concern to identify 'abnormal' ageing states such as dementia, medicine, through the surveillance of healthy populations, is also concerned to define 'healthy ageing'. However, I contend that medical constructions of old age are sociologically wanting, and lack substantial correspondence with the findings of social research in this area. Old age is predominantly alluded to in terms of decline. For instance, Gelder et al (1996) emphasise decline in physical capacity, intellectual function, increasing rigidity in attitude, loneliness, social dependency, and loss of social status and esteem, as prominent features of old age. Whilst I do not wish to deny that these 'problems' exist for *some* old people, careful reading of epidemiological and social research in this area (Falconer and Rose, 1991) reveals a rich variation amongst the elderly population, a point neglected in favour of a predominant cultural stereotype in this case. Acceptance of an 'inevitable decline' model of old age presents special problems in terms of the diagnosis of dementia. For instance, ICD-10 overtly claims that 'normal' cognitive decline occurs with ageing, and implicitly suggests that a degree of social incompetence is a necessary condition of old age (WHO, 1992):

> *The diagnosis of dementia is only warranted in the situation of demonstrable evidence of greater memory or other cognitive impairment than* would be expected due to the normal ageing process, and the symptoms cause impairment in occupational/social functioning. *(p. 327, my emphasis)*

POST-MODERN SOCIAL THEORY

Medical discourse, in both traditionalist and biopsychosocial forms, can be thought of as avowedly structuralist in nature (Box 3.1), insofar as:

- There is an attempt to provide a comprehensive set of theories by which to understand all health and illness states
- Scientific medicine is first and foremost concerned to establish cause and effect relationships between (mostly physical) agents and disease

---

Box 3.1   A definition of structuralism

Structuralism can be thought of as an attempt to discern regularities and laws relating to human conduct and the social world. It is evident in social theory in those attempts to explain the workings of society by recourse to a particular explanatory model. Similarly, structuralism is evident in psychology in those theories that suppose a structure to the human mind and consciousness.

- Medicine is guilty of reductionism in attempting to understand health and illness; scientific medical explanations constitute a kind of depth analysis in which the causes of disease are represented as hidden, or only 'knowable' through expert analysis
- Scientific medicine makes use of a number of theoretical devices (oppositions), principally that of normal versus pathological, in order to explain health and illness states
- Biopsychosocial medicine maintains the view of scientific medicine that the world possesses an orderly structure: illness is represented as being caused by separate but related biological, psychological and social factors.

Craib (1992) suggests that the biggest problem posed to structuralist theories in the social sciences is when they confront areas of social life that are inexplicable from within their circumscribed framework of interpretation. For instance, the use of Marxist economic categories in an attempt to explain issues of ethnicity and gender has been largely found wanting (Turner, 1989). I wish to argue here that the same limitations exist in relation to scientific medical explanations of dementia. Fox (1991) contends that the activity of deconstruction in the Derridan sense (Derrida, 1978, 1981) can be viewed as rooted in the loose alliance of theoretical approaches collectively subsumed under the banner of post-modernism. The main arguments of post-modern social theory as applied to our object of study are:

- It is impossible for scientific medicine (or any other discipline for that matter) to produce all-encompassing accounts of the human condition, including health and illness states.
- However, this claim does not deny the authenticity of scientific medical knowledge as one possible form of explanation. Rather, scientific medical theory creates its own world, and advances a particular 'world view' which, although valid in its own terms, cannot be seen as a 'superior' form of knowledge, and is therefore not universally valid.
- In these terms, scientific medicine can be viewed as presenting a partial and biased form of knowledge, as opposed to the discipline's own claims of objectivity and universality.
- Post-modernists question claims that the world is really as ordered and subject to regularities as disciplines such as scientific medicine argue. As opposed to conforming to regular patterns, it can be argued that health and illness states are infinitely variable in terms of their impact upon individual lives.
- In summary, scientific medical meanings can be viewed as a kind of construction: one particular representation of events from many that are possible in order to explain health and illness states.

Structuralist theories, particularly within sociology, received much criticism for the degree to which they failed to account for the personal actions of individuals. The need to retain some sense of the person is a recurrent theme in post-modern social theory (PMST). However, in terms of our object of study, this does not suggest that the starting point for any analysis of dementia should be located at the level of the individual sufferer. A common theme in PMST is the claim that people's identities are defined by powerful knowledge forms such as scientific medicine. The object of PMST is to illuminate how powerful knowledge forms can have an impact upon the individual (but not in any uniform or causal manner), defining an individual's identity, and mediating that individual's experience of the social world.

Following the points above, PMST would argue that a multiplicity of possible interpretations of dementia are possible, given the existence of multiple ways (as opposed to a single universal way) of understanding. Each interpretation is seen as valid in its own terms, but none can be seen as universal or superior to other knowledge claims. This point leaves PMST in danger of falling into a 'black hole' of relativism. How then, are we to judge between 'truth' claims, and claims to valid knowledge? The short answer is that we cannot – to do so would imply that we believe in one universal understanding of the world. Accepting this important point entails 'de-privileging' scientific medical understandings of the world, that is, dismissing claims that these world views are in some way superior to other views, e.g. 'lay understandings' of events. I contend that such a process gives voice to a number of theoretical claims previously dismissed as 'unscientific', or quackery, from within the rigid hierarchy of medical knowledge. The consequences of this theoretical open-mindedness may be to move beyond narrow, blinkered views of dementia, with one possible outcome being at least a more egalitarian relationship between professionals, lay carers and those experiencing dementia.

Deconstruction as theory and method

Norris (1991) argues that the texts of Jacques Derrida defy classification according to any clear-cut academic boundaries. They belong to philosophy insofar as they pose questions surrounding thought, language, identity and other long-standing themes of philosophical debate. However, he further suggests that Derrida's texts are unlike anything else in modern philosophy in that they represent a challenge to the whole basis of Western philosophy in refusing to grant it any kind of privileged status as a superior knowledge form. The starting point for deconstruction as a method is acceptance of the fact that each theory is ultimately dependent upon language for its articulation and dissemination, and that the language used possesses a certain underlying structure. Derrida (1978, 1981) argues strongly that the types of analysis that can be employed in interrogating literary texts are indispensable in the reading of any kind of theoretical text. As discussed by Husserl (1964), deconstruction aims to exploit the gap between a theory and events or phenomena that cannot be accounted for from within the confines of that particular theory. However, Norris (1991) indicates that deconstruction involves much more than simply challenging what is claimed within a theory (a common feature in many traditional critiques of scientific medicine). Translating the above points into a coherent analytical procedure, Flax (1990) suggests that deconstructive reading entails that readers:

- Are dismissive of claims that some forms of knowledge are inherently superior
- Are attentive to what is not articulated within a theory; this constitutes an equally significant part to that which is said
- Are suspicious when theories draw upon supposedly 'natural' categories or claim to represent the only authentic world view possible
- Start from the assumption that in order for a theory to appear 'complete', something must have been suppressed in order to sustain the appearance of unity.

Fox summarises the steps of deconstructive method thus, and for the purposes of this chapter, I have adopted this framework. Deconstructive reading entails identifying:

1. *Position* – the part of the theory that is given prominence within a text. An example from scientific medicine is diagnosing illness. However, in order to have any meaning, this part of the theory is dependent upon negation (below).
2. *Negation* – the opposite concept to (1); it is actually more important in making that theory work. Our example of diagnosing illness requires a definition of health in scientific medical terms. In order to have any meaning whatsoever, the term 'illness' must be juxtaposed to that of 'health'.
3. *Negation of negation* – this can be thought of as issues that have been concealed or neglected in order to make a theory appear plausible or 'complete'. In order to maintain the health–illness opposition, scientific medicine uses categories such as 'atypical presentation', and 'borderline case' to account for cases that disturb a clear-cut health–illness distinction.
4. *Deconstruction* involves exposing how a theory is given a false appearance of completeness, or plausibility, by exposing issues that cannot be accounted for from within the confines of a particular theory.

DECONSTRUCTION OF DEMENTIA

Derrida (1978, 1981) has suggested that the exploration of internal contradictions within a theory requires a detailed examination of how that particular theory is represented in text. The remainder of this chapter is thus concerned with exploiting the gap (*aporia*) between scientific medical views of dementia, and events or phenomena and experiences of individuals that cannot be accounted for from within the confines of the scientific medical position. The main issues that I have chosen to focus upon are interdependence, personhood and causation, which arise from my examination of the scientific medical texts cited above, and in many senses represent my own aesthetic interpretation of these texts. It is possible that another reader deploying the same method would choose to identify other key issues. I do not claim that the following analysis is comprehensive, or possesses any special theoretical significance. However, I do suggest that the main themes identified below represent areas of the experience from within the lives of people with dementia, their families and carers, which are poorly accounted for in terms of scientific medical theory.

Independence and dependence

Scientific medical theory clearly uses the dualism of dependence and independence in describing the lived experience of dementia. Dependency in the scientific medical view is almost exclusively described as loss of physical competence, as well as functional incapacity within social roles. This view perhaps replicates the way in which old age in general is culturally constructed within the Western world, and accounted for in sociological theory. Activity theory (Parsons, 1942) suggested that loss of social roles in old age, whilst all too common, represented a form of 'unsuccessful ageing'. Conversely, disengagement theory (Cumming et al, 1960) viewed the relinquishment of social roles as 'natural' and desirable. Political economy accounts argue that whilst dependency is a salient feature of old age, it is constructed and enforced upon older people in Western society, as opposed to being an essential feature of human ageing.

Deconstructing dependence and independence

I suggest that medical conceptualisations of dementia are guilty of selectively ignoring the relativity of the concept of dependency (Box 3.2), and treating as unproblematic the nature of the concept of 'power'. A belief system that accords people with dementia a passive and dependent role in the management of their own lives may result in regimens of 'care' that have the effect of actually enforcing dependency. The situation for all individuals in modern industrialised societies is that of highly complex interdependency in which a specialised division of labour renders individuals (including those who are supposedly independent) extremely vulnerable to changes in social systems.

> **Box 3.2** Dependence and independence – a deconstruction
>
> **Position** 'Dependence' in dementia arises as a consequence of pathological processes, which are causally related to various physical disabilities, loss of psychological competence and social incapacity.
>
> **Negation** 'Independence' exists in the absence of the pathological processes of dementia, and their sequelae.
>
> **Negation of negation** Independence cannot simply be equated to biopsychosocial capacity and competence (although these are significant elements). It is a wider concept entailing, amongst other things, freedom from normative constraints, cultural conventions, legal obligations, power and the possession of various forms of capital.
>
> **Deconstruction** Scientific medical ideas about dependence and independence obscure the fact that all people are essentially interdependent, regardless of physical, psychological and social capacity. Furthermore, the construction of people with dementia as passive and dependent may serve to legitimate regimens of care that deny choice, dignity and fundamental human rights.

Fennel (1986) asserts that where independence can be discerned, it can only be determined in relation to some understanding of human need. Such considerations are less than explicit in scientific medical discussions of dementia. However, embarking upon a quest for a universal definition of human need is futile; human needs in essence are culturally and socially specific, and relative to time and place, and are fashioned by what is collectively held as normative, fashionable and desirable at any given moment of human history.

Similarly, Hockey and James (1993) in discussing current representations of childhood and old age argue that Western industrialised societies have disguised the evident interdependence of all people, regardless of age, resulting in a collective mind-set which works to maintain the contrast between dependence and independence. In the context of the life course, Hockey and James (1993) identify that discourses of dependency have most impact on the life experiences of children and the elderly. For example, they suggest that similarities exist in the ways in which both the young and the old are subjected to regimes of control, often masked by the rhetoric of benevolence. There is consistent evidence from Robb (1967) and Meacher (1972), through to the present day, to suggest that these jeopardies are amplified for those made vulnerable through 'dementing illness'. This collective cognitive distinction underlies those social practices by which 'independent' adults are able to classify and define the old and the young as 'dependent'. In reality, dependency is multifaceted and represents a potentiality for any individual ('sick' or 'well') at any point in the life continuum. Therefore, it carries no single meaning and encompasses a range of different contexts. However, in Western societies, as Hockey and James (1993) identify, the category of 'dependency' is deployed in a narrow rather than a broad range of social contexts, and is used specifically to demarcate particular groups, especially those who have either lost or not developed social competencies or biological function. The apparently self-evident meaning of the term, however, conceals a number of assumptions. If independence and dependence are conceptually polarised, rather than seen as interconnected human conditions, their occurrence carries implications for ideas of power and status. For Hockey and James (1993), discourses surrounding ageing and disability are characterised by embedded metaphors of childhood, and furthermore, the metaphor of the dependent child provides a significant structure within which human dependency of whatever kind is understood. Such metaphors are maintained by recourse to verbal and visual imagery which portrays physical decline, dependency, marginality and passivity, as well as the 'natural' affinity between the old and the young. In summary, Hockey and James (1993) argue that the metaphorical transformation of the old and disabled into children can be understood as an ideological process, which both marginalises and disempowers its subjects.

In relation to scientific medicine and dementia, I contend that the concept of dependency is deployed in a meaningless sense, which takes no account of wider issues of human need. In scientific medical terms its use signifies a partial and biased representation of physical dependence and psychosocial 'incompetence'. However, the fact that psychosocial competence is both culturally and historically relative is not acknowledged in scientific medical accounts of dementia. The evident interdependence of all people in Western societies is therefore ideologically suppressed. For instance, political economy accounts of the medical-industrial complex in capitalist societies (McKinlay, 1984) argue convincingly that scientific medicine is a self-perpetuating enterprise, which generates its own ready market of medical need. Adopting this orientation towards dependency means that we can, with some validity, think of the individuals involved in the 'professional care sector' as dependent upon those for whom they provide care: dependent for career, employment, financial remuneration, etc. From the position of accepting such interdependence, Finch (1989) has hinted that relationships between carers and care recipients represent a form of reciprocation, an open acknowledgement of interdependency.

Maintenance and loss of personhood in dementia

Scientific medicine explicitly claims that the pathological changes associated with dementia inevitably involve a catastrophic disruption of personal biography, accompanied by alteration or loss of 'personhood'.

These claims are implicitly reflected in the diagnostic criteria reviewed above in which various losses of capacity and function are suggested as evidence of progressive and irreversible decline. However, the model of 'self' implicit in scientific medical definitions is an individualistic formulation; the 'self' is seen as an intrinsic property of individual consciousness.

Deconstructing biographical continuity and disruption

Hockey and James (1993) propose that the meaning of 'personhood' is neither fixed nor intrinsic, and is part of a particular cultural, (as opposed to natural) order of things (Box 3.3). They suggest that the concept of personhood often entails some notion of being 'complete'. However, it seems that the particular constituents of 'being whole' are culturally specific entities. Similarly, Mauss (1979) has argued that 'personhood' entails the identity that is socially constituted for an individual, not with respect to the individual's own sense of uniqueness, but by reference to a particularised set of cultural ideas about what is entailed in being fully human.

Hockey and James (1993) have argued that there is a conceptual link between dependency and personhood in Western industrialised societies, in which the denial, granting or withdrawal of personhood is contingent upon *perceived* dependency. In this sense discourses of infantilisation (considered above), occupy a pivotal role in sustaining the asymmetrical distribution of personhood for those who are 'dependent'. Given the centrality of highly valued individualism in Western cultures, the concepts of 'person' and

---

Box 3.3 Biographical disruption – a deconstruction

Position Biographical disruption occurs as a consequence of the progressive pathological changes of dementia, which inevitably entail fragmentation of the personality, and subsequent loss of social competence and participation, and ultimately loss of self identity.

Negation 'Maintenance of personhood' is possible, with the caveat that a person remains 'psychologically intact'.

Negation of negation The conditions of biographical continuity or 'maintenance of personhood' arise primarily as a consequence of one's social milieu, regardless of individual psychological integrity or pathological processes.

Deconstruction Affording primacy to individual pathological and psychological changes serves to present only a partial account of social identity, thus obscuring the fluidity and variation of the attribution of personhood throughout life, regardless of psychological or health–illness states.

'individual' are uniquely fused. In these terms, it can be argued that individualism is irreconcilable with human 'dependency', as in the Western context, the pursuit of individual freedom is the primary hallmark of personhood, and all those who, through 'dependency', are unable to aspire to this aim, are cast as less than full persons in the eyes of others.

In contrast, from a social constructionist position, Shotter (1963) asserts that personhood is created out of engagement in certain types of spoken discourse, as opposed to being wholly culturally constituted. A subjective sense of self is said to emerge via self-displaying discursive acts such as narration and declaration (speaking for oneself, or providing a commentary on events from one's own point of view). Similarly, both Coulter (1981) and Harré (1983) assert that selfhood is publicly manifested through various discursive practices such as the telling of autobiographical stories, taking on the responsibilities for one's own actions, expressing doubt, declaring an interest, decrying lack of fairness in a situation, etc. This latter model of the self is sharply at odds with the individualised version implicit in scientific medical theories.

Sabat and Harré (1992) differentiate between the *self* of personal identity, usually coupled with one's sense of personal agency (the degree to which we believe ourselves to be the authors and originators of our own actions), and the *selves* that are publicly presented, coherent clusters of traits we call 'personae'. Selves or personae are presented discursively by ensuring that public performances conform to the expectations of others in a given social situation. Each community has a repertoire of recognisable and acceptable person types. However, *self* can only be presented formally. It has no content, as it comprises a structural and organisational feature of one's mentality. Singularity of selfhood is manifested by the employment of discursive devices such as the first person pronoun 'I', as opposed to the use of generalised statements. In normal circumstances, each person may present a number of 'social selves' in a variety of social contexts. Since the *self* is a formal unity, it does not require the cooperation of any other person in order to exist. However, and more importantly, the existence of *selves* does hinge upon the formal cooperation of others. Our 'social selves' are only able to assume significance if they are recognised, responded to and confirmed by others around us. When scientific medical texts refer to a 'loss of self' in dementia, I contend that what is being 'lost' is the validation and acknowledgment of others, as opposed to the *self* (a structural and organisational feature of one's mentality). Sabat and Harré conclude that although dementia can result in a variety of cognitive and behavioural problems, it does not necessarily follow that the condition leads to 'loss of self', and furthermore, only indirectly contributes to loss of publicly presented 'selves'. The experience of people with dementia is one of double jeopardy, in that potentially, social misunderstandings can be seen to arise as a consequence of attempts to maintain both types of selfhood, and can from a medical position be interpreted as evidence of dementing illness. In this sense, interpreting the self-affirming behaviours of 'demented' people from a scientific medical standpoint assumes the quality of a self-fulfilling prophecy. Furthermore, following interviews with people with Alzheimer's disease, Sabat and Harré (1992) claimed that there was evidence that 'self' remained intact, even in situations where social participation and physical competence were no longer present. The maintenance of publicly presented 'selves' of those with dementia, however, was less evident. If others, for whatever reason, refuse to validate the identities of people with dementia, then their public personae are denied an existence. It is these discursive displays that appear as irrational from a medical standpoint (in which people with dementia are assumed to be confused and disoriented).

There is nothing new in the claim that accepting constructionist accounts of the self can result in a more valued status for those with dementia (Feil, 1972; Bleathman and Morton, 1988), see also Chapter 5. Supporting the discursively produced 'social selves' of people with dementia, regardless of value judgments about orientation towards shared realities, has the effect of both validating and valuing people as individuals. Kitwood (1993), in discussing a 'culture of dementia', argues that the validation of selves that arises from discursive exchanges between people with dementia is greatly undervalued by professional carers. In this light Kitwood argues that any attempt on the part of professionals to validate the social selves of dementia sufferers represents a favoured mode of practice. However, what of the consequences of adopting the implications of scientific medical discourse? Prior (1995), in a case study of psychiatric hospitalisation, has argued that retention of a strong sense of cultural identity, interaction with others who validate a publicly presented sense of self identity, and retention of social networks, are key features in mitigating the negative effects of institutionalisation, in the classical sense outlined by Goffman (1961). As well as the problem of institutional settings placing people with dementia in environments that may in themselves result in decline, Wardhaugh and Wilding (1993) in a discussion of 'corrupted care' (care ostensibly arranged for benevolent and therapeutic purposes, but which results in the abuse and degradation of the care recipients), ominously identify that one key precipitant of this process involves the neutralisation of normal moral concerns, so that people are cast as less than fully human. Thus, accepting the 'loss of self' hypotheses in the past may have provided implicit sanction for perpetrators of abusive treatment.

Nature, culture and dementia

Haimes and Williams (1994) suggest that the overarching dualism of nature and culture has been historically central to the development of the human sciences, and remains stubbornly resistant to resolution. At the minimum, they suggest, it represents an organising feature of debates about the proper province of the social sciences. In terms of the scientific medical view of dementia, the nature–culture debate serves to animate issues such as whether the diagnosis of dementia represents a discrete disease entity, as opposed to being an extremity of normal ageing. Roth (1994) points out that the normal–pathological debate has raged since Alzheimer published his original paper in 1907, fuelled by the high prevalence within 'normal' subjects of post-mortem features claimed by Alzheimer to be pathological. In broader terms, the question of whether dementia can be viewed as having a physiological or a behavioural basis can be seen as reflecting the nature–culture dichotomy. The scientific medical position as outlined above predictably opts for the 'nature' side of this argument, maintaining that dementia arises wholly out of physical pathological processes. Medical realities are thus embedded in versions of the natural world, and become subject to understanding through the premises of the 'hard' sciences. This formulation results in the idea that dementia can be objectively understood via diagnostic procedures. However, a significant problem exists in relation to the medical diagnosis of dementia. There is evident difficulty in establishing a correlation between supposed brain pathological changes and a person's 'clinical presentation'. Kitwood (1989) states that this failure is most apparent with those deemed to be suffering from moderate to severe dementia, some 80% variance existing between discernible pathological findings at post-mortem and the degree of clinical 'dementia' as measured in terms of behavioural and psychometric indices. Similarly, measures of cerebral atrophy attained by the use of non-invasive scanning techniques remain poor predictors of cognitive dysfunction. For Kitwood, this problem is compounded by the scientific medical assumption of a one-to-one correspondence between brain and mind. These disparities invite radical reinterpretation. It is possible to hypothesise that neuropathological changes may be coincidental, and not causative of dementia. The possibility that events in the social milieu and not individual pathological changes are responsible for the 'clinical picture' in dementia goes some way to undermining the dominant scientific medical position. Kitwood (1989) heavily subscribes to the 'culture' position in this argument about cause:

> It is now becoming clear that virtually all losses and difficulties in later life are socially constructed: that is, they are a consequence not of the ageing process itself, but also of the norms and collective arrangements that are taken for granted as applying to old age. (p. 1)

However, whilst it is true to say that scientific medicine remains committed to a neuropathological view of dementia, medical theories in recent years have gone further than simply offering crude ideas about causation. Roth (1994) identifies that two broad positions exist within the biomedical orthodoxy. Continuum theories argue that since a measure of cognitive decline, usually in the form of recent memory loss, is present (although to a variable degree) in normal ageing subjects, then patients suffering from Alzheimer's disease represent those drawn from the extreme end of the continuum. A second possible interpretation involves dismissing plaques, tangles and granular or vascular changes as of insufficient explanatory power to account for Alzheimer's disease. Therefore, it is suggested another element of unknown pathology must be present. Roth acknowledges that whilst it is possible to demonstrate a degree of correlation between 'pathological' changes and the outward signs of Alzheimer's disease, there is no single change that cannot also be found to some extent in the brains of healthy and mentally intact aged persons.

An alternative explanation favoured by Roth (1994) takes into account a 'threshold' effect. In threshold theories, the issue of 'reserve capacity' (of mental function) assumes significance. In short, in some individuals, it is claimed that a compensatory effect occurs in response to neuronal loss, as some people appear to have more in reserve than other 'vulnerable individuals'. However, once neuronal damage reaches a critical point, compensation fails, and outward signs of dementia appear.

Deconstructing nature–culture and dementia

Moving beyond the biomedical and constructionist positions (decon-structed in Box 3.4) to a large extent involves mediating between the

---

Box 3.4 Nature versus culture in dementia

Position Dementia arises as a consequence of physical causative agents. Dementia is objectively knowable by a process of medical diagnosis.

Negation Dementia is a constructed concept. The diagnosis of dementia is a social process which is not neutral and value-free as claimed, but reflects the cultural expectations placed upon the elderly in Western industrialised society.

Negation of negation Biomedicine presupposes the absence of psychological and social influence in the causation and diagnosis of dementia. Constructionist accounts conversely marginalise the role of physical and natural factors. Both positions therefore suppress possible interactions and interrelationships between biological and social factors.

Deconstruction Both the biomedical and constructionist accounts militate against complexity in the understanding of dementia. One possible object of study is the interaction between natural and cultural processes surrounding the conceptually complex phenomenon of dementia.

traditional oppositions within the social sciences of humanism and positivism. However, in terms of 'mental illness', this approach is not without precedent. Healy (1990) has argued convincingly that the traditional dichotomy between (organic) disorders of form and (functional) disorders of content, maintained by scientific medicine, is increasingly difficult to sustain. No clear criteria have ever existed in order to make this opposition justifiable. In particular, Healy argues, positivist psychiatry has failed to distinguish between the experience of mental illness and its supposed motives and causation. The model of mental illness proffered by Healy (1990) is implicitly underpinned by a philosophy of science that is concerned to show how the world can be understood in terms of complex multicausal models – the *scientific realist* philosophy of Bhaskar (1978). In place of direct causative relationships, the realist approach is concerned to demonstrate how a number of factors (both natural and cultural) can combine in specific circumstances to produce specific outcomes. Rather than being concerned to establish laws about the causation of, for example, dementia, such models focus upon tendencies towards the outcome of dementia. Healy's approach imitates contemporary neuropsychology, in which the proper object of attention is the individual's subjective description of their predicament, in contrast to 'scientific' psychiatry which aims to classify and interpret symptoms. The resultant model means that people diagnosed as 'mentally ill' must play a pivotal role in understanding and describing their own state. In the case of those diagnosed with dementia, this approach would certainly militate against the risk of self-fulfilling prophecy described by Sabat and Harré (1992). The therapeutic modality most appropriately suited to this model is therefore an assisted exploration of experience.

In terms of dementia, Kitwood (1989, 1990) offers a model incorporating the concepts of mind, brain and social interaction. Kitwood's focus is upon the *process* by which people come to be 'demented', in contrast to the approach of scientific medicine which is ultimately concerned with diagnosing and defining the state of dementia. In particular, Kitwood suggests that the psychological and social milieu, in which interactive events take place, assumes at least as great a significance as any potential neurological impairment. Following a series of semistructured interviews with family members, Kitwood claims that 'dementing illness' is intricately related to life history, life events and social relationships. One can appreciate, from this brief introduction to Kitwood's work, that he is dismissive of any simple, linear causal relationship between pathological changes and dementia. In contrast, he suggests that the variables involved are many, and interrelate in complex ways. The key ideas of Kitwood's approach are:

- That dementia is compounded from the effects of neurological impairment and interaction events which damage self-esteem and diminish personhood: a 'malignant social psychology', in Kitwood's terms (Table 3.1).

- Evidence of neurological impairment in individuals attracts 'malignant social psychology' as a response from others (the 'self-fulfilling prophecy' discussed above).
- Malignant social psychology experienced by elderly people who may be physiologically compromised may possibly *but not necessarily* result in further neurological impairment.

Kitwood's central point is that individuals are more affected by the psychosocial environment than has hitherto been acknowledged. The predominant cultural constructions of old age (as well as the material privations experienced by a significant minority of old people) in Western industrialised societies ensure that many losses are taken for granted as unremarkable in later life.

Table 3.1 Malignant social psychology	
Malignant social psychology	Example of interactive event
Treachery	Any dishonest representation or deception
Disempowerment	Any diminution or denial of sense of agency
Infantilism	Implying the mentality and capability of a child
Intimidation	Experiences with professional power and bureaucracy
Labelling	Framing or interpreting a person from within a diagnosis of dementia
Stigmatisation	'Demented' identity becomes the focal point of others and primary source of self-identity
Outpacing	Interaction that does not allow the 'demented' person time to respond
Invalidation	Refusal by others to validate the publicly presented selves of the 'demented'
Banishment	Physical exclusion from the human milieu on the basis of supposedly 'intolerable' behaviour
Objectification	Treatment of a person as a 'case' as opposed to fully human

From Kitwood (1990).

Commenting upon the institutional context of care provided to many 'demented' (and indeed older) people, Kitwood (1990) hypothesises that many of the 'malignant' social events outlined in Table 3.1 may be exacerbated by:

- 'Caring' professionals lacking intersubjective insight
- Competing priorities and the 'pressure of work' in busy settings
- A tendency not to believe people framed as 'demented', and therefore to deny personhood
- Psychodynamic processes within caregivers, rooted in socialised (Western) accounts of personhood and independence, and personal dread of ageing.

Thus, the multicausal model proposed by Kitwood takes account of interactions between a number of different tendencies, resulting in a succession of states which may be interpreted by others as evidence of dementia. I assert that there is a strong argument for researching dementia from the basis of Kitwood's position, given biomedicine's (*so far*) futile search for 'magic bullet' cures, as well as increasing evidence of promising psychosocial interventions.

CONCLUSION

The deconstructive reading of the biomedical position in relation to dementia offered within this chapter suggests that:

- Scientific medical practice discursively frames people with dementia as inevitably and progressively dependent.
- Scientific medical theory sustains the view that personhood is lost, and in doing so militates against the validation of the publicly presented selves of people with dementia.
- Scientific medicine, in its anxiety to maintain the 'doctrine of the lesion', suppresses the possible interaction of biological, psychological and social variables within the complex phenomenon of dementia. The mechanism of this suppression entails either discounting or minimising psychosocial accounts of dementia, as well as the intuitive insights of both lay and professional carers.

As a matter of conjecture, I tentatively advance the notion that accepting scientific medical discourse on dementia as the 'real truth' equates to working in a paradigm that allocates limited hope to those we call 'demented', reduces understanding of what is clearly a matter of complexity to the level of simplistic explanations, and through the power–knowledge relationship which is entailed within the medical model denies other possible understandings. It does not require a further exercise in abstract philosophical reasoning in order to argue that the scientific medical approach as I have outlined it can have detrimental effects for people with dementia and carers alike. In utilising deconstruction as a method, I am acutely aware of the charge of relativism levelled at this approach. For Fox (1991), deconstruction never ends: there is always a further opposition to be investigated, another silence made to speak. In this sense my interpretation is open to further deconstruction. Giddens (1990) has characterised deconstruction as 'playful'. However, I wish to contend that the approach entails neither the intellectually precocious pursuit implied by Giddens, nor does it involve falling into the 'black hole' of relativism; rather, I have attempted to give voice to further possibilities in understanding the lives of all people affected by dementia.

In the case of all of the apparent contradictions that I have explored, a singular theme to emerge is a call for greater complexity in understanding dementia in its widest sense. In offering this interpretation, I am not claiming that the resultant knowledge would lead to a complete understanding of dementia. Furthermore, I stringently distance my account from claims of privilege over other accounts of dementia (lay or professional). My tentative claim is this: that a deconstructive reading of the biomedical position has indicated potential fruitful areas for exploration (which in turn may lead to alternative understandings) which would possibly result in beneficial outcomes for people with dementia and carers alike. Specifically, the following areas may prove fruitful for exploration in moving towards a less restrictive paradigm of dementia:

• Acknowledgment of the highly complex nature of interdependence: inherently this approach invites acknowledgment of the problematic nature of 'power'
• A focus upon the social selves of people with dementia, however they are manifested
• An approach to investigating dementia that is prepared to move beyond the entrenched oppositions apparent within the natural and social sciences.

REFERENCES

American Psychiatric Association (1994) *Diagnostic and Statistical Manual of Mental Disorders*, 4th edn. Washington American Psychiatric Association.
Armstrong, D. (1987) Theoretical tensions in biopsychosocial medicine. *Social Science and Medicine* **25**, 1213–1218.
Armstrong, D. (1995) The rise of surveillance medicine. *Sociology of Health and Illness* **17**, 393–404.
Berrios, G.E. (1994) Dementia and ageing since the nineteenth century. In: Huppert, F.A. Brayne, C. O'Connor, D.W. (eds) *Dementia and Normal Ageing*. Cambridge University Press.

Bhaskar, R. (1978) *A Realist Theory of Science*. Hassocks: Harvester.

Bleathman, C. & Morton, I. (1988) Validation therapy with the demented elderly. *Journal of Advanced Nursing* **13**, 511–514.

Coulter, J. (1981) *The Social Construction of the Mind*. London: Macmillan.

Craib, I. (1992) *Modern Social Theory. From Parsons to Habermas*, 2nd edn. Brighton: Harvester Wheatsheaf.

Cumming, E., Dean, L.R., Newell, D.S. & McCaffery, I. (1960) Disengagement: a tentative theory of ageing. *Sociometry* **23**, 25–35.

Derrida, J. (1978) *Writing and Difference* (trans. Alan Bass). London: Routledge & Kegan Paul.

Derrida, J. (1981) *Positions* (trans. Alan Bass). London: Routledge & Kegan Paul.

Engel, G.L. (1977) The need for a new medical model: a challenge for biomedicine. *Science* **196**, 129.

Falconer, P. & Rose, R. (1991) *Older Britons. A Survey*. Centre for the Study of Public Policy. Glasgow: University of Strathclyde.

Feil, N. (1972) *Validation: The Feil Method*. Cleveland: Edward Feil.

Fennel, G. (1986) Structured dependency revisited. In: Phillipson, C., Bernard, M. & Strang, P. (eds) *Dependency and Interdependency in Old Age*. London: Croom Helm.

Finch, J. (1989) *Family Obligations and Social Change*. Cambridge: Polity Press.

Flax, J. (1990) *Thinking Fragments*. Berkeley: University of California Press.

Foucault, M. (1973) *The Birth of the Clinic: An Archaeology of Medical Perception*. London: Tavistock.

Fox, N.J. (1991) Postmodernism, rationality, and the evaluation of health care. *Sociological Review* **39**, 709–744.

Gelder, M., Gath, D., Mayou, R. & Cowen, P. (1996) *Oxford Textbook of Psychiatry*, 3rd edn. Oxford University Press.

Giddens, A. (1990) *The Consequences of Modernity*. Stanford University Press.

Goffman, E. (1961) *Asylums*. Harmondsworth: Penguin.

Haimes, E. & Williams, R. (1994) *Social Construction and the New Technologies of Reproduction*. Paper presented to the conference 'Constructing the Social'. University of Durham, April 1994.

Harré, R. (1983) *Personal Being*. Oxford: Blackwell.

Healy, D. (1990) *The Suspended Revolution. Psychiatry and Psychotherapy Re-examined*. London: Faber.

Hockey, J. & James, A. (1993) *Growing Up and Growing Old: Ageing and Dependency in the Lifecourse*. London: Sage.

Husserl, E. (1964) *The Phenomenology of Internal Time Consciousness*. Bloomington: Indiana University Press.

Kitwood, T. (1989) Brain, mind, and dementia: with particular reference to Alzheimer's disease. *Ageing and Society* **9**, 1–15.

Kitwood, T. (1990) The dialectics of dementia: with particular reference to Alzheimer's disease. *Ageing and Society* **10**, 177–196.

Kitwood, T. (1993) Towards a theory of dementia care: the interpersonal process. *Ageing and Society* **13**, 51–67.

Mauss, M. (1979) *Sociology and Psychology: Essays*. London: Routledge & Kegan Paul.

McKinlay, J.B. ed. (1984) *Issues in the Political Economy of Health Care*. London: Tavistock.

Meacher, M. (1972) *Taken for a Ride*. London: Longman.

Norris, C. (1991) *Deconstruction. Theory and Practice* 2nd edn. New York: Routledge.

Parsons, T. (1942) Age and sex in the social structure of the United States. *American Sociological Review* **7**, 604–616.

Prior, P.M. (1995) Surviving psychiatric institutionalisation: a case study. *Sociology of Health and Illness* **17**, 651–667.

Robb, B. (1967) *Sans Everything*. London: Nelson.

Roth, M. (1994) The relationship between dementia and normal ageing of the brain. In: Huppert, F.A., Brayne, C. & O'Connor, D.W. (eds) *Dementia and Normal Ageing*. Cambridge University Press.

Sabat, S.R. & Harré, R. (1992) The construction and deconstruction of self in Alzheimer's disease. *Ageing and Society* **12**, 443–461.

Shotter, J. (1963) *Social Accountability and Selfhood*. Oxford: Blackwell.

Turner, B.S. (1989) Ageing, status and politics in sociological theory. *British Journal of Sociology* **40**, 588–606.

Wardhaugh, P. & Wilding, P. (1993) Towards an explanation of the corruption of care. *Critical Social Policy* **37**, 4–31.

[WHO] World Health Organization (1992) *The ICD-10 Classification of Mental and Behavioural Disorders*. Geneva: WHO.

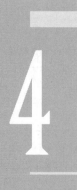

Ethical dilemmas in dementia care

Malcolm Goldsmith

KEY ISSUES

- How should a diagnosis of dementia be shared, and with whom?

- What do we mean by 'person'? To what extent does dementia destroy 'personhood' and to what extent do carers and others deny it?

- How can we utilise advancing technology while at the same time preserving privacy and autonomy?

- What are the boundaries of family responsibilities?

- Should people have the right to make decisions about their own death, and what authority should be given to advance directives?

- To what extent is society prepared to pay for the care of people who have dementia? Should the costs be borne corporately or individually?

INTRODUCTION

I first became seriously interested in exploring the ethical issues surrounding dementia when I heard a friend of mine, an Anglican priest, give a talk about his relationship with his mother who had been ill with Alzheimer's disease for over 10 years. For the last 6 years she had been in a near-vegetative state; she had not known him for 8 years, she had not spoken for 6 or 7 years and each time he visited her she was curled up in a fetal position on her bed. He visited her when he could, but lived several hundred miles away; his sister visited daily and caring for her mother had virtually taken over her whole life. Tragically, his sister had recently died after a brief illness, but his mother seemed to have no awareness of the fact.

He said that he had longed to kiss his mother good-bye, put a pillow over her face and bring the long illness to an end. After his talk, one listener said that she was appalled that a Christian minister could have said such a thing. She was relieved that she was not a member of his congregation. A second person said how wonderfully reassured she had been by his words; she said that she so often felt the same about her own mother, but thought that no-one else would ever have such awful thoughts, and was weighed down by feelings of guilt. To hear that someone else – and a priest as well-shared those thoughts was a moment of rare liberation for her. I was struck by the fact that people should have such different views. The more I have thought about these issues, the more I have realised that we live in a world of moral ambiguity, and we are struggling to find ways forward which are compassionate, sensitive and moral, and which allow us to act with integrity and conviction.

There are few areas of concern when thinking about dementia that do not throw up questions and that do not challenge assumptions and recognised ways of dealing with problems and people. As we learn more about the subjective experience of dementia, to what extent are our policies and approaches affected and influenced by this new knowledge? How do we understand the nature of being, or – put another way – how do we answer the question 'is there anyone in there?' when confronted by a person with dementia? What is truth, and how can it be communicated to people with dementia? How do we utilise technology so that it becomes an aid to supporting and affirming those who are ill rather than intruding upon their privacy and limiting their freedoms? What are the moral obligations of families, and how do we handle the tensions and ambiguities that arise amongst carers? How do we unpack and translate into social policy such fine words as 'autonomy', 'competence' and 'justice'? What about the differing approaches to future directives and living wills? What should be the role of the law? How are we to handle the complex arguments relating to assisted suicide, passive and active euthanasia, and what are these saying about how we understand and cope with suffering and dying? This minefield of ethical ambiguities was set out by Butler (1992) in this way:

> *Certain disorders provoke moral questions, even profound questions about the meaning of life itself. Such is dementia, especially in its advanced stages when it seriously jeopardises the faculties we ordinarily define as uniquely human: memory, personality, recognition, awareness, the capacity to love, even a sense of hope ... it is important to realise that, despite progress in our understanding of the central nervous system and its pathologies, including the dementias, we will not have solutions very soon. We must, therefore, confront considerable political, economic, moral, ethical and personal questions in the meantime. What does it mean for individuals to live under conditions that place them outside the usual criteria used to describe*

humanness? ... perhaps more difficult than dealing with the physical aspects of human disease and disorder is the struggle with different definitions of correct moral behaviour ... perhaps the greatest danger of all is to be found when, for economic reasons, battlefield triage is operative in peacetime, and only those least disabled and allegedly most likely to survive are cared for ... discussion of aging and dementia creates the need to consider ethics, values and the ultimate choices for action, since policy choices will have to be made, like it or not.

Modern dementia care rightly stresses the concept of partnership, of recognising our interdependence (Kitwood, 1997). Families and agencies seek to work alongside and together with the person with dementia, and seek to involve that person as fully as possible in the decisions that are being taken. This requires that we do not act as though there was no longer any 'person' hidden away within the illness, even though as the illness advances it may become more and more difficult to discover or engage with that person. It also requires that we make great efforts to hear what the person with dementia is seeking to communicate, and strive to find ways of communicating with them. It is important that dementia care is based upon this concept of partnership (Barnett, 1977), and that we seek to stress the *equality* of relationships, even though the person with dementia may be extremely vulnerable and dependent. The mind-set of equality and of partnership has enormous ethical implications. In the view of one professional, dangers occur when isolated individuals – be they a carer, a professional or the person with dementia – make major decisions without reference to others (Jacques, 1997).

SHARING THE DIAGNOSIS

Ethical issues are brought into focus the moment a diagnosis is made. Before that time there will almost certainly have been many ethical dilemmas, some acknowledged and worked through and others remaining unacknowledged. These will include issues such as the nature of personhood, the role and obligation of carers, and their own and other people's perception of dementia and whether it has stigma attached to it. When a diagnosis is made, however, there is the issue of whether to share that diagnosis with the person with dementia, and how it should be shared. McLean (1987) has described well some of the problems associated with making a diagnosis:

- *Overdiagnoses* are made sometimes when people with a non-dementing illness are diagnosed as having dementia
- *Misdiagnoses* occur when people who do have dementia are initially diagnosed as suffering from something else
- *Missed diagnoses* happen when doctors fail to recognise dementia in their patients.

When a diagnosis has been made, and we must accept the fact that making such a diagnosis is an extremely difficult task, – as Kitwood (1997) observes, 'it is notorious that GPs, clinical psychologists, psychiatrists and neurologists tend to differ in their opinions' (p. 26), – opinion is divided as to how important, indeed how possible, it is to share that diagnosis with the person with dementia. Arguments in favour of sharing the diagnosis include the fact that it might make it possible to identify symptoms and understand or explain unusual or embarrassing behaviour (Jacques, 1992); it may contribute to prognosis and thus help in the process of advance decision-making, and it may make possible the arrangement of social and psychological support interventions (Illiffe, 1992 Jacques, 1992; Kennedy and Rosser, 1993; Malcolm, 1993). Against this there is the rather nihilistic view that, since there is no cure, there is not much point in causing further distress by sharing a diagnosis, especially bearing in mind the possibilities of mistakes being made (Goldsmith, 1996). Many doctors think that sharing such news can have a harmful effect upon a patient; but whilst many carers seem content that the person with the illness does not know, people with dementia who have been given their probable diagnosis seem to welcome the increased control that such information brings (Cayton, 1995). There is then the problem of how often do you have to share the news if people forget what they have been told? Some professionals think that it is cruel to have to reiterate a diagnosis when each time the person hears it as though for the first time (Goldsmith, 1996).

There are ethical issues surrounding how the information is shared. Is it shared with the person with dementia alone, thus preserving that individual's self-determination? Is it shared with family members, rather than with the person with dementia or with the person together with a significant other? And how is the diagnosis shared? Does its communication take place over a number of sessions, or on one specific occasion? Is it reinforced by written information, and are relevant support structures and possible interventions ready at hand? Is there a follow-up a few days later, and if so, how is this handled?

General practitioners are often placed in extraordinarily difficult situations. There are often no support structures available locally for families after the reality and implications of such a diagnosis have sunk in. Little wonder, then, that the whole issue of sharing a diagnosis of dementia has been described as the 'doctor's dilemma' (Goldsmith, 1996). It is generally agreed that the role of the general practitioner and the primary care team does not end with the diagnosis but continues as the illness progresses (Brodaty, 1988; Philp, 1988; Haines, 1990; Jacques, 1992; Briggs, 1993). At least five roles have been identified (Downs, 1994):

- Providing information about diagnosis and prognosis
- Assessment of the carer's ability to cope
- Providing information about available services and benefits

- Helping with access to, and coordination of, a range of support services
- Providing emotional support to carers and patients.

Most of the literature suggests that general practitioners and primary care teams could do much better in both recognising and addressing the needs of people with dementia and their carers (Haley et al, 1992; McLean, 1993) and there is a great deal of anecdotal evidence to suggest that carers are not satisfied with the involvement of these key professionals (Brodaty et al, 1990). Downs (1994) writes that:

> [General practitioners] are notoriously poor at identifying people on their case load who have symptoms of dementia. This omission can be explained by GPs' lack of training in dementia, ageism, and therapeutic nihilism along with the difficulties intrinsic to establishing a diagnosis of dementia. (p. 9)

What does 'telling the truth' involve when speaking with people in the early stages of dementia? There is undoubtedly a great deal of deception in many cases, with families often insistent that the truth is not shared with the person who has been diagnosed. 'Having problems with your memory' is used to explain away many situations, and the outside professional may be caught up in a network of collusion, and may have serious questions to ask about whose integrity and best interests are at stake.

Ethical issues may emerge regarding testing, of which there are two main types: *diagnostic tests* for patients who display symptoms, the purpose of which would be to determine a definitive diagnosis; and *predictive tests* (presymptomatic) in relatives, to determine whether they are carrying the disease gene and hence may be prone to develop the illness at some future date. The extent of public awareness of such tests and their availability is a matter of conjecture. Should people be encouraged to be tested, should general practitioners be proactive? Or are such tests to be seen as possible resources in cases where families press, leaving general practitioners reactive? What are the factors that influence such decisions? Cayton (1995) explored some of the ethical issues involved in diagnostic testing and explained how it will require us to change our practices and attitudes. It will not be easy; it will take courage to seek a diagnosis and fortitude to live with the death sentence it brings', (Cayton, 1995); but a definite diagnosis from such testing allows people to take control of their situation, and can enhance their dignity.

STRUGGLING WITH PERSONHOOD

What is happening to a person who has dementia? It is relatively easy to explain what is, or might be, happening to the brain, but what is happening to the *person*? Is there still a real person in there, locked away in the midst of the illness? It all depends upon what we mean by 'person'! Some people reach the conclusion that the person whom they knew has long since disappeared, even though still breathing; whilst others believe that they can still detect signs of uniqueness and personality long after other people have become wearied by the effort of trying to sustain a relationship. Are people imposing a personality onto the one who has dementia long after he or she has ceased to have a personality, as suggested by Fontana and Smith (1989) in their essay on 'unbecoming', or are people denying a personality even when it is there? Is the experience of dementia one in which the person with dementia may be striving desperately to communicate with the 'outside' world, but is unable to do so because of the nature of the illness? There is increasing evidence to suggest that people with dementia are able to communicate for much longer than was previously thought possible, but such communication requires considerable effort and skill on the part of the person who does not have dementia (Killick, 1994; Goldsmith, 1996; Kitwood, 1997).

There is philosophical debate about what constitutes a person. Engelhardt (1996) has argued that people are 'persons ... when they are self-conscious, rational, and in possession of a minimal moral sense'. He goes on to accept the validity of 'conferred' or 'social' personhood for those who are not persons 'in the strict sense'. People may find it easier to cope with dementia if they are able to persuade themselves that the people so affected have somehow become less than real people, and Kitwood (1997) has identified various forms of 'malignant social psychology' surrounding the dementing process which include treachery, disempowerment, condemnation, intimidation, stigmatisation and outpacing (see Table 3.1).

There appears to be a great temptation for people to treat those with dementia as though they were somehow less than real people. It is probably a protective device, ensuring that those who look on are able to keep the reality of dementia at arm's length for, as Kitwood and Bredin (1992) observed:

> Professionals and informal carers are vulnerable people too, bearing their own anxiety and dread concerning frailty, dependency, madness, ageing, dying and death. A supposed objectivity in a context that is in fact interpersonal is one way of maintaining psychological defences, and so making involvement with conditions such as dementia bearable. (p. 270)

This section is headed 'struggling with personhood' deliberately, for it often is a very real struggle to maintain a conviction that within the shell of the person with dementia there is still a living person, who deserves and requires to be treated with dignity and honour. How many vulnerable people are abused by our withdrawing from the effort of establishing or maintaining a relationship with them? By seeking to impose our timetable, our world view and our understanding of reality, we undermine and often ignore their timetable, their world view and their understanding of reality. In so doing, we cease to treat them as human, and that is a real ethical problem. It is clearly brought home by Martin and Post (1992), who write:

> *The experience of dementia produces vulnerability ... he or she lives in a*
> *state of risk for physical and emotional harm resulting from impairment in*
> *judgement or from the callousness of those who do not wish to witness human*
> *frailty. Dementia produces an inability to reasonably interpret the physical*
> *and social world and leaves the sufferer vulnerable to abuse. Hence the*
> *impaired individual lives in a state of potential danger, regardless of whether*
> *the individual experiences the subjective feeling of fear. (p. 55)*

THE IMPACT OF TECHNOLOGY

Technology has brought great benefits to the care of people with dementia but, as in so many other areas, it is not without its problems, and it generates wildly conflicting reactions (Judd, 1997). The very effectiveness of technology raises problems, and opens up a number of ethical concerns. Surveillance is a good example. It is now possible to use remote controlled cameras and closed circuit television to monitor rooms, passageways, entrances and grounds. It is possible to 'tag' people with devices which mean that they are not lost wherever they might wander. It is possible to place electrical contacts under bedside mats so that we know when anyone gets out of bed. All these, and many others, are useful devices and can help us monitor the activities of people with dementia without the necessity of trailing them, thus allowing them a freedom which they might not otherwise enjoy. On the other hand, what are their limits, and how can we protect the privacy of these people? Is it not a violation of their space and their very being if such monitoring day and night takes place? To what extent can people give their assent to such procedures; indeed, is their consent always sought? There is a fine balance between freedom and protection and it is not clear that we always have it right.

There are also questions be to raised about the use of restraints, whether to protect the person with dementia or some other person. Berghmans (1996) has suggested that there is no scientific evidence that restraints protect patients against injuries; in fact, he argues, a number of reports show that such protective measures actually result in serious harm to the person with dementia. He goes on to suggest that every application of protective measures needs to be regularly evaluated on an individual basis. Among the questions to be considered should be:

- What is the background to the problematic behaviour?
- Why is the use of protective measures being considered?
- Are all the people who are involved sufficiently part of the decision-making process?
- Have alternative, less restrictive measures been examined?

- Is the person's legal position sufficiently safeguarded?
- Has informed consent been received, from the person with dementia or that person's representative?
- Is the situation being regularly monitored and revised?

A similar approach needs to be taken with regard to drugs. An increasing number of people are now arguing that we should be less concerned with controlling behaviour and more concerned with understanding and interpreting that behaviour. There is a marked difference in approach and attitudes between the two.

It can be argued that the increased use of technology can minimise risks related to forgetfulness or wandering, for example, and can help produce a safer environment for people with dementia, and in many cases this is clearly so. Technological aids to memory and compensatory devices have been discussed by Leikas (1994) and Pieper (1994). There have been important advances in the way that technology can be used within people's own homes, to enable them to continue to live independently. Technology can be harnessed to make the use of cookers more safe; it can be used to help with problems over keys, and in a whole range of everyday household tasks and equipment.

Problems arise more clearly when technology is transferred into a residential setting and is used to monitor residents and reduce staffing levels, but it can also serve to give greater freedom to residents and more autonomy. It is right that people should be concerned about the safety of people with dementia, but being overprotective can be intrusive and can fail to honour a person's autonomy. Conversely, being too lax may involve exposing people to unacceptable risks, either to themselves or to others. There is a fine moral judgment to be made in this area, as the risk of harm needs to be weighed against the moral costs and benefits of preventing harm; these matters were comprehensively discussed by Mary Marshall in a paper given at the annual meeting of the British Society of Gerontology in 1994 (Marshall, 1994).

ISSUES RELATING TO FAMILY CARERS

There are perhaps few areas of moral ambiguity that cause as much distress as those experienced by carers, particularly family carers. Carers often feel guilty, particularly female family carers (Gilbert et al, 1994; Berghmans, 1996). There is a difference, of course, between *feeling* guilty and *being* guilty. Many people feel guilty because they think that they have failed to live up to socially approved standards of care. The question about the boundaries of family responsibility is therefore now being raised all the more urgently (Woods, 1997). What, if any, are the obligations of families towards family members who become demented and are in need of care, support and assistance? Do grown children really 'owe' their parents something, for all the care and nurture that they presumably received when they were young? There is a growing body of opinion prepared to state categorically that the answer to such a question is 'No'.

It is important that carers care also for themselves and for other family members. Many daughters and daughters-in-law are placed in situations of enormous ambiguity when they have demands made upon them from their own or their husband's parents while at the same time they may be trying to bring up their own young, or maintain their own career. English (1979) argued that children do not owe anything to their parents, and any relationship between them ought to be on the basis of genuine friendship or love. She says that parents are the ones who chose to have children; the children did not choose to be born and therefore have no obligation to their parents simply on the basis of their existence. 'When friendship is absent the demands of reciprocity are absent as well ... filial obligation or debt can serve as a maleficent ideological warrant for the destruction of daughters' (English, 1979). Sommers (1986) follows a similar line, but differs from English in developing a concept of gratitude, both for the gift of life and also for the care bestowed in childhood. English is concerned with the quality of the relationship in the present, and that is all-important, whilst Sommers believes that there is a historic dimension to the idea of gratitude.

Use of the word 'gratitude' suggests that the sacrifices of parents do not have to be repaid in full, replicating the original offering, even if that were possible. Gratitude is a response on the part of those who receive to the generosity of those who have given. In the context of dementia care, obligations towards elderly parents based on gratitude do not have precedence over all other obligations. There may be a conflict with other obligations that are equally as strong or even stronger, such as the care of their partner or their children, or even their care of themselves. Even when children are genuinely grateful to their parents, such a sense of gratitude should not place unrealistic or even possibly destructive obligations upon them. The ethical responsibility of people towards those who are close to them, particularly to parents, should be seen as a matter of choice and not as an obligation. This is a difficult concept for many people to accept, especially for those who have been brought up within a moral environment which has stressed the commandment to 'honour thy father and mother' without exploring what this might mean or reflecting upon the moral ambiguities that it might create.

This is a difficult area and people will come to different conclusions; but having come to a conclusion many people may feel the pressure to project onto others their own viewpoint. Pluralism can be difficult to handle when it also involves sacrifice, guilt and a sense of powerlessness. If good dementia care involves the concept of partnership, then this can be difficult enough when all parties share a common set of assumptions and expectations, but when people are operating with differing convictions then it can be extremely stressful; a whole range of ambiguities suddenly emerge, and we may not have the resources to know how to handle them creatively. We are used in Britain to hearing that we live in a pluralist society, and most people can understand this when thinking about the mix of nationalities, religions or ethnic groups in society. Problems can arise, however, when the pluralism that exists within apparently homogeneous groups begins to emerge. This is not new: the loosening of class divisions, the impact of higher education and the emerging independence of women are all examples of how society has had to adapt to changing expectations and practices. We are now seeing similar tensions between generations, or between professions, and within generations and professions when it comes to expectations about the nature of the relationship between carers and people with dementia, and the relationship between family members when they are placed under stress. Very often these issues have not been thought about in any coherent way in advance, and it is only when the problem presents itself that ideas and positions become clarified, often causing feelings of guilt, anger, frustration or disappointment and bewilderment.

Ethical problems can also arise as the nature of relationships changes when a family member has dementia (Nolan and Grant, 1989; Pitkeathley, 1989). Not all these changes are for the worse for everyone – sometimes the illness can elicit a tenderness and a trust in the relationship that was perhaps not so clear or acknowledged before the illness. However, for many people the changing relationship is extremely stressful, and some people are not able to cope with it. The sexual relationship between husband and wife may change, one partner may be unhappy for it to continue, or one partner may wish to develop a relationship with someone else. The carer, particularly in cases of early-onset dementia, may ask whether it is morally acceptable to enter into an intimate relationship with another person while their partner is still living. Questions that generate considerable debate in contemporary society may be even more difficult to handle in the context of dementia. Some of these issues are highlighted by Carole Archibald in her study on sexuality and dementia (Archibald, 1994).

Considerable thought has been given to the nature of caring (Gadow, 1988; Martin and Post, 1992). A distinction can be made between *curing*. which involves the provision of services and interventions directed towards the goal of recovery, and *caring*, which can be thought of as a relationship between people which exists as an end in itself. Caring is not undertaken for any other end but that of expressing the nature of the relationship, it is about being there for the other person irrespective of the outcome. In the context of dementia care it has been described as the 'act of Sisyphus', forever rolling the rock uphill only to watch it fall again. However, such a view of caring is surely open to question. It may represent one stage in the caring relationship, but for many people what begins as a willing expression of a relationship can become, over time, a burden that prompts feelings of anxiety, anger, guilt and unhappiness. The concept of caring may shift from being a relationship that exists as an end in itself to becoming a subtle form of disempowerment and enslavement for the carer. Just what are the ethics of caring?

COMPETENCE AND ADVANCE DIRECTIVES

The competence of a person with dementia is not something that can be objectively measured. It has to be understood within a specific context, and in relation to a particular choice or decision which has to be made. This is of great importance in the field of dementia care. If people are to be involved in decisions relating to their own care, how competent are they to make such decisions? And how do we judge their level of competence? Where people are deemed not to be competent, others have to make decisions on their behalf. Who makes these decisions, and on what criteria the decisions should be based, are a matter for discussion and debate. It should also be remembered that some people did not act with a great degree of autonomy before they had dementia, so whilst it may be an important platform in dementia care in general, it cannot be assumed that autonomy is necessarily welcomed by everyone with dementia.

In recent years the idea of making some form of advance directive or 'living will' has been gaining acceptance. There are various types of directives (Box 4.1), and in most countries they are not legally binding upon physicians. There are many issues here that touch upon the autonomy of the person with dementia, the nature of personhood, the responsibilities of families and their relationships with professional bodies (Watson, 1994; Jacques, 1997). There are subjective elements, such as the degree of risk and the interpretation of intention.

DEATH AND DYING

If the area relating to the treatment of people with dementia is problematic, then the area relating to the withdrawing of treatment or of intervention that may cause death is even more so. Cecily Saunders, who pioneered work in hospice care in Britain, is quoted by Rinpoche (1992) as saying:

> We are not so poor a society that we cannot afford time and trouble and money to help people live until they die. We owe it to all those for whom we can kill the pain which traps them in fear and bitterness. To do this we do not have to kill them ... to make voluntary (active) euthanasia lawful would be an irresponsible act, hindering help, pressuring the vulnerable, abrogating our true respect and responsibility to the frail and the old, the disabled and the dying. (p. 375)

Box 4.1   Forms of advance directive

A *durable power of attorney* involves the appointment of someone who is given discretion and powers to make decisions in case of incompetence of a person with dementia.

A *living will* is a written document stating the limits of care that an individual wishes to receive in the event of falling ill and having no way of expressing such preferences at that time, either because of incapacity or because of incompetence. Whilst such statements can be of help in a general way, there are still problems with them and many ambiguous areas.

The *substituted judgment principle* is applied when decisions are made by others which are believed to reflect the views and wishes of the previously competent person.

Consent by a *tutor dative* (in Scotland) involves the appointment of someone who, in a legal capacity, may take medical decisions on behalf of a mentally incapacitated person, but this is an expensive procedure and requires a court involvement.

The *principle of necessity* can be used when a surgeon or physician believes that some intervention is in the best interest of the patient. Normally relatives or significant others are involved in any consultations, but they are not able to prevent such treatment as is deemed necessary from taking place.

However, most hospice patients suffer from cancer, and in such cases it is often possible to anaesthetise the pain and for the person to die with dignity. Can the same be said for dementia? May there not be some situations, for some individuals, where hastening death might be an act of mercy and personal integrity? Informed opinion is deeply divided. Religious opinion is also deeply divided, and so Kilner et al (1996) can produce a book of reflective essays on dignity and dying which emphasise the traditional, compassionate church view, whilst the theologian Kung has co-authored a more radical exploration of the subject (Kung and Jens, 1995), in which he quotes the Dutch theologian Kuitert:

> *The right to live and the right to die is the nucleus of self-determination; it is an inalienable right and includes the freedom to decide personally on when and how our end shall come, instead of leaving this decision to others or to the outcome of medical intervention. (p. 107)*

Battin (1992) confesses that answering the question 'ought euthanasia to be practised for persons with advanced dementia?' is not easy. She concludes that there are two eventual viewpoints, both of which are subjective. One is that of an uninformed public response and the other is that of an informed philosophical approach, and they will reach different conclusions. In her essay she surveys the three most common arguments for euthanasia in general – the arguments from autonomy, from mercy and from justice – and discusses what is problematic about each of them. She then moves on to a discussion of social policy and says that there are three principal positions. First, we can do what is possible to maintain and supply medical and supportive treatment for people with dementia until the end of their natural lives. Second, we can practise passive euthanasia on late-stage patients; by this she means providing maintenance and support but not life-saving medical treatment, thus allowing patients to die when infections or other potential fatal conditions arise. Third, we can practise active euthanasia on late-stage patients.

Battin (1992) claims that current social policy wavers between the first and the second alternatives, although the word 'euthanasia' is not used when discussing the second. However, as Watson (1994) makes clear, this is what is happening day by day:

> In common with other areas of terminal care of the elderly person with dementia, there are few clear guidelines about how action should be taken, and it is almost inevitably the case that nursing staff are left to make decisions themselves about feeding and hydration in the terminal stages of dementia. It is obvious from the literature on this area that nurses are faced with a great many ethical dilemmas. (p. 156)

This is a subject that is not going to go away. There is the need to safeguard and protect the vulnerable, but there is also the need to ensure that people are able, if they so wish, to determine the conditions under which life is no longer acceptable to them. There will always be those for whom it is ethically unacceptable to hasten death, whilst others argue that no-one would allow a pet dog to suffer in the way that some elderly people suffer. But how do we know if people are suffering? Can we be sure that we know what it is like for a person to be in an advanced stage of dementia? We know that it can be very distressing for the rest of the family, but what is it really like for the person involved? Are they aware, or have they long since ceased to have any awareness? This area of ethical debate is still in its infancy.

ECONOMIC ISSUES

An article in *The Times* (3 June 1996) revealed that about £10 per head for every person diagnosed as having Alzheimer's disease is spent on research in Britain; for those with heart disease the figure is about £109 per head; for those with cancer it is about £474; and for those diagnosed as having acquired immune deficiency syndrome (AIDS) it is £15 000. How money is raised, and what research is undertaken, is still very much a lottery, which means that there are few winners, many losers and a great deal of luck. How we decide what research needs to be undertaken and who should fund it is an area in need of urgent analysis and review.

There is also need for a greater recognition of the competing demands for funds by those committed to researching and providing high-technology medicine and those involved in providing care. What is the acceptable balance between the two, and upon what criteria are judgments made? Callahan (1992) comments that:

> Our society can get enthusiastic about finding a scientific cure for a fatal disease. It is far less zealous about providing the sustaining services necessary to help its victims endure their illnesses until such a cure is found. Its zeal to help family members and others cope with the social and psychological burdens of caring for the ill is even fainter. (p. 142)

Here, surely, is one of the great ethical issues of our day. To what extent is society prepared to pay for the care of people who have dementia? To what extent are *we* prepared to pay, for in the end it is a question about public attitudes towards illness and often towards ageing? Do we expect people to pay for their own long-term care, or should it be a governmental responsibility? With an ageing population and with current policy trends seeking to meet the needs of the frail elderly at home and within tight financial constraints (Challis et al, 1997) we are facing an enormous challenge to our welfare services and many questions are raised in the process. Cayton (1987) points out:

> It seems ironic that just as professionals and family caregivers, along with doctors and scientists are developing positive and constructive approaches to improving the quality of life of people with dementia, we have politicians and policy makers who seem to view older people as a burden on rather than an enrichment of our society.

Cassidy (1988) has written movingly and provocatively about hospice care. One does not have to share her religious faith to catch something of the vision of a new society that she has in mind when she writes:

> It is a particular form of Christian madness that seeks out the broken ones, the insane, the handicapped and the dying and places before their astonished eyes a banquet normally reserved for the whole and the productive. (p. 52)

The extent to which we, as a community, seek to provide and resource services to those members who are the most vulnerable and in need says something about the values and convictions of our society. In the end these are ethical issues; the raising of taxes and the distribution of resources stand or fall upon what society in general deems to be important and worthwhile. The way in which we resource the care of those who have dementia illustrates vividly our priorities and our convictions.

CONCLUSION

To take seriously the experience of dementia is to hold a mirror to our society and to see what kind of image it reflects. In so many areas the image is blurred, as though someone has breathed over the glass. Ethical ambiguity is so often used as an excuse to move slowly, not only in the areas where there is confusion and real questions, but also in areas where progress could be made much more speedily given the will.

Good dementia care centres on the individual, upon the person who has dementia; it affirms the personhood and the right of these people to be heard and to be treated as fully human beings. The very nature of the illness requires that people act together in various forms of partnership, but for all who are involved in dementia care, and for all who are concerned that we create and shape a more humane and caring society, some of the ethical issues outlined here need to be addressed as a matter of urgency.

REFERENCES

Archibald, C. (1994) *Sexuality and Dementia*. Dementia Services Development Centre, University of Stirling.
Barnett, E. (1997) Collaboration and interdependence: care as a two-way street. In: Marshall, M. (ed.) *State of the Art in Dementia Care*. London: Centre for Policy on Ageing.
Battin, M. (1992) Euthanasia in Alzheimer's disease. In: Binstock, R., Post, S.G. & Whitehouse, P.J. (eds) *Dementia and Aging: Ethics, Values and Policy Choices*. Baltimore: Johns Hopkins University Press.
Berghmans, R. (1996) *Dementia Care and Ethics – A Brochure for Informal Carers of Dementing Persons*. Draft paper produced by the Institute for Bioethics, PO Box 778, 6200 AT Maastricht, The Netherlands.
Briggs, R. (1993) Comment. *Geriatric Medicine* January, 40–41.
Brodaty, H. (1988) Minimal brain damage in the adult. II: Early dementia. *Patient Management* August, 127–150.
Brodaty, H., Griffin, D. & Hadzi-Pavlovic, D. (1990) A survey of dementia carers: doctors' communications, problem behaviours and institutional care. *Australian and New Zealand Journal of Psychiatry* 24, 362–370.
Butler, R. (1992) Foreword. In: Binstock, R., Post, S.G. & Whitehouse, P.J. (eds). *Dementia and Aging: Ethics, Values and Policy Choices*. Baltimore: Johns Hopkins University Press.
Callahan, D. (1992) Dementia and appropriate care: allocating scarce resources. In: Binstock, R.H, Post, S.G. & Whitehouse, P.J. (eds) *Dementia and Aging: Ethics, Values and Policy Choices*. Baltimore: Johns Hopkins University Press.
Cassidy, S. (1988) *Sharing the Darkness*. London: Darton Longman & Todd.
Cayton, H. (1995) Diagnostic testing: who wants to know? *Journal of Dementia Care* Jan/Feb
Cayton, H. (1987) The art of the state: Public policy in dementia care. In Marshall, M. (ed.) *State of the Art in Dementia Care*. London: Centre for Policy on Ageing.
Challis, D., von Abendorff, R., Brown, P. & Chesterman, J. (1997) Care management and dementia: an evaluation of the Lewisham Intensive Case Management Scheme In: Hunter, S. (ed.) *Dementia: Challenges and New Directions*. London: Jessica Kingsley.
Downs, M. (1994) *Dementia: A Literature Review*. Dementia Services Development Centre, University of Stirling.
Engelhardt, H.T. (1986) *The Foundations of Bioethics*. Oxford University Press.
English, J. (1979) What do grown up children owe their parents? In: O'Neill, O. & Ruddick, W. (eds) *Having Children: Philosophical and Legal Reflections on Parenthood*. Oxford University Press.
Fontana & Smith (1989) Alzheimer's Disease victims; the 'unbecoming' of self and the normalisation of competence. *Sociological Perspectives* 32, 1.
Gadow, S. (1988) Covenant without cure: letting go and holding on in chronic illness. In: Watson, J. & Ray, M.A. (eds) *The Ethics of Care and the Ethics of Cure*.

Gilbert, P., Pehl, J. & Allan, S. (1994) The phenomenology of shame and guilt: an empirical investigation. *British Journal of Medical Psychology* 67, 23–36

Goldsmith, M. (1996) *Hearing the Voice of People with Dementia.* London: Jessica Kingsley.

Haines, A. (1990) Diagnosis and management of dementia. *Practice Update* April, 744–749.

Haley, W., Clair, J. & Saulsberry, K. (1992) Family caregiver satisfaction with medical care of demented relatives. *Gerontologist* 32, 219–226.

Illiffe, S. (1992) What is the role of the general practitioner, – In: Bland, R et al (eds) *Diagnosis and Assessment.* Dementia Services Development Centre, University of Stirling.

Jacques, A. (1992) *Understanding Dementia.* London: Churchill Livingstone.

Jacques, A. (1997) Ethical dilemmas in care and research for people with dementia. In: Hunter, S. (ed.) *Dementia: Challenges and New Directions.* London: Jessica Kingsley.

Judd, S. (1997) Technology. In: Marshall, M. (ed.) *State of the Art in Dementia Care.* London: Centre for Policy on Ageing.

Kennedy, A. & Rosser, M. (1993) Management of dementia. *Practitioner* 237, 103–107.

Killick, J. (1994) Giving shape to shadows. *Elderly Care* 6, 3, May/June

Kilner, N., Miller, A. & Pellegrino, E. (1996) *Dignity and Dying: A Christian Approach.* Grand Rapids: Paternoster Press Eerdmans.

Kitwood, T. (1993) Frames of reference for an understanding of dementia. In: *Ageing and Later Life.* Buckingham: Open University Press.

Kitwood, T. (1997) *Dementia Reconsidered.* Buckingham: Open University Press.

Kitwood, T & Bredin, K. (1992) Towards a theory of dementia care: personhood and well-being. *Ageing and Society* 10, 269–287.

Kung, H. & Jens, W. (1995) *A Dignified Dying.* London: SCM Press.

Leikas, J. (1994) *Use of technical aids in the care of dementia.* Paper presented at the 10th Annual Meeting of Alzheimer's Disease International, September 1994, Edinburgh.

Malcolm, D. (1993) *Early Dementia and the General Practitioner.* Dementia Services Development Centre, University of Stirling.

Marshall, M. (1994) *Technology for people with dementia: some ethical issues.* Paper presented at the Annual Meeting of the British Society of Gerontology, London.

Martin, R.J. & Post, S.G. (1992) Human dignity, dementia and the moral basis of care giving. In: Binstock, R.H., Post, S.G. & Whitehouse, P.J. (eds) *Dementia and Aging: Ethics, Values and Policy Choices.* Baltimore: Johns Hopkins University Press.

McLean, S. (1987) Assessing dementia. Part 1: difficulties, definitions and differential diagnosis. *Australian and New Zealand Journal of Psychology* 21, 142–174.

McLean, S. (1993) Practical management of Alzheimer's disease. *Modern Medicine* (*Australia*) April, 16–27.

Nolan, M. & Grant, G. (1989) Addressing the needs of informal carers: a neglected area of nursing practice. *Journal of Advanced Nursing* 15 (5), 544–555.

Philp, I. (1988) Meeting carers' needs – an expensive task? *Geriatric Medicine* 18, 1173–1179.

Pieper, R. (1994) *Home adaptations of the demented elderly: Technical solutions, impacts on the care situation and implementation strategies.* Paper presented at the 10th Annual Meeting of Alzheimer's Disease International, September 1994, Edinburgh.

Pitkeathley, J. (1989) *It's My Duty, Isn't It? The Plight of Carers in Our Society.* London: Souvenir Press.

Rinpoche, S. (1992) *The Tibetan Book of Living and Dying.* London: Rider Books.

Sommers, C.H. (1986) Filial morality. *Journal of Philosophy* 83, 438–456.

Watson, R. (1994) Practical ethical issues related to the care of elderly people with dementia. *Nursing Ethics* 1 (3), 154.

Woods, R.T. (1997) Why should family caregivers feel guilty? In: Marshall, M. (ed.) *The State of Art in Dementia Care.* London: Centre for Policy on Ageing.

5

Towards a partnership in maintaining personhood

Jane Crisp

KEY ISSUES

- The prevalence of negative attitudes towards dementia increases the likelihood of our seeing people with dementia as less than human

- The qualities that we take to be essential to our status as human beings, and our ideas about what counts as a valid communicative interaction, determine whether we regard someone with dementia as a person or not

- The personhood of someone with dementia can indeed survive, despite the effects of their condition

- Caregiving behaviours can be developed that actively foster a sense of identity and worth in the person with dementia

- We need to develop strategies for understanding people with dementia better so that we can enter into their perspective and engage in a genuinely supportive partnership with them

INTRODUCTION

A major impediment to the survival of 'personhood' in someone with dementia is the prevalence of highly negative and stigmatising attitudes towards this condition. These attitudes influence caregiving practices, which in turn adversely affect the person in care and, indeed, may worsen the dementia.

How we define 'personhood' may well determine the degree of human status that we are prepared to give to someone with dementia. If we think of the self as some sort of inner essence, we may believe that this is capable of surviving the effects of dementia, or see it as being progressively eroded and finally lost. However, if we understand selfhood in constructivist terms, as something we actively produce throughout our lives, we are more likely to recognise and support the efforts of someone with dementia to continue constructing and maintaining an identity. The qualities and capacities that we take to be central to being human will also influence our attitudes towards people with dementia. The ability to reason and to recall facts accurately is compromised early in the dementing process, whereas the emotional, social and imaginative aspects of being human can survive virtually to the end. Hence our continuing to regard someone with dementia as a fellow human being will depend very much on our giving full value to these latter qualities.

The ability to engage in communicative interactions with others is also a major component of personhood, ensuring as it does our continuing membership of the human community. Again, our ideas about what constitutes communication will affect our estimate of what capacity for it survives in people with dementia. If we see communication in terms of a dynamic, two-way partnership we will be more ready to compensate for any problems caused by the other person's dementia and to recognise and value the significance of any interaction that does take place between us.

Helping people with dementia to maintain their personhood necessarily entails doing whatever we can to foster their sense of continuing identity and worth. Kitwood (1990) identifies the various harmful behaviours that carers often exhibit towards their charges. Reversing these gives us the following list of supportive behaviours: honesty towards the person with dementia, empowerment, treating them as an adult, encouragement, avoiding pejorative labels, acceptance, letting them set the pace, validation, inclusion, continuing to see them as a person rather than as an object.

Showing a willingness to interact with people with dementia is a way in which we can help support their sense of worth. Even if we have trouble understanding what they say, we can still acknowledge their existence through a friendly greeting; we can give value to the very fact of interaction itself; we can show them we are listening to and trying to understand them. Shared activities can also be seen as a form of interaction.

There are various established strategies for getting the general drift of a verbal communication being made by someone with dementia: listening for the feeling behind the words; responding to body language; and being alert to clues in the context. Knowledge of the person's past life may also provide us with clues to interpretation.

However, research on the changes in the language of people with dementia provides more specific strategies for interpreting what they are actually saying. The known tendency for a move to broader categories, for example, allows us to interpret the apparent misnaming of an animal as a 'dog' by recognising that the term now has the broader meaning of 'dog-like'. Such misnamings may also express an emotional response prompted by all members of the broader category. Other apparent misnamings can be made more intelligible by recognising the existence of links of likeness and links in common usage between the word used by the person with dementia and the word that would normally be used. Complementary strategies for doing justice to what someone with dementia is trying to say include focusing on what the person is achieving rather than on errors, and applying the criterion of appropriateness rather than strict accuracy.

By realising that broader categories of event or person are being drawn on to produce composite events or figures, we can learn to appreciate and make sense of the apparently confused and often fantastic confabulatory stories that people with dementia tell about themselves. Existing work on the life story suggests that these 'pseudo-reminiscences' may serve the same purposes as in all people in providing an ego-sustaining version or reconstruction of the past.

DOES PERSONHOOD SURVIVE IN SOMEONE WITH DEMENTIA?

It has become a basic tenet of caring for people with dementia that they should continue to be seen as human beings and treated with dignity (e.g. Sherman, 1991). This tenet is crucial to the perspective and practices advocated in this book, because considering that people with dementia are still endowed with personhood is a necessary precondition for conceiving of our relationship with them as anything approaching a real partnership – that is, as a mutual and cooperative relationship between two people who, despite any differences in health or capability between them, come together as fellow human beings.

However, the human status of someone with dementia is threatened not simply by the progressive effects of the condition but also by the negative way in which dementia tends to be perceived in our society and the influence of this on carers, caregiving practices and on the person diagnosed as having dementia. Our ideas about what constitutes being a person may well contribute to this problem, especially if the qualities that we see as essential to our humanity are those most seriously compromised by the dementing process. A closely related issue is whether we believe that people with dementia are still able to communicate or not. Do they still have something to say, despite the changes in their mental and linguistic abilities, and if so, how can we make sense of them? Once again, the idea of partnership is meaningless without the possibility of some sort of genuine communicative interaction between us.

The problem of negative attitudes towards dementia

The effect of negative attitudes on carers and caregiving practices

A major hindrance to seeing someone with dementia as a person is that dementia itself tends to be conceptualised in terms that make it difficult for carers to think of those for whom they care as still being fully human, especially if there is no pre-existing bond between them. Thus, even well-intentioned and otherwise helpful books for carers refer to dementia in their titles as 'a living death' and 'the loss of self' (Cohen and Eisendorfer, 1986; Woods, 1989). Such negative terminology effectively reduces people with dementia, especially those in the more advanced stages, to little more than physical shells now empty of whatever qualities once made them fully human. In consequence, their care is reduced to a matter of putting food into mouths and keeping bodies clean.

Even caregiving practices that recognise and conscientiously endeavour to cater for other needs that these people may have, risk undercutting their professed aims by implicitly reinforcing negative stereotypes about dementia. For instance, as Holden and Woods (1988) have noted, much of the vocabulary still routinely used of people with dementia (such as 'confused', 'attention-seeking' and 'demented') perpetuates commonly held and unhelpful perceptions of the condition and reinforces the stigma associated with it. Some 'therapeutic' programmes may have similar consequences. They may turn carers' principal interactions with people with dementia into attempts at remedying their perceived deficiencies and orienting them towards a normative version of reality, rather than social exchanges with a fellow human being whose similarities to us we recognise and whose differences from us we are prepared to accept (Shoham and Neuschatz, 1985). Thus, even though the stated aim may be to treat the person being cared for as a person, the vocabulary we use and the type of activities we offer may counteract this aim by indicating that we are primarily seeing these people in terms of their dementia and the consequent 'deterioration' and 'loss' of an earlier, more completely human self.

Despite the prevalence of these attitudes, close relationships can be maintained between people with dementia and those who care for them. Indeed, someone with dementia can continue to be treated 'as a person' right up to the end, as I and many other carers, both family and professional, know from personal experience. However, the general negativity about dementia adds to the already considerable burden of anyone who is endeavouring to maintain a relationship with a family member or friend with the condition. It also adds to the burden of the many professional carers who are striving to ensure that those in their care continue to be treated with respect by all those in contact with them.

The effect of negative attitudes on the person with dementia

The need for a change in the negative stereotypes of dementia becomes even more urgent if we take into account the impact these are likely to have on the sense of wellbeing and identity of the person most closely concerned – someone who has actually been diagnosed as having dementia. Indeed, the significance of this impact has been underlined by recent understandings of the dementing process as being caused not only by physical changes in the brain but by social and psychological factors as well. Representative of such recent understandings and of particular relevance to the current discussion is work by Maisondieu (1989), Kitwood (1990) and Sabat and Harré (1992).

The French psychogerontologist Maisondieu (1989) takes the most radical position in support of psychological causes of dementia over the more widely accepted biological causes. He argues that even though there are indeed plenty of people who are dementing, 'dementia' itself is no more than a construction of medical discourse. For him the key to the syndrome to which we give the label of 'dementia', and therefore the real plague of modern times, is a pathological fear of ageing and death. He sees people with dementia as being doubly affected by the consequences of this fear. Not only are they stigmatised for embodying the progressive losses associated with death, but fear of death is what has triggered their dementia in the first place. Unable to cope with the inevitability of their own mortality in any rational way, they resort to abandoning reason altogether. Hence the much sought-after means of preventing or curing dementia might best be found in a greater acceptance of ageing and death as a natural part of the life process. Whether or not one is prepared to accept Maisondieu's thesis in its entirety, the case for the need to change contemporary attitudes to death and dying is a compelling one, and particularly relevant to a condition that is all too frequently thought of as a form of 'living death'.

Kitwood (1990) does not go as far as Maisondieu in discounting the more orthodox biological explanation for dementia. He argues instead for a 'dialectic' model of the dementing process in which the affected person's initial 'neurological impairment' produces a change in the attitudes and behaviour of others which in turn causes a worsening of the impairment. A crucial factor therefore is the impact on the person with dementia of what Kitwood (1990) calls a 'malignant social psychology' (see Table 3.1). This is manifested in acts of treachery, disempowerment, infantilisation, intimidation, labelling, stigmatisation, outpacing, invalidation, banishment and objectification. Through these the person with dementia is progressively diminished and depersonalised, and the dementia is aggravated in consequence.

Sabat and Harré (1992) also argue for the contribution made to dementia by the attitude of others, and in terms that are if anything even more relevant to the concerns of this chapter. They draw explicitly on a constructionist theory of the nature of selfhood to challenge the assumption that dementia involves the 'loss of self' proclaimed by Cohen and Eisendorfer (1986) in the title of their book for carers. Drawing on detailed case studies, Sabat and Harré (1992) demonstrate that the self of personal identity, of a personal perspective on the world indicated by the use of 'I', 'my' and gestures that serve the same purpose, persists even into the later stages of dementia. The more public and social selves, the complementary roles or personae that are mutually negotiated in the course of our interactions with others, may indeed be lost. However, Sabat and Harré stress that this loss is neither an inevitable nor even a direct consequence of dementia itself. Rather, it is the negative response to dementia that prevents others from recognising or supporting the attempts of people with dementia to maintain their social identity.

The implications of how we define personhood

As the arguments summarised above indicate, the survival of the personhood of people with dementia may well depend on our continuing to treat them as a person. However, our capacity to do this is affected not only by our attitude towards dementia, but also by the ideas underlying that attitude as to what constitutes 'a person': that is, by our beliefs concerning the nature of personhood and the capacities and qualities that we deem to be essential to it.

The self as inner essence – kept or lost?

A 'self' that can be thought of as eroded or 'lost' during the dementing process is one that conforms to the way most of us tend to see the self, namely as an inner essence, a given set of qualities and characteristics, which are thought of as making up our 'true' identity. This 'inner self' is seen as being a personal endowment, something which we hope to be able to develop fully and to keep throughout our life but which in adverse circumstances may become stunted, hidden, betrayed or even lost.

Such a view can produce two different types of response to the changes that are symptomatic of dementia. On the positive side, it may encourage us to believe that the core elements of the self can and do resist the effects of dementia. Thus by recognising and responding to that core self, professional and family carers can help the person with dementia to maintain some sense of identity. This belief is central to some of the recent, more positive approaches to dementia care, such as the ELTOS method (enhancing life through optimum stimulus) outlined by Garrett and Hamilton-Smith (1995), and the adaptation of caregiving practices to the personality type of the person with dementia recommended by Khosravi (1993). The survival of core elements of identity is also borne out by the testimony of many carers. My experience with my own mother was that not only did many of her gracious social manners persist well into the dementing process, but many of her central interests and pleasures did too.

Her love of words, of gardens and of teddy bears remained virtually to the end of her life, and helped my father and me to interact with her and maintain a sense of rapport.

However, if we understand selfhood as an inner possession or essence, then the changes produced in someone by dementia are just as likely to be understood in the negative terms of progressive deterioration and eventual loss of an earlier 'true' self. Thus, my father and I might well have regarded my mother's loss of all memories of the novels of Jane Austen, which had long been her favourite reading and a constant point of reference, as the loss of a crucial element of her personality, instead of seeing her basic pleasure in language as persisting in the style of many of her comments and in her chanting of nursery rhymes. The view of the self as something that dementia can destroy underlies the oppositional rhetoric which I have discussed in detail elsewhere (Crisp, 1995a), in which the person with dementia is typically represented as having become radically different not only from 'normal' people but also from the person's own pre-dementing personality. It also manifests itself in the well-meaning advice sometimes offered to family members that a relative with dementia is 'no longer the person you knew and loved all those years'.

Insistence on the differences between us and the person with dementia, and between that person's former and present identity, may well be a response to the dread that the condition tends to inspire, and the corresponding need to distance ourselves from it. It may also be functional, helping family carers to cope with any feelings of threat, resentment, inadequacy or guilt; to deal with aggression or a lack of recognition from the person for whom they are caring; and to accept the need to commit that person to institutional care and to get on with their own lives.

Perceiving someone with dementia as no longer being a person is understandable and may sometimes be strategically useful. For example, family members may be unable to take on a partnership role in care, perhaps when an already indifferent or hostile relationship has been irrevocably damaged by the added burden of stress caused by dementia. However, such perceptions are clearly counterproductive in the many other cases where carers do desire to establish or maintain a partnership with someone with dementia, since they involve seeing sufferers almost exclusively in terms of what they have lost and so robbing them of any status as a 'whole' person.

The self as product of ongoing construction

Thinking of the self as a given core or essence, then, may or may not help carers to respond positively to the changes symptomatic of dementia. However, an alternative way of thinking about identity (and one that is consciously drawn on in the more positive approach to care taken in this book) is that it is not a given possession but something we are actively engaged in constructing throughout our lives. The value of this constructivist view, as Sabat and Harré (1992) demonstrate, is that it makes it possible for us to recognise that people who have dementia are still engaged in the process of defending, negotiating and reconstructing an identity for themselves. Moreover, as Kitwood (1990) and Sabat and Harré (1992) make clear, we are ourselves involved in this process through the way our behaviour towards people with dementia supports or denies their claim to possess a valid – and valued – human identity.

Central to being human – reason or feeling?

Regarding someone with dementia as still endowed with personhood depends very much on the assumptions we make about what constitutes the self. Closely related to these are the assumptions we make about what qualities are central to our human status. Indeed, how we estimate the capacities of people with dementia is directly related to the criteria we are using and the types of ability that they privilege. This point is borne out by Rigaux (1992) in her extended analysis of medical accounts of the condition, in which she demonstrates how different judgments about people with dementia can be correlated with the particular qualities or characteristics of being human to which these judgments implicitly appeal. As she notes, the standard medical and scientific texts on the condition give priority to the more obviously instrumental abilities of reasoning and remembering with accuracy. These are precisely the capacities that are earliest and most radically affected by the dementing process. When someone with dementia is judged by these criteria, as they are routinely in diagnostic tests, attention is drawn inevitably to what they can no longer do. As was the case with my mother, people with dementia may not know the name of the current leader of their country and they may not remember what year it is, how old they are or what they did yesterday. Whenever such criteria are uppermost in our minds, much of what the person with dementia says and does will tend to be seen as deficient in some way, as symptomatic of the dementia. Care becomes focused on counteracting these deficits and controlling these symptoms by means of therapy, drugs or physical restraints. Assessed predominantly in these negative terms, the person with dementia risks seeming less than fully human.

However, alternative, more psychologically oriented approaches to dementia tend to take into account the social, expressive, imaginative and even unconscious dimensions of being human, and consequently are more likely to see someone who is dementing as still a person. These approaches were fully represented at the first European *Psychotherapies of the Dementias* conference held in Strasbourg in 1994. The title of the conference is particularly significant, since the notion of psychotherapy is meaningful in this context only if people with dementia are recognised as having psyches. Thus, my own mother still enjoyed interacting with other people and formed close friendships with fellow residents and carers even after her dementia had reached the stage that required her admission to full-time professional care. She had opinions and feelings to express, even in the last stages: 'You see that woman – my, she's a horror'; 'I'm terrified, I don't know what to do'; 'Oh, what a beautiful morning' (sung when she was particularly enjoying herself). She had amazing confabulatory stories to tell me about herself (some of which I discuss later in this chapter), and (as I noted above) retained a facility with and pleasure in words virtually to the end: 'It's an in-between bird', she said, when I asked her if the bird we were admiring was big or little; she gleefully joined in and sometimes even initiated the old rhyming chants, 'Moses supposes his toeses are roses' and 'We'll weather the weather whatever the weather'. As Rigaux (1992) stresses (and as the positive experiences of many other carers, both family and professional, bear out), by valuing fully these other aspects of personhood we are in a better position to recognise and appreciate all the many ways in which the person we care for is still very much a fellow human being. Furthermore, we will be readier to think of care for people with dementia in terms of finding out what gives them pleasure and of striving to enhance their quality of life.

The issue of communication

If we are to believe that someone with dementia is still a person, then we are virtually obliged to believe also that people with dementia can and do communicate with others: that is, that they are still able to engage in some sort of two-way exchange that is meaningful to both participants and so can properly be called communication. Once we start thinking that what people say or do no longer makes sense, that their words and actions communicate nothing except the fact that they are dementing, we are effectively excluding them from any further membership of the human community. We are also exonerating ourselves from making any further effort to understand them. Conversely, if we do believe, as many carers fortunately do, that people with dementia still have ideas and feelings to be expressed, and that their words and acts are potentially communicative of these, we are much more likely to invest the time and energy necessary to understand them and to make an appropriate response. For instance, to make the point, as Cotrell and Schulz (1993) have recently done, that 'the perspective [of the person with dementia] is a neglected dimension of dementia research' is to believe that such a perspective exists, and can be obtained. It is to believe that people with dementia have something to tell us and deserve to be listened to, especially on a subject that so closely concerns them.

Does the capacity to communicate survive?

Given the obvious importance of believing that people with dementia do retain the ability to communicate, what evidence is there to support this belief? After all, dementia does produce significant changes in memory and language use, which do indeed interfere with the ability of people with dementia to communicate and of others to understand them. These changes have been well documented. Certain mental processes that we normally take for granted become progressively uncertain, e.g. recalling facts and events readily and accurately, remembering what was done earlier, distinguishing between what was done and what may have been read or fantasised about, finding the correct word for people and things. Later, people may repeat themselves endlessly, as my mother did when she was telling a favourite story about some impossible feat she claimed to have performed. Further, people may produce only fragmentary phrases or echoes of what was said, or even find producing speech virtually impossible, as happened to Wally, my mother's special friend and fellow resident. These changes can be disconcerting for carers, and do make it harder to listen to and carry on a conversation with someone with dementia. However, whether we continue to make the effort or not will naturally depend very much on our assumptions about how much capacity the person with dementia still has for communicating in any meaningful way with others.

The benefits of seeing communication as a partnership

As I have argued elsewhere (Crisp, 1995b,c), our estimate as to whether people with dementia do retain the ability to communicate may well depend on the assumptions that we make about how communication actually works, much as our estimate of their continuing personhood depends on how we define the qualities necessary for this. What is often referred to as the 'instrumentalist' model of communication (e.g. Penman, 1988) sees the meaning of what we say or write very much in terms of what the speaker or writer intends to communicate; these ideas or wishes are embodied in words and so transferred to others. If the spoken or written message is difficult for us to understand, the problem lies with the deficiencies of its originator. People with dementia are deemed to have lost the linguistic and mental abilities needed to produce a complete, correctly formed and meaningful message. However, the alternative constructivist model presents communication in very different terms, as a dynamic, two-way process of social interaction. Meaning, instead of being determined by the intentions of the speaker and simply transferred with differing degrees of success to the listener, is constructed through a process of active negotiation between them. Communication requires a partnership, and any problems that occur during the process are as much the responsibility of the listener as the speaker. As Ripich and Terrell (1988) note in their study of 'cohesion and coherence' in the speech of people with Alzheimer's disease, the judgment that someone's speech is incoherent or meaningless tells us as much about the listeners' problems in making sense of what they hear as it does about the nature of what is being said to them.

This more dynamic partnership model implicitly informs the belief in a continuing capacity for communication which underlies much of the work on interacting with people with dementia. For example, Bartol (1979) recognises the ways in which people endeavour to use language in their exchanges with others, and of the role of non-verbal aspects of communication in supplementing these. Khosravi (1993) provides telling accounts of dialogues, both verbal and non-verbal, with patients in advanced stages of dementia. All carers have a vested interest in consciously adopting this dynamic partnership model of language and communication. The advantages are twofold: a greater readiness to acknowledge the surviving communicative abilities of the person with dementia, and, as a result, a greater willingness to invest the time and energy that may be needed to maintain a communicative partnership with them.

Our success in establishing and maintaining a communicative partnership with people with dementia, however, will depend on our having the necessary means of coping with the obvious effects of their condition on their memory and on their use of language. We need to acquire strategies for understanding people with dementia and their perspective so that we can indeed respond positively and supportively to them. The success of many carers, both family and professional, in communicating with and making sense of people with dementia provides us with various strategies for enhancing our interactions with such people. These are outlined later in this chapter, together with some additional strategies which are the product of my own exploration of the language use of people with dementia. These offer a systematic and objective means of making better sense of what people actually say, including the apparently confused stories that they tell about themselves.

Different attitudes in practice: the example of 'wandering'

A practical illustration of the two different ways of looking at someone with dementia, and the consequences for care, is provided by attitudes to what is commonly referred to as 'wandering'. The subject is one that concerns me closely, since the designation of 'wanderer' was applicable to my own mother.

Wandering as a symptom

For those who subscribe to the standard medical model, wandering is a symptom of dementia, an aimless activity produced by deterioration within the brain. Wandering constitutes a problem for carers and, if the wanderer is in a home, for other residents. Indeed, as I discovered when I was seeking alternative accommodation for my own mother, many homes actually specify that they 'don't take wanderers'. The very term 'wanderer' as thus used implicitly reduces the person in question to a pathological category, and such behaviour to a disruptive manifestation of the effects of dementia.

Wandering as expressive of the person

For those who subscribe to the alternative, more psychologically oriented view of dementia, however, 'wandering' takes on a different set of meanings. Rather than being a mere symptom it becomes expressive of the person's habits and needs. For most of her earlier life my mother had spent hours of each day pottering about the garden, so I saw nothing strange about her continuing what had long been a favourite activity. Some of this behaviour may be semi-automatic, as indeed are any well-established habits, whether we have dementia or not. However, wandering may also be interpreted as being a strategic choice, an exercise of agency. A case in point is provided by Sabat and Harré (1992): they observed that one of the people they were studying wandered away from the day-care sessions in which she was involved whenever the activity centred on small group discussion. Given her problems with speech production this was not the random act it seemed to those who saw her behaviour in terms of her dementia, but 'a reflection of her grasp of the social situation and her rational decision not to embarrass herself'. Some residential centres, therefore, see wandering not as a problem but as a self-chosen and health-promoting form of exercise for which caring institutions should cater. Examples are Whare Aroha in New Zealand, with its enclosed landscaped garden and temptingly winding paths; and the custom-built Jardins d'Eleusis in France, with gently sloping ramps between the central recreation area and the upper storey which offer the more active residents the means of taking exercise indoors on days when it is too cold and wet outside. The crucial difference here is that the person who wanders is being seen and treated as a person and their activity is being regarded as a legitimate expression of that personhood.

MAINTAINING PERSONHOOD

A prerequisite of helping people with dementia to maintain their personhood is that we ourselves continue to see and to treat them as fellow human beings. As argued above, this depends on our developing a less negative attitude towards dementia by consciously subscribing to definitions of selfhood and humanness which will enable us to look beyond the effects of the condition and to recognise and value the surviving capacities of people with it. In the day-to-day practice of caregiving, however, our ability to support the sense of self of people with dementia, and to help them to maintain it, depends not only on our cultivating a more positive mental attitude but also on our being able to embody this attitude in our interactions with them. This chapter outlines two complementary sets of strategies for continuing to treat people with dementia as full human beings, and so help them to maintain their personhood. The first set of strategies involves ways of behaving towards people with dementia so that we can support their sense of identity and worth instead of contributing to the 'malignant social psychology' identified by Kitwood (1990). The second set of strategies involves ways of understanding what people with dementia are doing and saying so that we can enhance the quality of communication between us instead of contributing to its breakdown.

Fostering a sense of identity and worth

Kitwood (1990) usefully categorises the various all-too-common types of act through which carers may be robbing people with dementia of their personhood and thereby compounding the effects of their condition. His categories (see Table 3.1) not only provide us with an obvious list of 'don'ts', they also suggest alternative types of behaviour towards those for whom we care through which we can consciously nurture their threatened sense of personal identity and worth.

Honesty

Kitwood's category of 'treachery' applies to the tricking of someone with dementia as a means of getting them to do what we want. His example is of family members who pretend they are just going on a regular outing when really they are taking the person to be admitted to hospital. Instead, we might aim to be honest in our dealings with those with dementia, explaining as clearly as we can what we are doing and why, and giving them the chance to express their own views and feelings on the matter. We have a special responsibility to be honest with people who are cognitively impaired to ensure that we do not ourselves add to their confusion and to their problems in making sense of what is happening around them.

Empowerment

Kitwood (1990) notes how we disempower people with dementia by being overhelpful and so increasing their loss of everyday skills: feeding them, for example, in the interests of speed and efficiency, instead of giving them the extra time that they may need if they are to continue to cope by themselves. Instead we can foster their sense of agency, of 'having the power to do', by being less ready to assume that they are unable to do things and more sensitive to how we can help them to maintain their own performance of daily tasks.

Treating as an adult

Disempowerment is frequently compounded by infantilisation: people with dementia not only have everything done for them but they are treated and spoken about as if they were small children. I still feel angry when I recall the insensitive comment of an aide who had just been helping my mother get dressed: 'Bettie has been a very naughty girl this morning'. My mother was neither naughty nor a girl. She was nearly 90 years old, and given the stage of her dementia, it was to be expected that she might have problems putting her clothes on. The aide, however, had no such excuses for her attitude.

Encouragement

Kitwood notes how people with dementia are often intimidated by the impersonal and even bullying way in which tests and treatment may be administered to them, especially in a hospital environment. The alternative is to be sensitive to how confused or threatened someone may be feeling in these circumstances, and to behave towards them in a friendly, courteous and more encouraging manner.

Avoiding pejorative labels

Labelling someone as having Alzheimer's disease, or as being 'confused' or a 'wanderer', makes it all too easy to see that person in negative terms and to assume a progressive loss of capacities. This book follows a deliberate policy of using the term 'person with dementia' to ensure that the importance of the individual is stressed, rather than the condition.

Acceptance

Kitwood notes how readily labelling becomes stigmatisation: people with dementia are seen as different, 'alien' from us, and their company is avoided by others. Again, the alternative is to continue to recognise all the ways in which the person with dementia is still very much like us, despite the dementia. Interestingly, many of the symptoms of dementia (lapses of memory, uncertainty about whether we did something or merely thought about it, verbal slips) happen to everyone; the difference is in the frequency with which they occur. Where obvious differences do exist between what someone with dementia says and does and what so-called 'normal' people say and do, we can learn to accept these much as we are coming to accept other differences within an increasingly multicultural community.

Letting them set the pace

People with dementia are also diminished by what Kitwood (1990) calls 'outpacing': the failure to make allowance for the slower rate at which they can comfortably function mentally or physically. Again, we need to be more sensitive to their needs, letting them set the pace so that they can participate as fully as possible in what is happening.

Validation of their feelings and experience

By failing to understand or enter into the feelings and experience of people with dementia we deny the validity of their subjectivity. Such invalidation can be countered only if we make an honest attempt to understand their perspective on the world. The key here is being able to make sense of what they are saying, despite the changes in their use of language and their apparent confusion of fact and fantasy, past and present. Some practical strategies for doing this are outlined below.

Inclusion

People with dementia risk banishment from normal social contact with others: they are systematically ignored and left out of activities by family or fellow residents (as described by Jan Reed in Chapter 8) and are often literally banished to a separate part of the house or institution where they are living. Instead of excluding such people, we can learn to accept them as they are and find ways of including them in the daily life of the community. I still remember with pleasure the regular communal singsongs in which my mother and all the other residents and staff of the home participated, and the spirit of friendliness and common enjoyment that prevailed. I remember too with enormous gratitude the kindness of old family friends who continued to include my mother in afternoon tea parties, outings and picnics: all occasions which she was still capable of appreciating and responding appropriately to even when in an advanced stage of dementia.

Some specialised homes for dementia care are organised around this principle of inclusion. Residents are able to participate in the daily running of the place, much as they would in their own home, and are kept in contact with the larger community through trips out to restaurants and

---

Box 5.1　The French approach to inclusive care

The French *cantou* system has the underlying philosophy of making residents feel that they are 'at home by their own fireside'. A simple but telling illustration of this philosophy in action is the fact that the staff of the *cantou*-style wing of the residence for long-term care in Haute-Mitry, Nantes, successfully persuaded the health authorities to let them keep the old-fashioned brooms and mops with which those residents who liked to help with the housework were familiar, rather than replacing them entirely with more hygienic modern machines which would have prevented any such involvement. Larger establishments that are managed in an inclusive way include the Jardins d'Eleusis in Fontainebleau and in Lyon, under the direction of the psychogerontologists Dr Alfred Saillon and Dr Louis Ploton respectively, and the long-term care pavilion at the Hôpital Garderose in Libourne.

---

cinemas and seasonal festivals. Examples of such homes are the smaller, family-style units, with between 8 and 15 residents in care, known as *cantou* in France (Box 5.1).

A person, not an object

The tendency of all the processes of diminishment categorised by Kitwood (1990) is the eventual objectification of the person with dementia. Such individuals are no longer seen or treated as a valid person, but as an object, and a degraded one at that: 'a lump of dead matter, to be measured, pushed around, manipulated, drained, filled, dumped, etc.' (Kitwood, 1990). Ways of thinking about and behaving towards people with dementia that ensure their personhood is recognised and supported are the central theme of this chapter and a major concern of this book.

Fostering interaction

There are various ways in which we are able to foster the possibility of worthwhile interaction between ourselves and people with dementia, irrespective of how well they can communicate with us or we can understand them.

Acknowledge that they exist

Whether people with dementia appear to register our presence or not, there is still some point in letting them know that we are aware of them. Our naming them, our polite greeting tells them that they are visible to us as a human being with whom we are ready to interact. If they do not wish to respond, that is their right, but our effort has not been wasted. We have actually done two things: offered them the opportunity for an interaction, and, in so doing, told them that they do have an identity in our eyes.

Value the fact of interaction itself

A major advantage of the interactive model of communication is that it makes the very fact of interaction with another person a central part of the meaning of any communication activity. This is an especially important point to keep in mind when communicating with people with dementia. As Sabat and Harré (1992) note, people with dementia, like everyone else, rely on social exchanges with others to establish and maintain their sense of identity, but are less likely to meet with the cooperative response necessary for the construction of a valid identity. Hence a basic strategy is to keep reminding ourselves of the value that any interaction is capable of having. No matter how minimal the exchange, by engaging in it we are telling the person with dementia that he or she is still part of the human community, still a person with whom others are willing to interact. Even if the only response is an echoing of fragments of what you have said, this tells you that the person with dementia is acknowledging being spoken to and is attempting to respond. My father could almost always get a response from my mother, even during the final few days of her life: he would start to recite one of her favourite nursery rhymes and she would reply with a whispered echo of his words or even a picking up of the next line. Such an exchange may seem trivial, compared with the sophisticated discussions we could once have had with my mother, but its value to us was inestimable.

Show that we are listening

Given the value in the very fact of interaction, even if we are having trouble understanding what people with dementia are trying to express, we can still achieve something worthwhile by letting them know that we are listening to them, that we want to understand, and that we believe that they still have something worth saying. A smile, nods, an attentive stance, the repeating of a phrase that we do catch, all tell the other person that we are responding to the effort to interact with us.

Shared activity as interaction

It is worth remembering too that interactions can happen without words, through an exchange of nods or smiles or a touch of the hand. Doing something together is also a form of interaction: sharing a meal, hanging out the washing or laying the table. When my mother could no longer manage these routine household tasks, she still enjoyed handing me the pegs or carrying something for me.

Catching the general drift of a communication

During interactions with people with dementia there are many strategies that we can use to help us interpret the overall gist of what they may be trying to communicate to us. Some of these are described below.

Listening for the feeling behind the words

One well-known piece of advice is to 'listen for the feeling behind the words' (e.g. Bartol, 1979; Sherman, 1991). Tone of voice, posture and body language give clues to the emotional tenor of a message, even if little else is intelligible. If such clues suggest to us that the person is happy, agitated, excited or unhappy we know what general sort of response to make, and, depending on how well we know the person, may also be able to work out what is likely to have triggered the emotion.

Clues in the immediate context

The immediate context in which the interaction is happening may also provide us with clues to general understanding. For example, the shouts of another resident may be causing agitation, as anything that sounded rude and unmannerly (including the roar of the heavy-duty institutional vacuum cleaner) did in my mother's case.

Clues from their past

If we know something about the broader context of the earlier life of people with dementia, we may be able to recognise the relevance of what they are saying or doing by relating it to people or events in their past that may still seem present to them. As the research of Bohling (1991) has made clear, abortive verbal interactions with people with dementia are frequently the result of our failing to make an effort to discover what they are actually talking about. We persist with our own frame of reference rather than listening carefully in an attempt to identify theirs.

Strategies for interpreting what is actually said – the example of misnaming

The constructivist model of language sees the meaning of our communicative exchanges as a joint production, involving the interpretative skills of the listener as much as the mental and linguistic abilities of the speaker. Our failure to make sense of someone with dementia, therefore, may be due to our own lack of appropriate sense-making strategies, rather than to an inherent absence of sense in what the person is saying. This is similar to situations in which we fail to comprehend someone who is speaking a language or dialect with which we are unfamiliar. My own exploration into the possibilities of making sense of what people with dementia actually say was based on the assumption that these people might in effect be speaking a different language and that this might be one we could learn. With this in mind, I began to reread the considerable body of evidence on the changes in language associated with dementia, focusing not on what was going wrong with the use of words but instead on whatever was still working and how it worked. This evidence showed that even though the language of people with dementia is different in many respects from ours, it nonetheless still follows a system and obeys an underlying set of rules. This system and its rules provide us with an objective means of interpreting what is being said to us.

I have already outlined in detail elsewhere a set of interpretative strategies based upon recognising this system and its rules (Crisp, 1995c). What follows is a summary of the rules underlying one of the most characteristic problems associated with dementia – misnaming – and the simple interpretative strategies that can be based upon knowing these rules.

Moving to broader categories – from 'dog' to 'dog-like'

One well-documented aspect of the changed language use of people with dementia is a shift from narrower to broader categories. For example, a word like 'dog' which normally refers to a specific type of animal becomes used for a much wider range of small, dog-like animals (e.g. Schwartz et al 1979). Translating the word as 'dog-like' when it is used of animals other than dogs allows us to go beyond the obvious error and identify the meaning it has in terms of the speaker's altered language system. My mother applied the name 'bear' to a wide range of animals, but all of them were furry and ones of which she was especially fond. 'Bear' in her language now meant 'bear-like': 'cuddly and loveable creatures in the same category as the much-loved teddy bear that I always carry about with me'. 'Look at the dear little bear', she would say, pointing to such favourites as the hospital cat, or a sheep in a nearby field, or the little dog accompanying a visitor. Most of us are familiar with this sort of 'overextension' (as it is called) from our experience of how young children use 'dog' or 'horse' for a wider range of four-legged animals.

The broader category may have an emotional dimension

As the example of my mother's use of 'bear' shows, the broader mental category into which a range of items are being grouped may have an emotional dimension. This point is worth keeping in mind when, as often happens, someone with dementia apparently mistakes a relative for someone else. However, rather than being distressed by this apparent failure of recognition, we can make sense of it as an act of recognition of the person concerned as a member of the broader category, 'my family' and ask ourselves what additional significance putting the two people together might have. Thus, when my mother called my father by the name of her much-loved but now dead brother, she was acknowledging both her sense of kinship with him and her affection: both men were in the same category of close and dear male relations. Similarly, the elderly father with dementia who addresses his grown-up daughter as if she were his mother can be understood as expressing his sense both of the kinship between them and of the motherly care that the daughter is providing. In such cases, we can look beyond the apparent confusion that is a symptom of dementia and focus instead on the broader mental connections that make the 'misnaming' a meaningful one. Rather than seeing mother, grandfather or spouse as being so demented that they no longer know who we are, we can recognise them as people still capable of making an appropriate response to us and still knowing, albeit in broader terms, who we are.

Links of likeness

Research also shows that a large number of so-called misnamings are not random but are fairly closely linked with what would be the correct choice of word (e.g. Bayles and Kazniak, 1987; Mitchell, 1988). Many are linked perceptually: there is a similarity of some kind between the item being spoken about and the other item whose name it is being given. An extreme instance of this process was provided by my mother's insistence on identifying the hospital cat as a 'seagull'. When my father queried this, she indignantly replied, 'Of course it's a seagull – it's black and white!' The cat was indeed strongly marked in black and white, just like the blackbacked gulls which my mother regularly enjoyed feeding. Fortunately, such links of likeness are often more readily apparent, especially if we adopt the habit of looking for them.

Links in common usage

Another frequently occurring link is a semantic one: the word being used by the person with dementia is commonly associated with what we would consider the correct word. My favourite example of this is my mother's greeting to a much-loved carer, 'Hello, Redbreast!' The real name of this carer is Robyn, and the fact that she was wearing a red cardigan at the time provided an additional link of likeness which reinforced the appropriateness of my mother's choice of name for her.

The persistence of semantic links such as that between 'robin' and 'redbreast' also gives us a strategy for responding to the fragments of speech sometimes produced by people with dementia. We can ask ourselves what words would most often be used to make this fragment complete and test out our hunch on the speaker. The reaction will probably tell us whether we are on the right track or not. The fact that our brain stores words together that are commonly associated can also help us to understand the logic underlying even such apparently gross misnamings as 'hot' for 'cold'. The two words are stored side by side, as it were, and the person has retrieved not the word they needed but the one next to it. Even in this error, we can recognise that the person still has a mental and verbal system in place.

Focusing on achievement rather than deficit

Taken together, then, all the above examples demonstrate to us that people with dementia do still possess a mind and language, despite the implications of the word for their condition – 'de-mentia', losing one's mind. Although there are obvious changes in their thought processes and speech due to their condition, these still follow normal and recognisable rules. To help us conceptualise what is happening, we may think of it not as the sudden and total breakdown of an intact system that was operating before the onset of dementia, but rather as a matter of increasing play within the original system. As with an old car, the machinery is still working, but the connections are often rather 'hit and miss' because of the play that has developed between the adjacent parts. Nonetheless, the car itself is still capable of going, even if the rest of society regards it as no longer legally roadworthy, provided we understand and allow for that play.

Recognising that people with dementia do still have a mental and verbal system, and knowing the general rules by which this system now works, help us to understand what these people are trying to say to us, and so to interact more fully with them. More generally, this recognition allows us to move beyond seeing these people exclusively in terms of dementia, deficit and loss, and to focus instead on what they are still able to achieve – that is, on the qualities, capacities and emotions that proclaim their ongoing personhood.

Focusing on what is appropriate

A general strategy for focusing our attention on the achievements of someone with dementia is to apply the broader criterion of appropriateness to person and context rather than the more limiting one of 'right' or 'wrong'. Note, for instance, how appropriate the various types of 'misnaming' outlined above actually are, once we look beyond the obvious error and recognise its underlying logic. Note, too, the appropriateness of wandering off, rather than staying around for the oral activity which would show up one's deficits, as observed by Sabat and Harré (1992) in one of the people they were studying. My mother regularly failed to come up with the 'correct' name for her favourite fruit (bananas), yet her replies to my father when asked to identify what he was offering her were unfailingly apt: 'Something good to eat', for example (note the use of a broader mental category), or, 'You tell me, and then I'll tell you!'.

Making sense of the stories people tell about themselves

Focusing on what people with dementia are still capable of achieving and focusing on what is appropriate about what they say and do are strategies that help us to make sense of another characteristic aspect of the speech of people with dementia – confabulation or pseudo-reminiscence. These supposedly autobiographical stories which combine past and present, fact and fantasy indiscriminately are likely to seem muddled and incoherent, especially if we know enough about the speaker to realise how far the story departs from the literal truth. However, it is important to remember that the loss of the ability to distinguish between lived events and imagined ones is a symptom of dementia and so such stories are usually told us in good faith. Moreover, by drawing both on what we know about the shifts in the use of language and thought processes and on constructivist ideas about the life story, we can begin to understand the purposes such stories may serve for their teller and respond to them accordingly.

Broader categories and composite figures

A strategy for resolving much of the apparent confusion of such stories is to keep in mind the mental shift to broader categories and the general play within the system already mentioned. My mother's claims about having designed the hospital garden and organised the positioning of the rocks in the rockery, for instance, were literally false but became much more relevant when we thought of them in terms of the broader category of gardens. Just as one family member was linked with another, so too memories of all the gardens she had made were linked together in her mind. Elements of those earlier gardens and the one she was now walking in had become interchangeable. Many other apparently muddled stories about past events became more intelligible if we applied this principle to them. For instance, stories supposedly involving Willy, a pet sheep she had once owned, made much better sense when we realised that 'Willy' was a composite figure, a 'superpet' constructed from memories of all the pets she had had plus memories of other attractive pets seen on television, such as Mr Ed the talking horse.

The life story as ego-sustaining construction

Rather than seeing such stories as evidence of the mental confusion symptomatic of dementia, we can see them more positively as composite constructions through which people with dementia endeavour to make sense of their surviving fragments of memory and so sustain their threatened sense of identity. All those fragments of my mother's past gardening experiences, for example, had become woven into a coherent narrative about something that she had done – and in this very garden. In the process, an otherwise alien environment was remade into something familiar and capable of giving her feelings of belonging and worth.

As I have argued elsewhere (Crisp, 1995d), this view of confabulation is supported by recent work on autobiographical narrative which adopts a constructivist perspective (e.g. Hankiss, 1981; Tarman, 1988; Angrosino, 1989). According to this perspective, any story that we tell about ourselves is a construction designed to present us in a certain light in a particular set of present circumstances. It can never simply mirror the past. Issues of accuracy or distortion, therefore, become less relevant than the processes involved in constructing a version of one's life story and the functions that it serves. Especially relevant to the present discussion is Tarman's account of how older people in institutional care use autobiographical narrative to present themselves as being still worthy of regard in the face of the stigma associated with old age and dependence (Tarman, 1988). Rather than undercutting and devaluing the story told by someone with dementia by insisting that it is not true, we might instead ask ourselves what significance such a story might have for the teller. What sort of person is presented in the story? What claims on our interest or sympathy does it make? Do these stories express directly or indirectly the fears of people with dementia about what is happening to them, or do they serve to counteract the tellers' fears and present them as being still in charge of their own destiny? My own mother told me the significance of one of her favourite stories, in which she boasted of having slipped out of bed during the night and climbed the nearby mountain: 'It's nice to know that there are things that I can still do!' As Gerbeaud (1987) has put it, 'such narcissism is the life-buoy of an identity that is drowning'. Therefore, rather than snatching away such life-buoys that people with dementia have been able to construct for themselves, we would do better to acknowledge the general terms of the identity that the story aims to achieve for its teller, and to make clear to them that we value that identity: 'Yes, you have done a lot of things, and there are still things that you can do'.

CONCLUSION

The 'personhood' of someone with dementia can and does survive, provided we are prepared to enter into partnership with that person in their efforts to maintain a valid sense of identity. In practice, this requires taking stock of our attitude to dementia and our beliefs about what constitutes a person so that we can engage more positively with those for whom we care. It also requires developing various strategies for interacting and communicating with people with dementia so that we can play our part in helping them to maintain their sense of identity and worth, thereby ensuring that they remain active, and valued, participants in the human community.

The holding of conferences such as the *Psychotherapies of the Dementias* conference in Strasbourg in 1994, and the publication of books such as this, indicate that the survival of personhood in people with dementia is becoming increasingly accepted within the professional caregiving community. The focus of concern for the future, then, is how we as family and professional carers can enter more fully into a partnership with people with dementia to help them maintain their sense of identity and worth. The three areas that we need to address in the interests of such a partnership in practice are the development of more constructive attitudes and beliefs about dementia and the people with it; interaction with these people in ways that support rather than diminish their personhood; and learning whatever sense-making strategies may be necessary for us to enter into their perspective.

REFERENCES

Angrosino, M.V. (1989) The two lives of Rebecca Levenstone: symbolic interaction in the generation of the life history. *Journal of Anthropological Research* **45**, 315–326.

Bartol, M.A. (1979) Nonverbal communication in patients with Alzheimer's disease. *Journal of Gerontological Nursing* **5**, 21–27.

Bayles, K. & Kazniak, A.W. (1987) *Communication and Cognition in Normal Aging and Dementia*. Boston: College Hill.

Bohling, H.R. (1991) Communication with Alzheimer's patients: an analysis of caregiver listening patterns. *International Journal of Aging and Human Development* **33**, 246–267.

Cohen, A. & Eisendorfer, C. (1986) *Alzheimer's Disease: The Loss of Self*. New York: Norton.

Cotrell, V. & Schulz, R. (1993) The perspective of the patient with Alzheimer's disease: a neglected dimension of dementia research. *Gerontologist* **33**, 205–211.

Crisp, J. (1995a) She has Alzheimer's and they all suffer from it. In: Ferres, K. (ed.) *Coastscripts: Gender Representation in the Arts*. Brisbane: Australian Institute for Women's Research and Policy.

Crisp, J. (1995b) Dementia and communication. In: Garrett, S. & Hamilton-Smith, E. (eds) *Rethinking Dementia – An Australian Approach*. Melbourne: Ausmed.

Crisp, J. (1995c) Les conceptions de la demence: differents modeles de discours sur les dements. *Psychologie Medicale* **27**, 180–183.

Crisp, J. (1995d) Making sense of the stories that people with Alzheimer's tell: a journey with my mother. *Nursing Inquiry* **2**, 133–140.

Garrett, S. & Hamilton-Smith, E., eds (1995) *Rethinking Dementia – An Australian Approach*. Melbourne: Ausmed.

Gerbeaud, J. (1987) Role du narcissisme dans l'identite de la personne agee demente institutionalisee. *Psychologie Medicale* **19**, 1261–1262.

Hankiss, A. (1981) Ontologies of the self: on the mythological rearranging of one's life history. In: Bertaux, D. (ed.) *The Life History Approach in the Social Sciences.* Beverley Hills: Sage.

Holden, U. & Woods, R. (1988) *Reality Orientation.* Edinburgh: Churchill Livingstone.

Khosravi, M. (1993) *Aider et Accompagner le Malade d'Alzheimer.* Paris: Marabout.

Kitwood, T. (1990) The dialectics of dementia: with particular reference to Alzheimer's disease. *Ageing and Society* **10**, 177–196.

Maisondieu, J. (1989) *Le Crepuscule de la Raison.* Paris: Centurion.

Mitchell, D.B. (1988) Memory and language deficits in Alzheimer's disease. In: Dippel, R.L. & Hutton, J.T. (eds) *Caring for the Alzheimer Patient.* Buffalo: Prometheus.

Penman, R. (1988) Communication reconstructed. *Journal of Theory of Social Behaviour* **18**, 391–410.

Rigaux, N. (1992) *Raison et Deraison: Discours Medical et Demence Senile.* Brussels: DeBoeck.

Ripich, D. & Terrell, B. (1988) Patterns of discourse cohesion and coherence in Alzheimer's disease. *Journal of Speech and Hearing Disorders* **53**, 8–15.

Sabat, S.R. & Harré, R. (1992) The construction and deconstruction of self in Alzheimer's disease. *Ageing and Society* **12**, 443–461.

Schwartz, M., Marin, O.S.M. & Saffran, E.M. (1979) Dissociation of language function in dementia; a case study. *Brain and Language* **36**, 277–306.

Sherman, B. (1991) *Dementia with Dignity.* Sydney: McGraw-Hill.

Shoham, H. & Neuschatz, S. (1985) Group therapy with senile patients. *Social Work* **30**, 69–72.

Tarman, V. (1988) Autobiography: the negotiation of a lifetime. *International Journal of Aging and Human Development* **27**, 171–191.

Woods, R. (1989) *Alzheimer's Disease: Coping With a Living Death.* London: Souvenir Press.

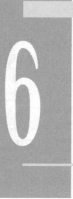

6

Communication in dementia care: a partnership approach

Anne Whitworth, Lisa Perkins Ruth Lesser

KEY ISSUES

- Dementia frequently results in a breakdown in communication
- Communication breakdown can be managed by working in partnership with carers
- Conversation analysis is a valuable tool in assessment and intervention
- Effective strategies can be developed to maximise communication

INTRODUCTION

The ability to communicate is central to social life, and the opportunity to engage in social interaction provides a powerful means for defining self, achieving self-esteem and maintaining relationships with others. The breakdown of communication in dementia has a devastating effect on both people with dementia and their families as the mechanism to maintain their relationship is compromised. Health-care professionals, in particular speech and language therapists, have an important role to play in providing advice and education to carers to help them keep the communication channels open.

This chapter begins with a brief examination of the effect of dementia on communication. Current practice in relation to working with carers is then reviewed and some limitations of generalised advice-giving are discussed. It is proposed that there is a need for work with people with dementia and their carers to be individually tailored, so allowing a focused partnership between family and therapist. Development of an assessment tool, the Conversation Analysis Profile for People with Cognitive Impairment

(CAPPCI) which promotes a partnership approach, is then described with illustrative data from a pilot study. It is argued that intervention needs to be client-led, incorporating the knowledge and skills that the carer has already developed, the communication strengths of the person with dementia and the therapist's professional knowledge of language and communication. The unique interaction between carers and people with dementia, their history and their needs, drives the partnership approach to intervention.

COMMUNICATION AND DEMENTIA

In dementia, communication can be compromised by a breakdown in language processing, a breakdown in motor speech production, or a breakdown in other cognitive processes. Particular constellations of deficits have been associated with different forms of dementia (e.g. Hodges et al 1991; Randolf et al, 1993; Snowden, 1994), although it is important to recognise that there is a huge amount of variability within diagnostic categories which group studies may obscure (Perkins et al, 1996).

Communication deficits

Breakdown in language processing

Considerable research has been undertaken to examine how language processing breaks down in dementia, with the bulk of work in this area focused on dementia of the Alzheimer type. Areas that have been addressed include semantics (meaning), syntax (grammar), phonology (the sound system) and pragmatics (use of language in context).

Breakdown of semantic processing has been reported as a feature of dementia of the Alzheimer type (e.g. Chertkow and Bub, 1990), dementia with Lewy bodies (Perkins et al, 1996) and multi-infarct dementia (e.g. Fischer et al, 1988), and it is the cardinal feature of semantic dementia (Snowden et al, 1989) in which there is selective impairment of semantic memory with relative sparing of other components of cognitive function. The consequences of a semantic impairment include word-finding impairments, with either inability to find the word or incorrect selection of a word that is similar in meaning to the target (e.g. 'cat' for 'dog'), difficulty in defining words, and comprehension difficulties, with particular confusion between words that are similar in meaning. In contrast to semantic processing, syntactic and phonological processes appear to be relatively well preserved for both comprehension and production in dementia of the Alzheimer type until later in the disease process (Whitaker, 1976; Schwartz et al, 1979; Appell et al, 1982; Kempler et al, 1987).

Pragmatic ability has been researched through analysis of the ability of the person with dementia to produce different forms of discourse, including picture description, story-telling, procedural discourse and conversation. Since all of these different types of discourse require very different skills and researchers have addressed a wide range of different discourse features, it is difficult to summarise research in this area concisely. Ehrlich (1995) suggests that the discourse of people with dementia of the Alzheimer type

> ...*may be marked by fewer substantives, more circumlocutions and digressions from the topic. This profile of 'empty' speech in discourse is also characteristically egocentric and concrete with ideational perseverations, and either excessive speech or little or no speech in later stages. (p. 151)*

Discourse ability is not an independent language process but is dependent on other linguistic and cognitive processes. Breakdown in these areas will clearly have implications for the person's ability to produce discourse. Recent work has also recognised the importance of understanding discourse abilities not as solely attributable to the deficits of the person with dementia but also in terms of the interactions in which they are displayed, since the communication partner can greatly influence the ability of the person with dementia to produce discourse (Sabat, 1991; Ramanathan-Abbott, 1994; Ramanathan, 1997).

Breakdown in motor speech production

Some forms of dementia are associated with impairments in the mechanics of speech production which can severely compromise communication. Neuromuscular weakness and impaired neuromuscular control can result in dysarthric speech characterised by poor articulation and impaired control of volume and prosody (i.e. those aspects of speech conveyed by variation in pitch, loudness and duration, such as intonation). Dysarthria, which refers to a group of speech disorders resulting from impaired control and flexibility of the speech apparatus, is a primary feature of Parkinson's disease (which can occur in association with dementia with Lewy bodies and Alzheimer's disease) and Huntington's chorea. It also frequently occurs in multi-infarct dementia and in the later stages of dementia of the Alzheimer type.

Breakdown in other cognitive processes

Although other cognitive deficits in different forms of dementia, for example, psychotic symptoms and deficits in memory and attention, are well documented (Hart and Semple, 1990), there has been little work on the impact of these deficits on communication. Bayles and Kaszniak (1987) stress that in dementia the ability to communicate is affected by more than just the speech and language deficits. They propose that communication is impaired because ideation (the formation of ideas) is impaired as a consequence of memory deficits. In order to understand the impact of dementia on communication, further research is required to explore the relationship between communication breakdown and coexisting cognitive deficits.

The impact of the environment on communication breakdown

Lubinski (1991) has proposed that in addition to the changes in cognition, emotion and communication seen in dementia, learned behaviours may also arise as a consequence of the perceptions or beliefs of others. In particular, a commonly held perception of incompetence associated with dementia will influence the social and communication opportunities available to the person with dementia. Lubinski (1991) proposes that learned helplessness and a cycle of incompetence can be triggered by the diagnosis of dementia. Learned helplessness occurs when people believe that events and outcomes are independent of their actions and that any further action is futile. The stereotyping of helplessness in dementia by caregivers may lead to overgeneralisation of incompetency, thus restricting the opportunity to demonstrate intact skills and promoting dependency. Carers in the environment do not expect the person to perform with competence and may give feedback concerning both actual and potential failure. Such a perception will be influenced by the carer's own reactions and difficulties in coping and may be reflected in such behaviours as reducing social outings or visitors to the home, assuming the role of main communicator, or not informing the person with dementia of relevant daily affairs. Similarly, the structure of the environment, which may be highly controlled, sends cues to people with dementia that they are no longer expected to behave or interact competently. An example of this may be seen in seating a person with dementia in front of the television, away from the area of main family activity. Together, these social and environmental cues help set up minimal expectancies in people with dementia from both themselves and significant others in the environment. Skills cannot be maintained when there are reduced opportunities to perform them. This reduction in demonstration of skills reinforces the stereotype of helplessness and so the cycle of incompetence is maintained.

Communication plays a key role in the learned helplessness cycle. It is a primary tool through which the competency of people with dementia is both judged and reflected back to them (Fig. 6.1).

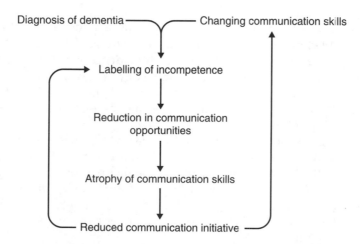

Figure 6.1   Cycle of incompetence as applied to communication. Adapted from Lubinski (1991).

The impact of communication breakdown on people with dementia and their carers

For the population with communication impairments, the compromised ability to engage in social life results, from a psychosocial perspective, in a handicap that is acutely experienced in virtually every aspect of daily living (Kagan and Gailey, 1993). As the mechanisms for maintaining their relationship are systematically eroded, communication impairment has consequences for both the person with dementia and the carer. Given the many facets to communication breakdown in dementia explored above, identifying the source of these and then maintaining effective communication between people with dementia and their carers, both family and professional, is regarded as central when working with this population.

The absence of positive communication is both well-documented and far-reaching in its implications. In a survey of family members caring for people with dementia of the Alzheimer type (Orange, 1991), almost half of the respondents noted a change in their relationship with the person with dementia as a direct result of their relative's communication problems, reporting feelings of frustration, loneliness, guilt, embarrassment and social isolation. A reduction in the quality of life for all involved is clearly present and often reflected in high levels of stress within the family. Increased carer stress as a direct result of communication problems experienced with people with dementia has been extensively reported (Rabins, 1982; Poulshock and Deimling, 1984; Kinney and Stephens, 1989; Rau, 1991; Stephens et al, 1991). Unfortunately, however, it is still unclear which aspects of the breakdown in communication have the most impact on families, as this information is often grouped together with other measures and is not investigated in greater depth (Ripich and Ziol, 1996). Muir (1996) does, however, report research evidence which suggests that 'the loss of meaningful interactive and conversational skills is more distressing to carers than the developing of behaviours upon which many professionals focus their attention, e.g. "aggression", wandering and incontinence' (p. 222).

Maintaining people with dementia in their own homes is often closely linked to communication patterns with family carers. Sanford (1975) followed up 50 admissions of patients whose relatives or friends could no longer cope with them at home. The person principally involved with home support was interviewed and causes of inability to cope were identified. Only 50% of the sample could accept the inability of their relative to communicate.

The quality of care received by people with dementia from professional carers may also be influenced by their communicative effectiveness. Ekman et al (1994) reported that in a geriatric clinic, nursing staff spent less time on care activities with people with dementia than with non-demented patients with the same degree of dependence. In a follow-up interview study (Ekman et al, 1994), 50% of the nursing staff reported that they spent less time because they did not have to communicate with patients with dementia. These staff also reported that they never or very seldom spent time just talking with patients with dementia. Sixteen of the 21 professional carers interviewed described mostly negative reactions to patients with dementia when they had concomitant communication disorders. Comments included: 'When you cannot get into contact with the patient you feel insufficient, without hope, dissatisfied or burned out. Care seems meaningless. You lose your commitment.' (p. 169). The findings of this study suggest that poor communication influences commitment to that individual and, subsequently, commitment to the quality of care to that individual (Ekman et al, 1994).

Involving carers in the management of communication in dementia

The value of involving carers in the management of their relatives with dementia is undisputed, providing the basis for one of the key approaches used by speech and language therapists in addressing communication breakdown. As highlighted by Muir (1996), management approaches that involve carers have a number of facets, including assessment incorporating the carer, provision of information, support counselling, advice and education.

Assessment using information provided by the carer can provide wide-ranging information on real-life communication which is not picked up by direct assessment of the person with dementia. Muir (1996) proposed that involving carers in assessment can help the identification of strengths and preserved skills as well as weaknesses and needs, thus providing a learning experience for the carer. Assessment of the carer's own attitudes and perceptions of the change in communication is also valuable in establishing a baseline for intervention. Morris (1996) reported several advantages in using spouses or close family members as informants of behavioural change. He suggested that spouses are sensitive to even mild impairment, provide more reliable reports of cognitive difficulties than the person with dementia, and have a level of premorbid knowledge against which to compare changes.

It is also important to acknowledge, however, that the carer may not always be the most accurate observer, as reported by Orange (1991):

> *Family members are influenced ... by a number of factors that may prejudice their perceptions of real communicative change ... They include, but are not limited to: (1) the many years of intimate contact that may limit objectivity; (2) the caregiver's understanding of what constitutes real change in functional communication skills; and (3) the subtle adjustments caregivers may make in their interactive style that anticipates and minimises the expression of communicative disturbances. (p. 169)*

Provision of information about the nature of the communication process and the ways in which communication can break down in dementia is also a key part of intervention with carers. Providing the carer with an understanding of the often bewildering changes observed in the relative can be a powerful tool in reducing anxiety and stress. Brodaty and Peters (1991) found that a 10-day intensive education and support programme with follow-up resulted in a reduction in carers' psychological stress and an increase in the time that patients remained living at home.

The provision of support and counselling for carers is also an important aspect of management to reduce stress. It is important for the carer to have the opportunity to talk with someone at a time when there is a deterioration in communication with the person who has often been their key conversational partner. As noted by Muir (1996), 'the emotional responses, anxiety and preoccupation of the carer are likely to further diminish communication with the sufferer, unless they are addressed' (p. 237). Support may be provided through involvement in a carers' support group which may also function to provide information. Alternatively, individual counselling may be offered either by the speech and language therapist or other key professionals working with the family (providing that they have the necessary skills), or by a professional counsellor.

Finally, advising carers on how to enhance communication with the person with dementia is an area of intervention which has received considerable attention by professionals working with this population.

Facilitating communication involves the development of strategies that the carer is advised to integrate into daily situations to avoid or manage difficulties in communication. Shulman and Mandel (1988) and Clark and Witte (1989) describe communication training of relatives and friends of older people living in institutional settings. The latter study stresses the importance of recognising that modification of lifelong patterns of verbal interactions are difficult to effect without emotional support and practical skills development training. A number of studies have reported the success of teaching strategies to professionals working with people with dementia. Post et al (1994) described the evaluation of a training programme for nursing-home staff working with people with Alzheimer's dementia (AD) and reported that 'educating these carers in communication skills enhances their control over the social interaction and increases their satisfaction with communicating with the AD-affected person' (p. 63).

The emphasis on training carers to enhance communication with the person with dementia is demonstrated by the numerous comprehensive lists of strategies reported by, for example, Bayles and Kaszniak (1987), Mace and Rabins (1987), Dodd et al (1990), Enderby (1990) and Orange (1991). The advice given may be of a non-linguistic nature, e.g. distracting the person with dementia by engaging in other activities or reducing conflicting stimuli. It may also include more linguistically specific strategies related to modifying the communication partner's language input. For example, advice may be given to use right-branching sentences rather than left-branching ones (i.e. put important information at the end of a sentence rather than at the beginning to reduce demands on memory), or to change open-ended questions to closed ones which only require 'yes' or 'no' as an answer.

A major limitation of existing lists of strategies is that they are in a generalised form and are not tailor-made for the individual. The same list of general strategies is therefore applied to a range of clients and communication partners who may experience very different difficulties in communication. This practice is contrary to the claim that any management programme must be individualised and based on a thorough assessment of the individual's difficulties and strengths (Woods, 1994). Maxim and Bryan (1996) state:

> Research is now taking us to the stage where we can describe different patterns of impaired and retained abilities which suggest that different dementias and stages of dementia require different types of advice to carers. (p. 38)

While supporting the notion that the population with dementia is heterogeneous and requires differential advice, however, it is suggested here that it is not enough to direct advice on the basis of the diagnosis and the stage of the disease with which the person with dementia has been labelled. Instead, advice needs to be individualised. This is because, even within groups of people with the same diagnosis and severity of disease, the exact pattern of cognitive impairment can vary greatly. In addition, the diagnosis and severity do not provide information about the communicative environment of the person with dementia which, as discussed above, makes a significant contribution to the extent of communication maintenance or breakdown. Post et al (1994) state:

> The experience of dementia must be appreciated in the words of the AD-affected individual rather than in the words of the professional or through the filter of theories about the stages of dementia. The person evolves through the disease, not in a linear way but in a way that leads to different experiences and different needs for communication techniques as the process unfolds.
> (p. 62)

There is increasing recognition of the benefits of an individualised approach to management (e.g. Orange et al, 1995; Muir, 1996). Three issues relating to this are highlighted below.

Recognition of the spontaneous development of strategies by carers

Carers do spontaneously accommodate their communication when talking with people with dementia. This may take the form of a reduction in semantic and syntactic complexity and increased stress on salient items. This has been shown by Kemper et al (1994), who found that carers spontaneously used these strategies to facilitate the performance of their spouses with probable Alzheimer's dementia on a communication task. However, carers may not be aware of their behaviour and may therefore be inconsistent in their strategy usage, reducing its efficacy (Tanner and Daniels, 1990). How such strategies differ between individual dyads has not yet been studied in detail. Teaching of general strategies does not, however, take into account the knowledge and skill that the communication partner may have already developed.

Valuing the existing knowledge and skill of the carers empowers them, facilitating a proactive role in intervention which builds on the information that they have provided. Orange (1991), who has conducted a comprehensive study of strategies used by carers, also stresses the value of including family members' observations. Furthermore, Perkins (1995a) has shown that in conversations with people with aphasia, different conversational partners may develop different strategies with the same person with aphasia, reinforcing the importance of engaging the carer in planning intervention. An individualised approach allows the knowledge and skill of carers to be fully utilised. It allows intervention to be client-led, driven by the issues important to the person with dementia and the carer rather than by the preconceptions of the professional.

Recognition of a range of communication problems

The use of a general list of communication strategies fails also to attend to the wide range of problems other than language which can affect communication. Other behavioural changes that may arise in dementia – for example, deficits in memory and attention or psychotic symptoms – need also to be considered with respect to their impact on communication. Owing to the often central nature of such features to the communication impairment, it is necessary to address the relationship between other presenting cognitive problems and the interaction that takes place between the communication partners involved. This highlights the need to liaise with other professional groups, such as psychiatrists, psychologists and day-centre staff. There is a need to consider all sources of interactional difficulties rather than focusing on only those arising from overt linguistic impairments.

Evaluation of strategies

To date, virtually no empirical data about the effects of modifying variables in communication with people with dementia have been reported (Bayles and Kaszniak, 1987). The current procedure of providing non-individualised strategies does not permit such evaluation. Studies that have shown the effectiveness of carer training (e.g. Shulman and Mandel, 1988; Post et al, 1994) have used increased knowledge of the carer and reduced carer stress as outcome measures (or indicators) rather than evaluation of change in communication between the person with dementia and the carer. An individualised approach should facilitate evaluation of training in strategy development, since it will result in appropriate targeting of strategies. Comparison of their use in communication before and after the intervention should then provide a relevant measure of the outcome of the intervention.

This review of current practice in working with carers highlights the need for a methodology that will assist in maintaining effective communication between people with dementia and their key communication partners, and one that works closely with those involved to identify effective strategies. An individualised approach is required, which can recognise the range of possible communication problems, the spontaneous development of strategies by carers, and the need for careful evaluation of those strategies.

WORKING IN PARTNERSHIP WITH CARERS

The importance of working closely with carers, both as informants of communication difficulties and active participants in facilitating effective

communication, is paramount. The assessm
dementia should be shared between three pe
dementia, the carer and the professional – in thi.
language therapist. Whilst the first two contribute i
the interaction that takes place within the family, the .
therapist's experience in interpreting information on
the light of family subjectivity is a necessary elemen
involvement of the carer in planning and participating in
and use of strategies is also a pivotal aspect of a partnershi,
carer's initial and continuing participation in any interv.
given the carer's integral role and the commitment required
is to be effected.

The authors of this chapter have developed a partnershi
designed both to characterise the interaction taking place be
person with dementia and the carer, and to implement strate
interventions, based on a method of analysing conversation
approach looks directly at the interaction between the partners, as of
to the deficits only of the person with dementia, and works closely
those involved to identify effective strategies, being client-led rather
clinician-led. It is an individualised approach, which recognises the rar
of communication problems that can arise, the spontaneous developme
of strategies by carers and the need for careful evaluation of those
strategies. The assessment tool used in the approach, the Conversation
Analysis Profile for People with Cognitive Impairment (CAPPCI) (Perkins
et al, 1997), was developed as a resource for speech and language
therapists for use with people with generalised cognitive impairment, as in
dementia, and their key communication partners or family carers.

Conversation analysis profile for people with cognitive impairment

The specific objectives of the CAPPCI are:

- To determine the carer's perception of the current conversational abilities of the person with dementia
- To determine the strategies being employed in interaction and their success
- To assess change from premorbid styles and opportunities of interaction
- To capture the relationship between the carer's perceptions and what actually occurs in a sample of conversation.

ation analysis was selected as the framework for the CAPPCI on
sis of a number of features which are valuable to the assessment
ordered interaction (Lesser and Milroy, 1993). These are discussed

use of everyday conversation

nversation analysis uses everyday conversation as data which provides
analysis with high validity, since it is everyday conversation with
rers that is ultimately the target of intervention. It also looks directly at
e interaction between the person with dementia and the carer, not at
rtificially construed communication such as would commonly occur
between the person with dementia and the professional in a clinical
situation. The use of everyday conversation also allows the social role of
language to be addressed.

The joint responsibility of both conversational partners

Conversation analysis focuses on conversation as a collaborative
achievement (Schegloff, 1982) thus stressing successful communication as
the joint responsibility of both conversational partners. This emphasis
demonstrates that interaction is more than the addition of the two
partners' contributions; an essential component is the collaborative
construction of the discourse. Ramanathan-Abbott (1994) describes how
the narrative ability of a woman with dementia of the Alzheimer type
differed greatly with two different conversational partners, demonstrating
that the ability of the person with dementia to produce extended and
meaningful speech is, in part, interactionally produced.

A data-driven approach

Conversation analysis is a data-driven approach, emphasising the
description of observable behaviour and seeking evidence of communicative success or failure from the sequential context, i.e. the responses of
the conversational partners. This approach permits the therapist to move
away from prescriptive judgments of appropriacy based on subjective
judgments of what is normal. As highlighted by Jane Crisp in Chapter 5
with respect to 'accuracy', the person with cognitive impairment does not
have 'normal' interactional resources, but deviation from what is normal
does not necessarily equate with failure or communicative ineffectiveness
(Perkins, 1995a, b). It is important to value the interactional strengths that
exist between the person with dementia and their carer rather than
focusing only on deficit and loss of abilities.

A minimally obtrusive assessment tool

The use of everyday conversation as the data for conversation analysis provides a minimally obtrusive assessment tool. It makes few demands on the person with dementia and it can therefore be used for people who are not able to cooperate with formal assessment.

The CAPPCI comprises an interview conducted with the carer, and an analysis of a sample of conversation between the carer and the person with dementia. These combine to provide an overall profile of the interaction between the person with dementia and the carer, from which intervention can proceed. The interview seeks to elicit information from the carer about the current conversational abilities of the person with dementia. It solicits information on the conversational management procedures of initiation, turn-taking, topic management and repair, as well as examining the impact of speech, linguistic and other cognitive impairments on the interaction. For each question, the conversational partner is asked to indicate the frequency with which a behaviour occurs. If the frequency meets the criterion of potentially differing from what would be expected in normal conversational management, three further probes are provided to elicit information about the strategies used to manage the behaviour, the response to or outcome of the strategies, and how much the informant considers the behaviour to be a problem.

The interview also elicits information on premorbid and current interactional styles and opportunities, enabling a comparison to be made between the two periods. Such information includes communicative style; people with whom the subject communicates; situations in which communication takes place; topics of conversation; non-verbal communication skills; and hearing status. With the onset of communication impairment, opportunities for interaction are often reduced (Lubinski, 1991; Kagan and Gailey, 1993), an important factor to consider in the analysis of the handicap resulting from dementia. Knowledge of premorbid styles is also important to understand the change that has taken place in communication and to ensure the suitability of treatment goals (Green, 1984).

Complementing the interview is a sample of conversation recorded between the person with dementia and the carer at home. Around 10 minutes of the conversation are transcribed and a conversation analysis is undertaken to look for evidence of the behaviour, the subsequent conversational management and the strategies reported by the carer during the interview. This allows an evaluation of the accuracy of the carer's perceptions as well as providing an opportunity to observe strategies not reported by the carer.

Finally, a summary profile collates information from all parts of the CAPPCI and provides both a starting point for collaborative intervention and a baseline from which any subsequent change can be measured.

Components of intervention based on the CAPPCI

The CAPPCI allows exploration of a number of key issues which can directly inform the intervention process and which embody the principle of partnership between the person with dementia and the carer.

Identification of current conversational management

Both intact ability and impairment of conversational management between the person with dementia and the carer are captured, first, by the carer's rating of the frequency of a behaviour and, second, in the analysis of the conversational sample. Comparison of the findings of the conversation analysis to the carer's frequency rating can indicate whether or not the carer has a realistic picture of the conversational abilities of the person with dementia, providing important information for establishing the starting point of intervention. It is from this information that the therapist may draw conclusions about whether the carer may be overestimating or underestimating the person's abilities. If overestimation of abilities gives rise to breakdown in conversation, stemming from poor understanding of the cognitive changes that have taken place in the person with dementia, education may be necessary. If underestimation of abilities is occurring, this may be promoting a learned helplessness cycle, and discussion to promote a more accurate and positive perception of the person's interactional abilities may be helpful.

The carer's perception of the problem

The interview also establishes a rating of problem severity for all impaired behaviours. The relationship between this rating and that for frequency requires careful interpretation. The problem severity rating will be influenced by the strategies upon which the carer draws. For example, where a carer has developed successful strategies, a particular aspect of impaired conversational management may not be perceived as a problem. The problem severity rating may also indicate the level of acceptance that the carer has reached. A high problem severity rating may be indicative of a lack of acceptance, which the therapist may wish to address in management. A low problem severity rating may reflect that the carer has accepted the cognitive changes. In the piloting of the CAPPCI, a common report was that a behaviour that had been a major problem in the past was no longer a problem because the carer had learned to accept it. Although this may be considered a positive feature from a management perspective, it is important to consider whether, as a consequence, the carer is underestimating the person's abilities which may, once again, be feeding into a learned helplessness cycle.

The carer's strategies

The carer's strategies and their outcomes will have a large impact on the maintenance of successful interaction. Qualitative information about strategies is elicited in the interview and also identified from the analysis of the sample of conversation. The conversation analysis permits validation of the carer's report and allows exploration of how the person with dementia responds to the strategies employed. The conversation analysis may also identify strategies that the conversational partner uses but has not reported.

In participating in the interview, the carer's awareness is heightened of positive steps that the carer is already undertaking to deal with difficulties. The therapist, in management, can positively reinforce productive strategies. In certain instances no further intervention may be warranted. In areas where strategy use is not found to be successful, the therapist and carer can work together to identify possible alternative approaches.

Comparison of premorbid and current interactional styles and opportunities

The CAPPCI also provides information on the change in interactional styles and opportunities of the person with dementia. It provides the therapist, first, with a wider picture within which to interpret the findings of the analysis of current conversational abilities. For example, lack of initiation in conversation will differ in significance between someone who premorbidly had a quiet, passive interactional style and someone who had a talkative, dominant style. Second, it allows assessment of the degree of change with which the carer has to deal. Analysis of change in interactional opportunities (people, situations and topics) has management implications in considering possible modification of the interactional environment.

In summary, the CAPPCI is designed to provide accurate information on the specific conversational strengths and weaknesses of the person with dementia, the carer's knowledge and perception of these, and the strategies already being employed by the conversationalists. This provides a basis for the therapist to develop rationally motivated intervention which is client-led and incorporates both the knowledge and skills already developed by the carer and the communication strengths of the person with dementia.

The following case study describes the findings of the CAPPCI for a man with dementia and his wife, and the implications of these findings are discussed in relation to a partnership approach to intervention.

Case study

Background information

Mr L is a 67-year-old man who has a 2-year history of cognitive impairment and a 15-year history of Parkinson's disease. Mr L's impaired cognitive abilities have been putatively diagnosed as resulting from cortical damage associated with Lewy bodies. He lives at home with his wife. He has received speech and language therapy services, with the more recent focus of intervention being on improving intelligibility, in particular volume control, associated with the Parkinson's disease.

A pilot version of the CAPPCI interview was conducted with Mr L's wife and a conversation analysis undertaken on a sample of conversation between Mr and Mrs L recorded at home.

Identification of current conversational management

The ratings given by Mrs L for each of the areas of conversational management are shown in Figure 6.2. A range of impairments in conversational management were identified in the interview with Mrs L. High levels of manifestations of memory, linguistic and articulation and prosodic impairments were reported in conversation. Mrs L also reported impaired turn-taking with failure to respond when spoken to, delayed responding and reliance on minimal turns to participate in conversation (i.e. short turns which do not contribute further content to the conversation, e.g. 'mmm ...' 'yes'). On the positive side, she reported that he retained the ability to initiate conversation and showed awareness of the need not to interrupt other people when they were speaking. In relation to topic management, Mrs L reported that her husband was able to introduce new topics and maintain topics. He did, however, fail to orient

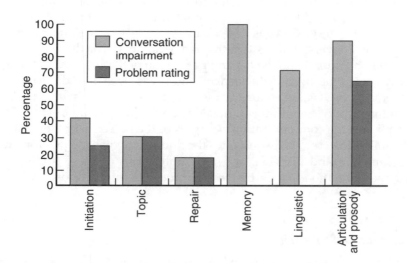

Figure 6.2 Profile of current conversational abilities for Mr L.

others to new topics that he introduced and he repeatedly introduced the same 'favourite' topics. She also reported the occurrence of topics based on hallucinations. Ability to handle repair in conversation (i.e. to clarify when difficulties of understanding or hearing arose) was reported as relatively preserved, although it was reported that Mr L was sometimes unable to clarify his own turn successfully when asked to do so.

Carer's strategy use

Mrs L was able to identify a large number of strategies to manage the problems that she and her husband face in conversation and to describe the outcome of these strategies. Confirmation of these strategies was obtained from the conversation analysis and further strategies which Mrs L had not reported were also identified. Examples of the strategies used are given in Table 6.1. These strategies relate to Mr L's failure to respond during conversation reported in the interview and noted in the conversation.

Table 6.1 *Strategies reported and observed to deal with failures to respond in conversation*

Strategy	Outcome
Strategies reported in interview When Mr L fails to respond, Mrs L: 1. repeats comment or question 2. rephrases 3. backtracks	Usually Mr L responds but sometimes Mrs L has to give up
Strategies identified from conversation analysis When Mr L fails to respond, Mrs L: 1. rephrases question, changing from an open to a closed question 2. provides more information 3. changes direction of the conversation 4. waits and allows more time 5. cues with a word 6. repeats the question	Mr L responded following all strategies

Carer's perception of problems

The problem severity rating of the changes in Mr L's communication (Fig. 6.2) showed that there was no one-to-one link between the level of conversational impairment and the problem rating. Thus, although memory and linguistic abilities were highly impaired, these deficits were not perceived as a problem by Mrs L. This can be accounted for by the large number of successful strategies that she reported for this area. In contrast, the area of articulation and prosody was considered to be a more severe problem; although Mrs L was able to report a number of strategies for this area, they were not deemed to be successful. Impaired conversational management in turn-taking, topic management and repair were all considered to be a problem by Mrs L. The strategies reported by her for these areas were seen as having variable success. The conversation analysis, however, revealed that Mrs L had a larger range of strategies than those that she had reported and often these were successful in maintaining a supportive interaction.

Changes from premorbid interactional style and opportunities

Exploration of the changes undergone in Mr L's interactional styles and opportunities since the onset of his communication difficulties (Fig. 6.3) revealed that his communicative style, the people with whom Mr L now communicated and the situations in which he now communicated were maximally affected, with a moderate reduction seen in the range of topics used by Mr L.

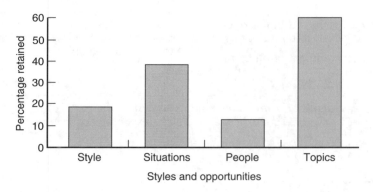

Figure 6.3 Profile of retained interactional styles and opportunities for Mr L.

Implications from the CAPPCI for intervention

Many implications for interventions arise from these findings. Completion of the CAPPCI interview offered Mrs L an opportunity to discuss in detail her experience and feelings in relation to the changes in communication with her husband. Mrs L was able to demonstrate her awareness, during the interview, of a large number of strategies that she spontaneously employed. The conversational data both supported her reports and identified further strategies that were not reported.

Through discussion of the range of strategies employed and their often differing outcomes, Mrs L can be made more aware of how she may engage different strategies at different times. For example, in managing Mr L's difficulties with topic, Mrs L at times used a confrontational approach ('What are you talking about?'), while also employing a strategy of listening patiently on those occasions when Mr L repeated topics. As the outcomes of these strategies were different, Mrs L's attention could be drawn to this with a view to managing the conversation differently at different times. By providing specific evidence through the conversational data, the therapist has a data-driven base from which to demonstrate the different and/or additional strategies. There were also instances noted when a behaviour was still rated as a problem despite an apparently successful strategy. For example, in the case of Mr L's hallucinations, Mrs L referred to this as Mr L's 'dreaming', to which Mr L responded with laughter and agreement. Whilst such a strategy did not aim to reduce the behaviour, Mr L was not threatened by this approach to a potentially distressing topic and conversation was able to continue both about and around it. This may warrant further discussion to explore why Mrs L rated the behaviour as a problem of some concern for her.

Use of the CAPPCI also provided evidence as to which area of intervention should be given priority. While memory deficits were a major component of Mr L's dementia and clearly affected conversations between him and his wife, they were not regarded as a problem by Mrs L, a factor no doubt related to her employment of successful strategies. Consequently, with the exception of reinforcing existing strategies, memory deficits are unlikely to take a major focus in intervention. In contrast, Mr L's poor intelligibility represented a considerable problem for Mrs L and her husband, despite the extent of speech and language therapy input that he had received. Conversational evidence, however, revealed the successful employment of strategies by Mrs L that she had not reported, for example, requests for repetition that allowed Mrs L to interpret his second attempts. Discussion between Mr L, Mrs L and the therapist will determine the extent to which impaired speech will be the focus of intervention. Such discussion would benefit from attention being drawn to the positive strategies that were being employed in conversation. This may help to reduce the degree to which the speech impairment is considered a problem.

The level of agreement between Mrs L's reporting and the conversational evidence also has implications for management. First, her awareness and current management (where successful) should be reinforced, and, second, areas of conflict should be discussed with a view to exploring further possibilities. For example, Mrs L reported that her husband did not have difficulties initiating repairs on his own errors, but the conversational sample showed that he did. This could be drawn to Mrs L's attention with explicit examples.

Changes were noted between Mr L's premorbid and current interactional styles and opportunities. Even though Mr L was still able to talk about many of the topics in which he engaged before the onset of cognitive impairment, his increased social isolation shifted the focus of his interaction primarily to his wife, potentially placing greater stresses on both of them. Discussion of these factors with Mrs L would ensure that she had an understanding of the changes that had occurred and their implications for both Mr L and herself, and would potentially lead to constructive outcomes such as identifying other services in the community or key personnel who might enable Mr L's interactional opportunities to be expanded.

In addition to driving intervention, the CAPPCI permits quantification of a number of facets of intervention. It therefore forms a basis for evaluating the efficacy of working with Mr and Mrs L.

CONCLUSION

This chapter has advocated an approach to the management of communication in dementia that stresses the need for individualised assessment. It has outlined a method that can facilitate this through the medium of conversation analysis. This contributes to a partnership approach to intervention which draws upon the knowledge and skills of the person with dementia, the carer, and the speech and language therapist. It is anticipated that the CAPPCI will facilitate research into a number of areas important to the development of effective communication intervention with people with dementia and their carers. Three potential areas include firstly, the effectiveness of interventions for changing interaction; secondly, longitudinal studies of the change in conversational management with the progression of dementia; and thirdly, the insight and views of the person with dementia into changes in communication.

In relation to the first area, Rau (1991) has highlighted the lack of objective data supporting the effectiveness of communication-focused interventions with carers. It has been suggested in this chapter that this deficiency arises partly from the lack of a methodology to investigate changes. The CAPPCI has the potential to address this issue by comparison of both interaction and carers' perceptions of interaction before and after intervention. Further research is required to investigate the effectiveness of an individualised approach to intervention. Secondly, while a number of research studies have explored the longitudinal changes in linguistic and cognitive functioning with the progression of dementia, to date there is limited information on the changes in conversational management over time – see Hamilton (1994) for an exception. Exploration of this area should provide insight into how support and advice can best be provided to accommodate the cognitive changes faced by the person with dementia and the carer. Thirdly, because of the cognitive changes in dementia, it is frequently assumed that people with dementia are unable to take an active part in their own management. Rau (1991) suggested that information about how people who carry a diagnosis of early dementia feel about themselves and how they perceive others' reactions to them could be extremely useful in carer education. Use of an allied assessment for people with aphasia, Conversation Analysis Profile for People with Aphasia (Whitworth et al, 1997) has successfully been used with people with aphasia as well as with their carers. Investigation of the use of the CAPPCI interview with people with mild dementia is warranted. Should the CAPPCI prove to be a constructive method of collecting information from people with dementia, this has important implications for empowering them to take a more proactive role in their own management.

Acknowledgements

This work was supported by grants received from the Parkinson's Disease Society (U.K.) and the Nuffield Foundation. Many thanks are extended to the patients and carers who contributed to these projects.

REFERENCES

Appell, J., Kertesz, A. & Fisman, M. (1982) A study of language functioning in Alzheimer's patients. *Brain and Language* 17, 73–91.

Bayles, K. & Kaszniak, A. (1987) *Communication and Cognition in Normal Aging and Dementia.* Boston: College Hill.

Brodaty, H. & Peters, K.E. (1991) Cost effectiveness of a training program for dementia carers. *International Psychogeriatrics* 3, 11–23.

Chertkow, H. & Bub, D. (1990) Semantic memory loss in dementia of Alzheimer's type. What do various measures measure? *Brain* 113, 397–417

Clark, L.W. & Witte, K. (1989) Dealing with dementia in long term care. Mini seminar presentation for annual Convention of New York State Speech, Language, Hearing Association, Kiameshi Lake, NY, cited in Clark, L.W. (1995) Interventions for persons with Alzheimer's disease: strategies for maintaining and enhancing communicative success. *Topics in Language Disorders* 15, 47–65.

Dodd, B., Worrall, L. & Hickson, L. (1990) *Communication: A Guide for Residential Care Staff.* Canberra: Australian Government Publishing Service.

Ehrlich, J.S. (1995) Studies of discourse production in adults with Alzheimer's disease. In: Bloom, R.L., Obler, L.K., De Santi, S., & Ehrlich, J.S. (eds) *Discourse Analysis and Applications: Studies in Adult Clinical Populations.* Hillsdale: LEA.

Ekman, S.L., Norberg, A., Viitanen, M. & Winblad, B. (1994) Care of demented patients with severe communication problems. *Scandinavian Journal of Caring Sciences* 5, 163–170.

Enderby, P. (1990) Promoting communication in patients with dementia. In: Stokes, G. & Goudie, F, (eds) *Working with Dementia.* Bicester: Winslow Press.

Fischer, P., Gatterer, G., Marterer, G. & Danielczyk, W. (1988) Non specificity of semantic impairment in dementia of the Alzheimer's type. *Archives of Neurology* 45, 1341–1343.

Green, G. (1984) Communication in aphasia therapy: some of the procedures and issues involved. *British Journal of Disorders of Communication* **19**, 35–46.

Hamilton, H.E. (1994) *Conversations with an Alzheimer's Patient*. Cambridge: CUP.

Hart, S. & Semple, J.M. (1990) *Neuropsychology and the Dementias*. London: Taylor-Francis.

Hodges, J.R., Salmon, D.P. & Butters, N. (1991) The nature of the naming deficit in Alzheimer's and Huntington's disease. *Brain* **114**, 1547–1559.

Kagan, A. & Gailey, G.F. (1993) Functional is not enough: training conversation partners for aphasic adults. In: Holland, A.L. & Forbes M.M. (eds) *Aphasia Treatment: World Perspectives*. London: Chapman & Hall.

Kemper, S., Anagnopoulos, C., Lyons, K. & Heberlein, W. (1994) Speech accommodations to dementia. *Journal of Gerontology* **49**, 223–229.

Kempler, D., Curtiss, S. & Jackson, C. (1987) Syntactic preservation in Alzheimer's disease. *Journal of Speech and Hearing Research* **30**, 343–350.

Kinney, J.M. & Stephens, M.A. (1989) Care giving hassles scale: assessing the daily hassles of caring for a family member with dementia. *Gerontologist* **29**, 328–332.

Lesser, R. & Milroy, L. (1993) *Linguistics and Aphasia: Psycholinguistic and Pragmatic Aspects of Intervention*. London: Longman.

Lubinski, R. (1991) Learned helplessness: application to communication of the elderly. In: Lubinski, R. (ed.) *Dementia and Communication*. Philadelphia: BC Decker.

Mace, N. & Rabins, P. (1987) *The Thirty-Six Hour Day*. Baltimore: Johns Hopkins University Press.

Maxim, J. & Bryan, K. (1996) Language, cognition and communication in the older mentally infirm. In: Bryan, K. & Maxim, J. (eds) *Communication Disability and the Psychiatry of Old Age*. London: Whurr.

Morris, J. (1996) Plenary session on neuroimaging, neuropsychology and neuropathology. Lancet Conference: *The Challenge of the Dementias: Towards a Better Understanding of Cognitive Impairment*, Edinburgh.

Muir, N. (1996) Management approaches involving carers. In: Bryan, K, & Maxim, J. (eds) *Communication Disability and the Psychiatry of Old Age*. London: Whurr.

Orange, J.B. (1991) Perspectives of family members regarding communication changes. In: Lubinski, R. (eds) *Dementia and Communication*. Philadelphia: BC Decker.

Orange, J.B., Ryan, E.B., Meredith, S.D. & Maclean, M.J. (1995) Application of the communication enhancement model for long-term care residents with Alzheimer's disease. *Topics in Language Disorder* **15**, 20–35.

Perkins, L. (1995a) Applying conversation analysis to aphasia: clinical implications and analytic issues. *European Journal of Disorders of Communication* **30**, 372–383.

Perkins, L. (1995b) An exploration of the impact of psycholinguistic impairments on conversational ability in aphasia. *International Journal of Psycholinguistics* **11**, 167–188.

Perkins, L., Lesser, R. & McKeith, I. (1996) Language as a possible diagnostic medium for dementia with Lewy bodies (poster presentation). Lancet Conference: *The Challenge of the Dementias Towards a Better Understanding of Cognitive Impairment*, Edinburgh.

Perkins, L., Whitworth, A. & Lesser, R. (1997) *Conversation Analysis Profile for People with Cognitive Impairments (CAPPCI)*. London: Whurr.

Post, S.G., Ripich, D.N. & Whitehouse, P.J. (1994) Discourse ethics: research, dementia and communication. *Alzheimer Disease and Associated Disorders* **8**, 58–65.

Poulshock, S.W. & Deimling, G.T. (1984) Families caring for elders in residence: issues in the management of burden. *Journal of Gerontology* **39**, 230–239.

Rabins, P.V. (1982) Management of irreversible dementia. *Psychomatics* **22**, 591–597.

Ramanathan, V. (1997) *Alzheimer Discourse: Some Sociolinguistic Dimensions*. London: Lawrence Erlbaum.

Ramanathan-Abbott, V. (1994) Interactional differences in Alzheimer's discourse: an examination of AD speech across two audiences. *Language in Society* **23**, 31–58.

Randolf, C., Braun, A.R. & Goldberg, T.E. (1993) Semantic fluency in Alzheimer's, Parkinson's and Huntington's disease: dissociation of storage and retrieval deficits. *Neuropsychology* **7**, 82–88.

Rau, M.T. (1991) *Impact on families*. In: Lubinski, R. (ed.) *Dementia and Communication*. Philadelphia: BC Decker.

Ripich, D. & Ziol, E. (1996) A survey of service provision to the cognitively impaired elderly in the USA. In: Bryan, K. & Maxim, J. (eds) *Communication Disability and the Psychiatry of Old Age*. London: Whurr.

Sabat, S. (1991) Turn-taking, turn-giving and Alzheimer's disease: a case study in conversation. *Georgetown Journal of Language and Linguistics* **2**, 161–175.

Sanford, J.R. (1975) Tolerance of debility in elderly dependants by supporters at home: its significance for hospital practice. *British Medical Journal* 3(5981), 471–473.

Schegloff, E.A. (1982) Discourse as an interactional achievement: some uses of 'uh huh' and other things that come between sentences. In: Tannen, D. (ed.) *Georgetown Roundtable on Language and Linguistics 93*. Georgetown: University Press.

Schwartz, M., Marin, O. & Saffran, E. (1979) Dissociations of language function: a case study. *Brain and Language* **7**, 277–306.

Shulman, K.I. & Mandel, E. (1988) Communication training of relatives and friends of institutionalised elderly patients. *Gerontologist* **28**, 797–798.

Snowden, J.S. (1994) Contribution to the differential diagnosis of dementias. I: Neuropsychology. *Reviews in Clinical Gerontology* **4**, 227–234.

Snowden, J.S., Goulding, P.J. & Neary, D. (1989) Semantic dementia: a form of circumscribed cerebral atrophy. *Behavioural Neurology* **2**, 258–271.

Stephens, M.A., Kinney, J.M. & Ogrocki, P.K. (1991) Stressors and well-being among caregivers to older adults with dementia: the in-home versus nursing home experience. *Gerontologist* **31**, 217–223.

Tanner, B.B. & Daniels, K.A. (1990) An observation study of communication between carers and their relatives with dementia. *Care of the Elderly* **2**, 247–250.

Whitaker, H.A. (1976) A case of isolation of the language function. In: Whitaker, H. & Whitaker, H.A. (eds) *Studies in Neurolinguistics II*. New York: Academic Press.

Whitworth, A., Perkins, L. & Lesser, R. (1997) *Conversation Analysis Profile for People with Aphasia (CAPPA)*. London: Whurr.

Woods, B. (1994) Management of memory impairment in older people with dementia. *International Review of Psychiatry* **6**, 153–161.

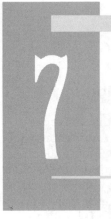

This is your life: research paradigms in dementia care

Kevin J. McKee

KEY ISSUES

- Much of the research on quality of care has examined the person with dementia only in relation to the care professional's presence or the family carer

- When describing the 'user's views', much research is limited to the views of the family carer rather than those of the true user, the person with dementia

- The concepts of 'quality of care' and 'quality of life' have been conflated, to the detriment of the person with dementia

- Residential and community care have been constructed as opposites, whereas they share many common features

- Future research on quality of care must examine the relationship between the person with dementia, the care professional and the family carer, and be sensitive to the influence of the care environment

- Future research on quality of life must address the nature of life for people with dementia over and above the quality of care received, and must provide a vehicle for the voice of the person with dementia to find expression

THIS IS MY LIFE (1)

Quality of care and staff–patient interaction

In July 1987, I took up a post as a research fellow at the University of Edinburgh. The project on which I was engaged was an examination of job satisfaction among nurses and the quality of care received by patients in psychogeriatric wards in Scottish hospitals. At the time, there was considerable discontent among nurses with regard to their working conditions, and to the limitations that a paucity of resources imposed upon the quality of care they could provide. Discontent was felt to be particularly rife within psychogeriatric nursing, perceived as the 'Cinderella' of the nursing profession.

I had recently graduated with a PhD in psychology. During the process of gaining my first and second degrees, the nearest I had come to old age or older people as a topic of study was during a brief introduction to the sociology of old age. In my PhD on the psychology of heart disease, I had occasionally interviewed men over 60 years old who had suffered a heart attack. My recruitment to the Edinburgh project was evidently not because of my intimate knowledge of mental health issues related to ageing and older people. During my BSc, such topics had been superficially mentioned within a course on clinical psychology, perhaps half a lecture buried within a 4-year degree. The project team felt that I was of potential value, partly because I was a psychologist (to balance the team's abundance of sociologists), and partly because my research training to date had provided me with skills relating to semistructured interviewing and questionnaire design and a knowledge of doctor–patient communication.

The Edinburgh project had two phases. The first phase has little relevance to this chapter, and was concerned with establishing the morale of nursing staff in psychogeriatric wards in Scottish hospitals (Gilloran et al, 1994). From this phase, hospitals were selected as fieldwork sites for the second phase of the project. Selection was made on the basis of ward morale profiles: hospitals with either uniformly high or uniformly low morale across all wards were of interest, as were hospitals whose constituent wards could be found at both the top and bottom of a morale 'league table'. The subject of this second phase was the quality of care that was delivered to psychogeriatric patients. It was thought that a difference between wards in terms of the quality of care delivered might be explained by differences in morale, amongst other variables. This, indeed, proved to be the case: job satisfaction and quality of care were found to be linked, with both influenced by the manner of ward and hospital management (Robertson et al, 1995).

The major task confronting the project team was the measurement of quality of care, a concept noted for the difficulty inherent in its definition.

In a paper published on the manner by which the project team set about measuring quality of care, Gilloran et al (1993) stress the overlap between the concepts of quality of care and quality of life for individuals in institutional settings. The authors then go on to describe the issue of quality of life measurement as 'like a dog's favourite slipper, well-chewed, continuously worried, yet remaining undefeated' (p. 269).

Quality of care was eventually measured as a result of a combination of different assessments. One assessment involved observational sweeps of the ward at 20-minute intervals. During these sweeps, the observer would establish the location and activity of each patient and each member of staff. On the basis of the data collected, the daily life of patients and staff could be constructed. Analysis of the data suggested a daily life consisting of large periods in which patient activity was minimal, combined with brief periods of frenetic staff–patient interaction, structured around key nursing tasks.

A second assessment concentrated on these tasks. Feeding, bathing and toileting of patients constituted the periods within which care delivery was most concentrated. After a comprehensive review of the literature and extensive discussion, the concept of quality care was disaggregated by the project team into six indicators: patient choice, information provision, promotion of independence, staff supervision, conversation and privacy. An operational definition for each indicator was agreed upon by the project team, so that during observational data collection each indicator could be scored as to its presence or absence when care was provided. Given the need for detailed observation of the care process, it was impossible to assess the care provided for every patient on the wards. A selection of six patients for observation from each ward was therefore made. All patients had been given a dependency rating, based upon the behaviour rating scale of the Clifton Assessment Procedures for the Elderly (CAPE) instrument (Pattie and Gilleard, 1979). Patients were selected for observation so as to represent a range of dependency scores, and matched for their scores across wards.

A third assessment concentrated on periods of unstructured time. The same six patients on each ward who were observed during feeding, bathing and toileting were also each observed for three periods of 20 minutes. The three periods were timed for mid-morning, mid-afternoon and mid-evening, respectively, when staff and patient activity was not structured by essential care processes. Observation of these periods concentrated on the interaction between staff and patients. Each minute, the observer recorded for a given patient the nature of any interaction with staff. Conversation was coded as to whether it contained a greeting, or instrumental, social or personal details. Touch was also noted, and its task or social function content. Finally, the initiator of the interaction, staff or patient, was noted. The analyses of these assessments have appeared in two publications to date (Gilloran et al, 1995; Robertson et al, 1995), and have been described in the project team's final report (McGlew et al, 1991).

THIS IS MY LIFE (2)

Family carers and the breakdown of care of people with dementia

Immediately after starting on the Edinburgh project, I was given a list of relevant literature I should track down and read. At the top of the list were classic studies of institutional life, such as those by Goffman (1961) and Wing and Brown (1970), and more recent studies specifically focusing on quality of life in residential homes, such as that by Hughes and Wilkin (1987). Another work at the top of the list was Chris Gilleard's *Living with Dementia* (Gilleard, 1984), a comprehensive examination of the family care of older people with dementia living in the community. The book provided me with an excellent working knowledge of dementia, its impact on the person with the condition, and on the caregiver of the person with dementia. *Living with Dementia* was the work that best prepared me for my first contact with individuals with dementia, and the extraordinary alterations the disease can manifest in the mental and physical life of a person. The work also acquainted me with the concept of 'caregiver'. The family caregiver is not a new phenomenon (e.g. Abel, 1994), but as Twigg (1992b) has pointed out, the concept of the 'caregiver' or 'carer' has a recent currency. Use of the term was virtually unknown in the UK in the 1970s but it is now ubiquitous in gerontological and health and social care research. *Living with Dementia* is a seminal work from a period in which the concept of a family carer came to be considered central to the world of the person with dementia. This was powered in a large part by the shift in emphasis during the 1980s and 1990s from institutional to community care for people with dementia.

It therefore felt as if I was adrift on the *Zeitgeist* when I took up a research post at the University of Dundee in July 1991, managing a project on factors associated with the maintenance and care of demented elderly people in the community. The study, funded by the Scottish Home and Health Department, emerged from concerns about the rising proportion of older people in the population, and the impact this demographic change would have on health-care costs and on the families caring for older people in the community. The study was particularly concerned with the additional economic and social burden that accrued when an older person had dementia over and above the other health frailties associated with later life.

The project was longitudinal in design. It examined the association between baseline variables (characteristics of the person with dementia and of the carer, service use, and carer perceptions) and subsequent institutionalisation during a 2-year follow-up period, concentrating on a group of people with dementia and their carers. This group was compared

with an age- and sex-matched group of older peop
and their carers.

People over 65 years old with suspected dementi
primary health care teams (PHCTs) in the city of I
time, people matched for sex and age with the p
dementia were drawn from the practice list. The
interviewed by myself to confirm the presence of dementia, or confirm its
absence in the comparison group. The interview was structured around a
diagnostic schedule incorporating the Medical Research Council
minimum data set (MRC, 1987). In addition to using the interview
information, case notes (when available) for the people with suspected
dementia were reviewed by a consultant in old age psychiatry to exclude
non-dementia causes of apparent dementia.

A further criterion for inclusion in the study was that the person with
dementia should have contact at least once a week with a relative living
nearby. This family member was identified by the older person whenever
possible, but in circumstances where the older person had advanced
dementia, the family member was approached directly after having been
identified by the PHCT. All family supporters participated in a structured
interview that covered psychological, social and financial aspects of their
caregiving status and sought their views about services.

After a period lasting on average 2 years, the family supporters of both
samples were contacted again and interviewed. The whereabouts and
wellbeing of the relative with dementia were established, and relatives still
living were assessed for progress of dementia. The study found that a
model incorporating four factors assessed at baseline best explained the
subsequent pattern of institutionalisation. These four factors were the
carer's willingness to continue caring, the carer's perceived need for a
careworker, the carer's report of the level of behavioural problems posed
by the person with dementia, and the person with dementia's score on the
Mini-Mental State Examination (MMSE) (Philp et al, 1997).

By the end of 3 years, I had interviewed 228 older people, half of whom
had dementia. In the first phase of data collection, interviews were carried
out in the older people's homes, and I became extremely familiar with the
road system of Dundee as I drove to various housing estates and small
cottages to recruit my sample. By the second phase of the study, I became
acquainted with many of the residential and nursing homes of Dundee, to
which a considerable number of the older people had relocated during the
2-year period between the initial interview and follow-up. In all, 45 older
people had died, and 56 were now living in residential settings. Forty-
nine of this latter figure were from the original sample of people with
dementia. Analysis of the data collected during the project can be found
elsewhere (Philp et al, 1995; McKee et al, 1996; McKee et al, 1997; Philp et
al, 1998).

...IS IS MY LIFE (3)
Hindsight and reflection

When I reflect on the research publications that emerged from the 6 years I spent working within the field of dementia care, the overwhelming impression that now presents itself is the absence from that output of the people with dementia. This is not to say that the published papers are poor, but rather that the research output is limited in its perspective owing to the nature of the input.

Essentially, my work to date on dementia care has been embedded within two dominant research paradigms: the *paradigm of the professional perspective*, and the *paradigm of the family carer*. Both in their way are perfectly valid, but both in their way also exclude the subjective experience and voice of the person who is, allegedly, at the centre of the enquiry: the cared-for person. Unless research questions become more related to this currently intangible cared-for person, the value of such enquiries will be constrained by the discourses within which the questions are constructed. In the case of the paradigm of the professional perspective, the operating discourses are, among others, those of organisational psychology and the sociology of work, health-care management, nursing practice and pathophysiology. In the case of the paradigm of the family carer, the constraining discourses are, among others, those of clinical psychology, social care practice and social policy. These discourses have, to date, constructed the cared-for person, and particularly the person with dementia, as an object that predicates the need for research. However, the research, when realised, fails to recognise people with dementia as the subject of enquiry, with their own agency and experiences.

The paradigm of the professional perspective

The Edinburgh project is an exemplar of a study conceived and executed within the paradigm of the professional perspective. Within this paradigm, people with dementia are represented largely as a series of numbers that chart their position on a journey of terminal decline, or are defined by membership of a given category of disability. The people in the long-stay wards who were under observation for the Edinburgh study were selected on the basis of their severity rating on the behavioural dependency scale of the CAPE. They are manifested in a data set in terms of their location on the ward and behaviour, and in respect of the care received and their communication with members of staff. Certainly, the data construct a notion of observed life on the ward, and care given. Yet there is still an absence that would give such data greater resonance – the lived existence on the ward, and the subjective meaning of the care received. An argument could be made that the evidence collected concerning staff activity no more manifests the lived experience of the staff than it does that of the person with dementia. Whilst this is true, the methodology of the Edinburgh project was developed through focus groups with nursing staff, and intensive piloting with feedback sessions with staff. Furthermore, part of the data collection involved interviews with key ward staff and the hospital and health board management. Ultimately, the providers' views were sought and incorporated into the data set, and guided and informed the analysis and interpretation of the data.

For care workers as opposed to academics, there will be a greater attendance to how a given set of statistics manifest as a pattern of individual behaviour, a necessary prerequisite for the provision of individualised care and personalised interaction. Nevertheless, there is real danger even here that the perspective that will be legitimated is entirely that of the professional – the collector, collator and interpreter of numbers – and that the subject of study will have no voice in what kind of data are collected, nor the manner in which they are utilised. The paradigm of the professional perspective can thus apply to both academics and care workers.

It has been argued by Gilloran et al (1995), that the Edinburgh project is an example of a patient-centred approach to the analysis of quality of care. Yet the 'patient-centred' construct seems to me to exist as a continuum as opposed to a single position. At one end of the continuum, an evaluation of the quality of care is patient-centred if data is collected – as in the Edinburgh project – using a methodology that is informed by the principle that what is important for the patient is paramount. However, even with this principle enshrined, no attempt was made to assess the users' views. As stated by Gilloran et al (1993), in the Edinburgh project 'we decided not to canvass ... the views of the users, either patients or their relatives, on the quality of care received ... the high level of dependency of the majority of our patient populations would make such a task difficult (p. 271). Given the precise research questions being addressed in the study, and the limitation on project resources, this is a reasonable decision to take. However, it does make the study only loosely patient-centred.

At the other end of the patient-centred continuum are studies that attempt to elicit the users' views through interview and questionnaire (e.g. Philp and Ghosh, 1992; Koch et al, 1995; Porter, 1995; Owens and Batchelor, 1996). Again, the importance of seeing 'patient-centredness' as a continuum is underlined when it is considered that the use of methods such as patient satisfaction questionnaires may provide only a limited insight into the users' views (Williams, 1994). Although no doubt constructed with reference to the views of patients as elicited through interview, the final questionnaire is an extension of the researcher's conception of patient satisfaction. Semi-structured interviews provide greater freedom for patients to make their views known (e.g. Powell et al, 1994), but even here there is an imposition of the researcher's interpretation on the raw data of the patient's views (Smith, 1995). Methodology such as grounded theory (Glaser and Strauss, 1967; Strauss and Corbin, 1990) offers perhaps the greatest hope of obtaining the true essence of the users' views, since theoretical insight and interpretation follow, rather than precede, data collection. Theorists such as David Armstrong have argued that patients' views are inevitably a manifestation of the medical gaze, and that it is therefore futile to seek their true essence (Armstrong, 1984). While Armstrong makes a strong theoretical case, when one returns to the pragmatic necessity of measuring quality of care and quality of life, it is still perhaps preferable to seek an unreachable essence than to ignore its existence.

When it comes to eliciting the views of the person with dementia, further issues become pertinent. For a long time, the accepted case was that dementia rendered the subject incapable of presenting a coherent view of the world. This perspective has since been challenged by a series of studies in which researchers have worked intensively with people with dementia in order to understand their world view (e.g. Sabat and Harré, 1992; Cheston, 1996; Golander and Raz, 1996). The debate has revolved around the issue of 'personhood' (Kitwood and Bredin, 1992; Jenkins and Price, 1996) and the validity of the self offered by the person with dementia relative to the self that is accepted or imposed by the agents (nurses, carers) of the prevailing authorities. The contrasting positions in this argument are reflected in the (superficially, at least) conflicting perspectives that inform two of the key therapeutic interventions, reality orientation (Folsom, 1968) and validation therapy (Feil, 1993).

The argument as to whether or not the concept of self has any validity in the person with severe dementia is beyond the scope of this chapter. However, research has surely demonstrated that people with dementia, as patients on long-stay wards or as residents in nursing homes, clearly manifest a social identity that makes their lives far more than the passive receipt of nursing care (Cheston, 1996; Henderson and Vesperi, 1995). With hindsight, it is ultimately the conflation of quality of care with quality of life that most limits the relevance of the Edinburgh project and other projects of its kind to the professional perspective. If care is life, then all aspects of life can be reduced to interactions between patients and nurses or doctors. All behaviour, all vocalisations are understood in relation to the professional presence, and potential dimensions of independent existence are ignored. The concept of quality of life, even when operationalised within the paradigm of the professional perspective, allows for the possibility of someone with dementia being a 'person'. Such a person lives in a community which, even if limited by four walls and a locked door, still contains social networks and interpersonal relations. The concept of quality of care, however, reduces the person with dementia to no more than a patient or resident within a ward or a home.

I am still proud of the work that I carried out within the Edinburgh project. I believe that the project's methodology and findings were valuable contributions to research into quality of care in long-stay wards for older people. At the same time, the project's findings in no way overlap with my memories of the people with dementia who were part of my life for the 6 months of data collection. The project's methodology failed to capture the life of these people over and above the care they received as patients.

The paradigm of the family carer

The Dundee project is an exemplar of a study conceived and executed within the paradigm of the family carer. In such a paradigm, our experience of the person with dementia is mediated and moderated by the assessment instruments of the care professionals, and by the family carer's symptoms and sentiments. The people with dementia are represented by their profiles on Activities of Daily Living and Instrumental Activities of Daily Living scales (Porter, 1995), and are manifested in terms of MMSE and CAPE scores. We come to know these people in terms of the caregiver burden they elicit, the service use for which they are the trigger.

The theoretical model adopted by the Dundee team, of the breakdown of family care of people with dementia, located the breakdown within the dynamics of the family itself. Given the research literature available at the time (e.g. Levin et al, 1984; Gilhooly, 1986; Brodaty et al, 1990) and the prevailing political ethos of family responsibility, such a model was entirely justifiable. However, it meant that from the outset, the vast majority of the data collected pertained to the psychosocial profile of the family carer. Interviews with the carer could last for up to 3 hours in duration, and much of that time would be spent in eliciting the carer's perceptions of their relative. In contrast, the interview with the person with dementia would last no more than 30 minutes, and consisted entirely of a test of cognitive ability. The grant-awarding body also required that an intelligence test, involving subsections of the Wechsler Adult Intelligence Scale (WAIS), should be performed. Since this additional assessment could take up to an hour, a second visit was required specifically for this purpose. To my knowledge, the WAIS data have never been analysed or utilised.

In the paradigm of the family carer, the issue of the subjective experience of the person with dementia is especially complicated. The person with dementia as a research object is no longer one of a number of people being cared for in a uniform fashion, but a member of a care dyad. The person with dementia is inseparable from the family carer. One would imagine that this would increase the opportunity for the person with dementia to become a fully realised research subject, being an equally prominent member of the dyad. However, because that dyad is accessed only through the stories and perceptions of the carer, the person with dementia once again disappears.

The problems of assessing the users' views, as discussed above, are even more pertinent here. Whereas the conflation of quality of care and quality of life was a central issue for the paradigm of the professional perspective, within the paradigm of the family carer the significant problem is the conflation of the family carer as user with the person with dementia as user. While it is, ostensibly, the people with dementia who 'use' the social and health-care services, that use is moderated by the family carers according to their perceptions of the needs of the person with dementia. In a sense, the family carer becomes synonymous with the person with dementia, and the use of services brought about by the person with dementia become the service use of the family carer. The 'user's view' of the community care of people with dementia has been extensively documented (e.g. Lawton et al, 1995), – but it is not the person with dementia, the 'true' user, whose views are recorded, but those of the carer. While the carer's views are important, the very act of their assiduous documentation makes the silence imposed on the person with dementia even more profound. The paradigm of the family carer has become such a dominant entity in community care research that the person with dementia has become entirely absorbed within its discourse. The person with dementia exists only as an adjunct to the family carer: merely a catalyst of the relative's assumption of the carer role; the metamorphosing entity that provides the relative with the driving narrative whereby the carer's role is defined and expressed.

Within the theoretical framework that located family dynamics as the cause of the breakdown of care, the Dundee project failed to identify the social forces acting on the care dyad. The relationship between the carer and the person with dementia was the object of investigation; divorced from the biomedical discourse that creates the concept of dementia (Gilleard, 1996; Koch and Webb, 1996), the political rhetoric of family responsibility, and the lay representations of senility and decline. Ultimately, the breakdown of care was seen as the rational decision-making process of a given individual, with its attendant psychosocial predictors. In the Dundee project (McKee et al, 1996), the four main predictors of the breakdown of care were:

- The severity of dementia as measured by the MMSE.
- The carer's perceived need of help with the personal care needs of the person with dementia
- The level of problem created for the carer by the person's overall behavioural disturbance
- The carer's willingness to continue caring.

The Dundee project was carefully conceived, and adds valuable information to the research literature on the breakdown of family care of the person with dementia. Yet the answers obtained are a result of the questions asked, and in the case of the Dundee project, the questions asked were entirely within the paradigm of the family carer. The answers provided are therefore limited to enabling risk assessments for the breakdown of family care, and psychological interventions to reduce carer stress and improve carer coping. The person with dementia is broken down into a series of variables that affect, to various degrees, the carer, service use and the likelihood of the continuation of care. At the end of the project, the person with dementia is operationalised as an outcome measure: the person is recorded as being in the community, at risk of going into care, in care, or dead.

My personal experiences of this fieldwork led me to question my research role. When assessing the cognitive status of the person with dementia, I felt as if I was a heartless magician, demonstrating to these people the growing insubstantiality of their memory, providing them with an explicit display of the shrinking limits of their minds. I found the work distasteful in the extreme. While the information I gathered may have been integral to answering the research questions posed by the project, I left each home that I visited convinced that the information I had collected told me next to nothing about the 'true' nature of dementia. It was clear to me that whilst dementia may well have an organic basis, measurable through clinical assessments, its essential form was the myriad social displays enacted before me when I entered the homes of ordinary people. Dementia, as well as being a pathological state, existed most forcefully and meaningfully as a constellation of relations: between the mind and body of the person with dementia; between the person with dementia and the carer; between the family group with dementia and the external social world. Kitwood (1990) has described the social relations through which dementia is realised as a 'malignant social psychology'; these include infantilisation, intimidation and stigmatisation (see Table 3.1). These social relations allowed me to enter a person's world, ask a series of demeaning questions, and reduce that person to a series of depersonalised scores. The same relations removed the validity of the expressions of the person with dementia, and replaced it with the views and perceptions of the family carer. Ultimately, these relations would allow family carers – themselves able to make 'decisions' only so far as the available biomedical and social care discourses permitted – to discharge the responsibility of care onto others, and thereby remove the person with dementia – now categorised as 'at risk' – from their home.

In many ways, my experience on the Dundee project reflected that of the Edinburgh project: I had entered each project with a notion that I would be growing closer to an understanding of dementia, and yet I left each project feeling that what I had learned of dementia was not to be found in the output of my professional work. Within the research paradigms that I had adopted, the projects had been successful. Yet it was apparent to me that it was time to seek out a new research paradigm.

THIS IS THEIR LIFE

Having worked in both residential and community settings, I was struck by the similarity in the observed life of people with dementia in the two environments. The rhetoric of community care would have it that the community provides a far more enriched environment for the older person – and indeed for people with dementia – than do long-stay institutions. From my experience, I could not see any clear evidence for such an assertion.

The principle that 'community is better' is based on a few assumptions that lack supporting evidence. The first assumption, the alleged cheapness of community care in comparison with long-stay accommodation, has been refuted by Victor (1991) with her calculation of the astronomical hidden costs of unpaid informal care provided by the community. The second assumption is that the quality of care provided by family carers is better than that provided by nurses. While it is likely that the emotional content of the relationship between the family carer and the person with dementia is greater than that between nurse and patient, this in no way determines the quality of the care provided. As Kitwood (1990) argues, intending to give good care does not mean that good care is in fact delivered. Being able to deliver good care depends upon having the requisite skill base, which most family carers do not possess. The caregiving relationship is often an imposition on the life of the family carer, something that has to be dealt with in addition to the normal demands of life. Pressures can build up, which mean that the circumstances in which the relative delivers care are less than ideal.

A third assumption concerning community care is that being cared for by a family member is the desired option of most older people. As Christina Victor has noted (Victor, 1991), there is remarkably little evidence available regarding this issue. Once again, it seems that the 'user's views' are felt to be largely irrelevant. The small amount of research in this area suggests that there are conflicting beliefs among older people. While residential care is clearly not a preferred option, older people are also adamant that they do not wish to be a 'burden' to their family (Salvage et al, 1989; Groger, 1995). Inadequate research on the 'user's view' in this area means that our understanding of exactly how older people perceive and respond to the challenges of late life is entirely unsophisticated. The choice between professional or family care, for instance, will be informed by beliefs concerning the importance of independence, the value of privacy and a personal 'home' (Gurney and Means, 1993), and the meaning of the 'institution'.

A great part of the problem in the debate on the relative merits of residential and community care is that the two environments have been – partly through political expediency and partly through cultural representation – constructed as opposites. The stigma that has always been attached to institutional life, in particular the negative value of the idea of the asylum, is manifested in and reinforced by images of an existence that is the antithesis of family home life. These images are prevalent in literature and film, and are endorsed by the scientific community in the extensive research showing the impoverishment of life in such environments (Kenny, 1990; Nolan et al, 1995; Koch and Webb, 1996). The sterile, uniform lifestyle enforced within the 'institution' is structured through the removal of rights from the institution's inhabitants, and the allocation of control to the professionals who manage and maintain institutional life. Autonomy and dignity are stripped away. For the person with dementia, the mental death within the ageing physical shell is mirrored by the shrivelling of life within the hull of the institution. In addition, for the person with dementia, this is a containment unto death. Life within such a place therefore presages physical death, and psychological research has consistently demonstrated that when an event is contingent upon another, the event that carries the predictive information (in this case, institutionalisation) takes on the psychological meaning of the event that it predicts (in this case, physical and spiritual negation) (Mackintosh, 1995). It is rare for research to present a picture of institutional life that does not conform to this overwhelmingly dark metaphor of the 'total institution', see Higgs et al (1992) for one example.

When such a negative image is contrasted with the rosy caricature of the grandfather or grandmother being cared for by a loving spouse or by loving children and grandchildren in the warmth of the home environment, one becomes aware of how powerfully a constructed reality can influence reasoned thought (Blaikie, 1994). For whilst the diametrical opposition of the constructions of home and institution can lead to only one conclusion – that 'home is where the heart is' – one forgets that the grounds on which one should make such a judgment (the quality of life of people with dementia) lack any supporting evidence. On this issue, reason has been hijacked by compelling propaganda, and it is too readily forgotten that an 'institutionalised' way of life can be found outside stereotypical institutions, that is, it can just as easily be found within the community (Higgins, 1989).

Quality of life is a notoriously difficult concept (Farquhar, 1995a). A quick scan of the research on this subject, indicates that whereas medical conditions – health and illness – play a prominent part in the realisation of the concept, the older person with dementia is rarely the subject of enquiry (Farquhar, 1995b). Much of the early work on quality of life sought to impose values of what was important for a life to be 'good'. More recently attempts have been made to conceptualise quality of life as a relative concept, and to assess the 'user's views' in order to establish the parameters on which quality of life can be judged. One of the more successful attempts to measure the user's view of quality of life is that of the Schedule for the Evaluation of Individual Quality of Life (SEIQoL) (McGee et al, 1991). The short version of this scale, the SEIQoL-DW, has been used to assess quality of life in family carers of people with dementia (Coen et al, 1996). Whilst this work is important in itself, it clearly falls within the paradigm of the family carer. When it comes to the issue of the quality of life of the person with dementia, the quality of life research literature either mutates into quality of care literature, or abruptly dries up, with merely a handful of notable exceptions such as Berlowitz et al (1995), and further work with SEIQoL (Coen et al, 1993).

Whilst it is understandable that the size of the challenge of conceptualising the quality of life of a person with dementia might inhibit the research community from addressing the issue, the current political climate and the imperative of demographic change clearly require this issue to be tackled with urgency. Every day, people with dementia are living in worlds not of their making, in which their capacity for making life-course preferences is not even considered. If it is accepted that quality of life is a relative concept, then that is a starting point from which people with dementia can be compared with people like themselves in order to determine the living environment that most improves the quality of their existence. To my knowledge, only one paper to date has attempted to compare the quality of life of people with dementia who live in the community with those who live in institutions (Shepherd et al, 1996), but even in this paper the community setting chosen is residential accommodation, and the concepts of quality of care and quality of life are to some degree conflated. One study cannot hope to address all of the key questions in such an important issue. More studies are needed to establish whether our prejudices are correct, and the quality of life for people with dementia within residential settings is poorer than for those in the community. Even given such a result, it is time that the palpably false opposition of community and residential care is deconstructed (Higgins, 1989).

Community care and residential care of people with dementia seem to me not to be opposites, but rather to share common features. Although the paradigm of the professional perspective and the paradigm of the family carer would have us think otherwise, in both residential and community settings the person with dementia is in the centre. Without this person, the family carer and care professional become redundant. In the residential setting, the next most dominant person is the professional carer, the nurse. The family carer is here a marginal figure, and it is only recently that attempts have been made to integrate family members into the care of people with dementia living in long-stay accommodation (Duncan and

Morgan, 1994; Laitinen and Isola, 1996). When one looks at the community setting this situation is reversed, with the family carer occupying the dominant position beside the person with dementia, while the care professional – social worker, or district or community psychiatric nurse – has the minor role. It is usually only with repeated visits that the care professional in the community is accepted by the family carer as a member of the household who 'shares' the care work (Twigg, 1992a).

Described in such terms, it becomes clear that what one is observing when comparing community and residential care is not an opposition, but rather two ends of a continuum, representing the range of possible contexts within which the person with dementia can live. If it is accepted that self-harm and self-neglect are far too high a price to pay for allowing the person with dementia total autonomy, then it is inevitable that the person with dementia must always be cared for, within this continuum. It is a continuum of care where a care triad (care professional, family carer, person with dementia) will tend to obtain, although this triad is often reduced to its component dyads from the point of view of practice and research paradigms. The nature of the triad – the strength and importance of the links between the members – varies along the spectrum of care from community to residential settings. The notion of a continuum helps also to break down the artificial division between community and residential settings, in so far as it highlights the shadings between the various environments within which one finds a person with dementia living: own home, family home, day care, respite care, sheltered housing, residential community, residential home, nursing home, hospital.

IS THIS YOUR LIFE?
Emergent issues

While the paradigms of the professional perspective and the family carer will always have their place, the new constructions of the continuum of care and the care triad show up such paradigms for their limitations. Research must address the uniqueness of each care context, and the corresponding arrangement of the care triad, in order to understand both the predictors of and the outcomes of care. It is important, however, to emphasise again the distinction between quality of care and quality of life. It is undoubtedly the case, as Gilloran et al, (1993) claim, that the quality of care for a person with dementia will have a powerful impact on that person's quality of life. This notion is in line with Lawton's (1983) 'environmental docility' hypothesis, which holds that as an individual's cognitive and physical competence is compromised, the environment will become increasingly influential. However, care is the central theme of this continuum for only so long as one focuses on the care triad. At the level of the *individual*, at the level of the person with dementia, this is a continuum of *life*, and so there will always remain questions that must be asked which go beyond the more superficial notion of care. In all probability, the variance in the nature of life *within* each care environment is greater than the variance in the nature of life *between* environments. As such it is unlikely, when comparing people with similar severity of dementia across environments, that one would obtain a significant difference in their elicited quality of life. However, the issue of quality of life is important to retain, for there is far more to such a concept than simply a numerical scale along which individuals can be located. Quality of life is not just about obtaining a relative score, but also about fundamental questions relating to the meaning of life and the subjective sensation of being, and it is here that we still have so much to learn with respect to the person with dementia. In respect of this, I disagree with the assertion by Kitwood and Bredin (1992) that 'personhood' should be seen in social rather than individual terms. Whilst personhood may manifest itself at the level of the social, to describe personhood purely at the social level creates a danger that people with dementia will be understood once again only in reference to their environment. Although there may be several years of living with dementia without the need for care, there is within the construct of a social personhood the implicit requirement that we see the person with dementia in a relational frame, and we therefore find ourselves once more on the slippery slope that leads us into the paradigm of the professional perspective or the family carer. Thus, while Kitwood's work is on the whole commendable, his conceptual approach to dementia is to some degree culpable of adding to the conflation of care with life.

I have briefly addressed above the new research agenda for dementia care, which should focus on the changing arrangement of the care triad across the continuum of encompassing care environments. When it comes to the issue of the quality of life of the person with dementia, two main research agendas need to be further developed. First, what form does life take for the person with dementia? In our adoption of the paradigms of the professional perspective and the family carer, we have already developed the methodologies for capturing the structure of life for the person with dementia (Gilloran et al, 1993; Bottorff and Varcoe, 1995; Lawton et al, 1995; Birchall and Waters, 1996; Martichuski et al, 1996). However, this structure has always been understood in relation to external carers, and in relation to carer activities. What is needed is research that, whilst cognisant of the fact that the observed life is occurring within a care environment, also acknowledges that the observed life has a structure and an internal momentum in and of itself. This kind of research is exemplified in work by, amongst others, McIsaac (1995), Reed (Reed and Macmillan, 1995; Reed and Payton, 1996) and Powers (1995). Here, it is the interaction between people with dementia that is important – what the structures of the observed relationships tell us about the content of these relationships, and how these relationships are in and of themselves a life, informed by but separate from the immediate care environment. This research naturalises the observed world of the person with dementia. We recognise the similarities between the world of the person with dementia and the world of the person without dementia, in a way that we were previously prevented from doing by the prevailing discourse that defines the person with dementia purely as a patient in receipt of care. This research dares to ask the same questions of the world of the person with dementia as has been asked about the world of those without dementia (Gubrium and Sankar, 1994). We had hitherto assumed that such questions are meaningless in the meaningless world of the person with dementia. Again, we are finding that our assumptions are wrong.

A second line of research seeks a way to make manifest for us all the internal, lived world of the person with dementia. Such work is not interested in the judgment of quality, nor confined to the therapeutic discourse, but rather sets out through narrative, life story and grounded theory methodology to make tangible the inner life of the person with dementia (Gubrium, 1993; Cromwell, 1994; Buchanan and Middleton, 1995; Cheston, 1996; Golander and Raz, 1996). This is perhaps the most difficult research task of all. Yet, if there is one research agenda that could generate the greatest challenge to the overwhelming weight of stigma that besets a person with dementia – the double stigma of agedness and mental illness – then it is surely this agenda. Whilst research in this area can take a variety of forms, the central thesis of this work is that the person with dementia has a voice, and that given persistence and skill, this voice can be elicited.

CONCLUSION

It is possible that we are at the beginning of a new research partnership, one in which the position of the researcher is understood in relation to the person with dementia, the care professional and the family carer. Perhaps we have finally realised that the research that pronounces 'This is Your Life' is far less valuable than research that enquires 'Is This Your Life?' In making this plea for more positive and empowering work to be the agenda for the future in dementia care research, I do not for one moment wish to suggest that dementia is anything other than the most dreadful affliction that can beset a person, and one which, in its final stages, is an entirely dehumanising death. Neither do I wish to seem insensitive to the needs of the family carers, for such people daily make efforts and sacrifices that defy the imagination. Yet this is precisely why our imagination is too readily switched off: confronted by the constellation of indignities attendant on dementia, we scarcely want to believe that human life is still present.

The essential argument I have made here is that unless we ask the correct questions, we cannot know the content or quality of life that persists within the world of the person with dementia. If, as I suspect, there is a connection, and not a discontinuity, between the worlds of those with dementia and the worlds of those without, and if there is the slightest possibility that a kernel of tranquillity persists at the heart of the chaos of dementia, then we have been culpable in the past of a hideous sin: that of denying humanity to those who, in their vulnerability, are perhaps most human. In so doing we have probably not only exacerbated that vulnerability, but also heightened the terror of the experience.

REFERENCES

Abel, E.K. (1994) Family caregiving in the nineteenth century: Emily Hawley Gillespie and Sarah Gillespie, 1858–1888. *Bulletin of the History of Medicine* **68**, 573–599.

Armstrong, D. (1984) The patient's view. *Social Science and Medicine* **18**, 737–744.

Berlowitz, D.R., Du W., Kazis, L. et al (1995) Health-related quality of life of nursing home residents: differences in patient and provider perceptions. *Journal of the American Geriatrics Society* **43**, 799–802.

Birchall, R. & Waters, K.R. (1996) What do elderly people do in hospital? *Journal of Clinical Nursing* **5**, 171–176.

Blaikie, A. (1994) Photographic memory, ageing and the life course. *Ageing and Society* **14**, 479–497.

Bottorff, J.L. & Varcoe, C. (1995) Transitions in nurse-patient interactions: a qualitative ethology. *Qualitative Health Research* **5**, 315–331.

Brodaty, H., Griffin, D. & Hadzi-Pavlovic, D. (1990) A survey of dementia carers: doctors' communications, problem behaviours and institutional care. *Australian and New Zealand Journal of Psychiatry* **24**, 362–370.

Buchanan, K. & Middleton, D. (1995) Voices of experience: talk, identity and membership in reminiscence groups. *Ageing and Society* **15**, 457–491.

Cheston, R. (1996) Stories and metaphors: talking about the past in a psychotherapy group for people with dementia. *Ageing and Society* **16**, 579–602.

Coen, R., O'Mahony, D., O'Boyle, C. et al, (1993) Measuring the quality of life of dementia patients using the schedule for the evaluation of individual quality of life. *Irish Journal of Psychology* **14**, 154–163.

Coen, R.F., O'Boyle, C.A., Lawlor, B.A. & Coakley, D. (1996) *Individual Quality of Life Factors Distinguishing Low Burden and High Burden Caregivers of Alzheimer's Disease Patients.* Paper presented at the 10th European Health Psychology Conference, Dublin, September 4–6.

Cromwell, S.L. (1994) The subjective experience of forgetfulness among elders. *Qualitative Health Research* **4**, 444–462.

Duncan, M.T. & Morgan, D.L. (1994) Sharing the caring: family caregivers views of their relationships with nursing home staff. The Gerontologist **34**, 235–244.

Farquhar, M. (1995a) Definitions of quality of life: a taxonomy. *Journal of Advanced Nursing* **22**, 502–508.

Farquhar, M. (1995b) Elderly people's definitions of quality of life. *Social Science and Medicine* **41**, 1439–1446.

Feil, N. (1993) *The Validation Breakthrough: Simple Techniques for Communicating with People with 'Alzheimer's-Type Dementia'.* Baltimore: Health Promotions.

Folsom, J.C. (1968) Reality orientation therapy for the elderly mental patient. *Journal of Geriatric Psychiatry* **1**, 291–307.

Gilhooly, M.L.M. (1986) Senile dementia: factors associated with care-givers' preference for institutional care. *British Journal of Medical Psychology* **56**, 165–171.

Gilleard, C.J. (1984) *Living with Dementia.* London: Croom Helm.

Gilleard, C.J. (1996) *Psychosocial Aspects of Mind and Dementia.* Paper presented at the British Congress of Gerontology, Manchester, July 3–5.

Gilloran, A.J., McGlew, T., McKee, K. et al (1993) Measuring the quality of care in psychogeriatric wards. *Journal of Advanced Nursing* **18**, 269–275.

Gilloran, A., McKinley, A., McGlew, T. et al (1994) Staff nurses' work satisfaction in psychogeriatric wards. *Journal of Advanced Nursing* **20**, 997–1003.

Gilloran, A., Robertson, A., McGlew, T. et al, (1995) Improving work satisfaction amongst nursing staff and quality of care for elderly patients with dementia: some policy implications. *Ageing and Society* **15**, 375–391.

Glaser, B.G. & Strauss, A.L. (1967) *The Discovery of Grounded Theory*. Chicago: Aldine.

Goffman, E. (1961) *Asylums*. New York: Doubleday.

Golander, H. & Raz, A.E. (1996) The mask of dementia: images of 'demented residents' in a nursing ward. *Ageing and Society* **16**, 269–285.

Groger, L. (1995) Health trajectories and long term care choices: what stories told by informants can tell us. In: Henderson, J.N. & Vesperi, M.D. (eds) *The Culture of Long Term Care*, pp. 55–69. Westport: Bergin & Garvey.

Gubrium, J.F. (1993) *Speaking of Life: Horizons of Meaning for Nursing Home Residents*. New York: Aldine.

Gubrium, J.F. & Sankar, A., eds (1994) *Qualitative Methods in Aging Research*. Thousand Oaks: Sage.

Gurney, C. & Means, R. (1993) The meaning of home in later life. In: Arber, S. & Evandrou, M. (eds) *Ageing Independence and the Life Course*, pp. 119–131. London: Jessica Kingsley.

Higgins, J. (1989) Defining community care: realities and myths. *Social Policy and Administration* **23**, 3–16.

Higgs, P.F., MacDonald, L.D. & Ward, M.C. (1992) Responses to the institution among elderly patients in hospital long-stay care. *Social Science and Medicine* **35**, 287–293.

Hughes, B. & Wilkin, D. (1987) Physical care and quality of life in residential homes. *Ageing and Society* **7**, 399–425.

Jenkins, D. & Price, B. (1996) Dementia and personhood: a focus for care? *Journal of Advanced Nursing* **24**, 84–90.

Kenny, T. (1990) Erosion of individuality of care of elderly people in hospital – an alternative approach. *Journal of Advanced Nursing* **15**, 571–576.

Kitwood, T. (1990) The dialectics of dementia: with particular reference to Alzheimer's disease. *Ageing and Society* **10**, 177–196.

Kitwood, T. & Bredin, K. (1992) Towards a theory of dementia care: personhood and well-being. *Ageing and Society* **12**, 269–287.

Koch, T. & Webb, C. (1996) The biomedical construction of ageing: implications for nursing care of older people. *Journal of Advanced Nursing* **23**, 954–959.

Koch, T., Webb, C. & Williams, A.M. (1995) Listening to the voices of older patients: an existential-phenomenological approach to quality assurance. *Journal of Clinical Nursing* **4**, 185–193.

Laitinen, P. & Isola, A. (1996) Promoting participation of informal caregivers in the hospital care of the elderly patient: informal caregivers' perceptions. *Journal of Advanced Nursing* **23**, 942–947.

Lawton, M.P. (1983) Environment and other determinants of well-being in older people. *Gerontologist* **23**, 349–357.

Lawton, M.P., Moss, M. & Duhamel, L.M. (1995) The quality of daily life among elderly care receivers. *Journal of Applied Gerontology* **14**, 150–171.

Levin, E., Sinclair, I. & Gorbach, P. (1984) *The Supporters of Confused Elderly Persons at Home: Extract from the Main Report*. London: National Institute of Social Work Research Unit.

Mackintosh, N.J. (1995) Classical and Operant Conditioning. In: Mackintosh, N.J. & Colman, A.M. (eds) *Learning and Skills*, pp. 1–18. London: Longman.

Martichuski, D.K., Bell, P.A. & Bradshaw, B. (1996) Including small group activities in large special care units. *Journal of Applied Gerontology* **15**, 224–237.

McGee, H.M., O'Boyle, C.A., Hickey, A. et al (1991) Assessing the quality of life of the individual: the SEIQoL with a healthy and a gastroenterology unit population. *Psychological Medicine* **21**, 749–759.

McGlew, T., Robertson, A., Gilloran, A., McKee, K., McKinley, A. & Wight, D. (1991) *An Empirical Study of Job Satisfaction Among Nurses and the Quality of Care Received by Patients in Psychogeriatric Wards in Scottish Hospitals*. Final report, Scottish Home and Health Department.

McIsaac, S. (1995) *Identity Maintenance Amongst Confused Residents Within Institutional Settings*. Paper presented at the British Society of Gerontology Annual Conference, University of Keele, September 15–17.

McKee, K.J., Philp, I. & Armstrong, G. (1996) *Predicting the Breakdown of Family Care of People with Dementia*. Paper presented at the 10th European Health Psychology Conference, Dublin, September 4–6.

McKee, K.J., Whittick, J.E., Ballinger, B.B. et al (1997) Coping in family supporters of elderly people with dementia. *British Journal of Clinical Psychology* **36**, 323–340.

[MRC] Medical Research Council (1987) *Report from the MRC Alzheimer's Disease Workshop*. London: MRC.

Nolan, M., Grant, G. & Nolan, J. (1995) Busy doing nothing: activity and interaction levels amongst differing populations of elderly patients. *Journal of Advanced Nursing* **22**, 528–538.

Owens, D.J. & Batchelor, C. (1996) Patient satisfaction and the elderly. *Social Science and Medicine* **42**, 1483–1491.

Pattie, A.H. & Gilleard, C.J. (1979) *Manual of the Clifton Assessment Procedures for the Elderly*. Sevenoaks: Hodder & Stoughton.

Philp, I. & Ghosh, U. (1992) Community care services: views of patients attending a geriatric day hospital. *Health Bulletin* **50**, 296–301.

Philp, I., McKee, K.J., Meldrum, P. et al (1995) Community care for demented and non-demented elderly: a comparison study of financial burden, service use and unmet needs in family supporters. *British Medical Journal* **310**, 1503–1506.

Philp, I., McKee, K.J., Armstrong, G. et al (1997) Institutionalisation risk amongst people with dementia supported by family carers in a Scottish City. *Aging and Mental Health* **1**, 339–345.

Porter, E.J. (1995) A phenomenological alternative to the 'ADL research tradition'. *Journal of Ageing and Health* **7**, 24–45.

Powell, J., Lovelock, R., Bray, J. et al (1994) Involving consumers in assessing service quality: benefits of using a qualitative approach. *Quality in Health Care* **3**: 199–202

Powers, B.A. (1995) From the inside out: the world of the institutionalized elderly. In: Henderson J.N. & Vesperi, M.D. (eds) *The Culture of Long Term Care*, pp. 179–196. Westport: Bergin & Garvey.

Reed, J. & MacMillan, J. (1995) Friendship – the proper focus of care? *Reviews in Clinical Gerontology* **5**: 229–237.

Reed, J. & Payton, V.R. (1996) Constructing familiarity and managing the self: ways of adapting to life in nursing and residential homes for older people. *Ageing and Society* **16**: 543–560.

Robertson, A., Gilloran, A., McGlew, T. et al (1995). Nurses job satisfaction and the quality of care received by patients in psychogeriatric wards. *International Journal of Geriatric Psychiatry* **10**: 575–584.

Salvage, A.V., Vetter, N.J. & Jones, D.A. (1989) Opinions concerning residential care. *Age and Ageing,* **18**, 380–386.

Sabat, S.R. & Harré, R. (1992) The construction and deconstruction of self in Alzheimer's disease. *Ageing and Society* **12**: 443–461.

Shepherd, G., Muijen, M., Dean, R. et al (1996) Residential care in hospital and in the community – quality of care and quality of life. *British Journal of Psychiatry* **168**, 448–456.

Smith, J. (1995) Semi-structured interviewing and qualitative analysis. In: Smith, J.A., Harré, R. & Van Langenhove, L. (eds) *Rethinking Methods in Psychology*, pp. 9–26. London: Sage.

Strauss, A.L. & Corbin, J.A. (1990) *Basics of Qualitative Research: Grounded Theory Procedures and Techniques*. Newbury Park: Sage.

Twigg, J., ed. (1992a) *Carers in the Service System*. London: HMSO.

Twigg, J., ed. (1992b) *Carers. Research and Practice*. London: HMSO.

Williams, B. (1994) Patient satisfaction: a valid concept? *Social Science and Medicine* **38**: 509–516.

Wing, J. & Brown, G. (1970). *Institutionalism and Schizophrenia*. Cambridge University Press.

Victor, C. (1991) *Health and Health Care in Later Life*. Milton Keynes: Open University Press.

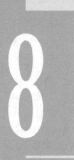

8

Keeping a distance: the reactions of older people in care homes to confused fellow residents

Jan Reed

KEY ISSUES

- Some older people who are confused live in nursing and residential homes with people who are not confused. Whilst there is a debate about the value of such integrated living, there is little research to support this strategy, or conversely to suggest that it is not helpful

- Some arguments suggest that the 'normalising influence' of older people who are not confused is beneficial to those who are

- Results of a study which looked at older people moving into care homes and followed them up for 6 months after the move suggest that older people who are not confused are ambivalent about the presence of those who are confused: some people enjoy adopting a helping role, while others try to avoid these residents

- Both helping and avoidance are strategies that maintain a distance between residents, and signal to visitors that those who are not confused are different from those who are

- These approaches are often adopted in an ad hoc way, and this can have negative consequences for people who are confused, as fellow residents may be inconsistent in their manner and behaviour

- Integrated care may need to be managed more carefully, with staff alert to the problems of relationships between residents

INTRODUCTION

The study reported in this chapter sought to understand the experiences of older people moving into care homes, privileging their voices, and making their views central to debates on care provision; it was not intended to explore the issues of 'confused' and 'non-confused' residents living together. By listening to the participants in the study, however, a number of issues developed in importance, some of which had not been anticipated. One of these issues was the importance of relationships with other residents, and related to this was the issue of the presence of residents who were 'confused'. The way in which participants talked about these residents suggested that the dynamics of this relationship could have significant consequences for their care, and for any therapeutic interventions the staff may try to make. Some of the benevolent attitudes expressed by residents were potentially supportive and therapeutic, but there was an undercurrent of paternalism which could lead to problems, and some residents expressed hostility, anger and impatience which could potentially be damaging to residents who were confused. It became evident that this range of reactions were a way of keeping a distance from people who were confused, and a way of maintaining an identity as a non-confused person. In other words, participants in the study were very eager to point out differences between them and confused residents because they were concerned that people would think that they were confused, or because they were worried in case they were. Pointing out differences was a way of reinforcing a 'non-confused' identity, both to themselves and others.

When I was asked to write this chapter, I and my colleagues thought that this would be an opportunity to place our data more firmly in the context of what had already been written about the issue of 'mixed' residential care, i.e. in settings that cater for older people both with and without cognitive problems. Surprisingly, however, literature searches did not yield a great deal of material. A 'historical' literature search, starting with a relatively recent paper that was vaguely relevant and chasing up the references in it, yielded some information, but this was largely confined to the late 1970s – it seemed as if we were coming to a debate which had long since been closed, but it was difficult to find out what the conclusion had been. In addition the literature was not framed in the way that we had expected it to be. We had expected there to be some work looking at the impact of mixed care on each group, and hoped that some of it would be ethnographic work, which would fit in with our perspective. What we found instead, was limited material about the pros and cons of specialised care, evaluating this mainly in terms of clinical outcomes. In a study from the USA (Webber et al, 1995), for example, special care units were compared with integrated nursing homes in terms of patient outcome, and little difference was found. This study looked at process and quality of life measures as well, but again it was difficult to identify differences between the two types of care.

Part of the problem may lie in the wide variation in specialised facilities for people with dementia, noted by Ohta and Ohta (1988), and also because of the lack of clarity about their function. There is a suspicion, voiced by Webber et al, (1995), and also by the US Congress Office of Technology (1992), that although there are claims made for the efficacy of special units, there is little evidence to support them, and the provision of such units is a development more strenuously marketed than evaluated.

Ohta and Ohta (1988) make an interesting point about special care units (SCUs) when they discuss the 'primary beneficiaries' of such units. In their study they found that while some SCUs clearly emphasised the benefits to people with dementia, others were just as likely to stress the benefits of segregation for those who did not have dementia – in other words that the specialised facility had the primary advantage of protecting the quality of life for those who were not cognitively impaired. Meacher (1972) in his discussion of the history of 'separatism' in the care of older people with mental health problems, reports a long-established concern with the effect of confused older people on those who are not confused. He goes back to discussions from the beginning of the twentieth century where concern was raised about 'the cruelty of requiring sane persons to associate, by day and by night, with gibbering idiots' (Preston-Thomas, 1901).

Some of this thinking is evident in policy in the UK today, in the maintenance of a system that assumes that older people are more comfortable living with others who have similar needs. In the Burgner report (Burgner, 1996), for example, it is confidently asserted that 'elderly people with few nursing needs would not be comfortable in a home where dependency levels are much greater and nursing needs are therefore paramount' (p. 68). Care provision, then, becomes more and more like an 'escalator of care' (Davison and Reed, 1995) which older people step on to when they need support, and which carries them on to further support as their needs increase. As Eley and Middleton (1983) point out, however, it is very difficult to get off this escalator – services are provided on the assumption that older people will inevitably decline in health and functioning, and are structured on the assumption that the best way to meet these changing needs is to move people from facility to facility as their needs increase. The SCU – or Elderly Mentally Infirm (EMI) unit, as it is called in the UK – for people with dementia fits into this model as the last step on the escalator.

The escalator model, in its more positive interpretation, is arguably a way of ensuring that specialised care is provided for people as they need it, and there is also some evidence that this is a motivation for some policy-makers. The Royal Commission on the Law Relating to Mental Illness and Mental Deficiency (1957), for example, argued that, 'Many old people could be protected from further mental deterioration if they could be given the security and attention provided in this sort of [specialised] home early enough, and might not need to be admitted to hospital' (Cmnd 169, para. 628).

In a negative interpretation, however, this model can be seen as a way of gradually removing people from view, for progressively placing them in more and more restricted and less 'normal' environments, for putting an increasing distance between 'us' (the healthy) and 'them' (the sick). Douglas (1991) has eloquently described the ways in which we try to protect ourselves against the contamination of death and disease through the creation of boundaries, and some writers in the field of dementia care have pointed out similar dynamics in the way that we treat people with dementia.

Kitwood (1990), for example, has talked about 'malignant social psychology', the way in which people with dementia are treated as not human (see Chapter 3). This type of treatment serves to maintain a distance between people with dementia and others, but it compounds and reinforces a loss of 'personhood'. Sabat and Harré (1992) have also talked about the social construction of dementia, and argued that a sense of self is still retained by people with dementia, but the public self – the self that is socially mediated and validated – can be lost if others fail to acknowledge it. In other words, even if a person with dementia still retains a sense of self, this may be negated by the attitudes and behaviour of others who ignore or demean it. The possible rationale behind this is explored by Kitwood (1993) when he argues (and it is worth quoting him in full, given the force with which he expresses his view) that:

> It is as if a radical divide has been made between 'us' (the cognitively intact and fundamentally sound members of society) and 'them' (the damaged and deficient). The 'problem' of dementia is attributed to 'them' while 'we' are let off the hook. The dementia sufferer is thus a kind of alien, and caregiving tends to be viewed as action by superiors – a modern version of old-time charity.
> Matters look very different when 'the problem' of dementia is seen as something that belongs to us all, whether or not we have cognitive impairments. The damage and deficits that 'we' bring come clearly into view, and behind that the ageism, fear, greed and hypocrisy endemic in society. (p. 53)

This discussion has focused implicitly on the relationships between people with dementia and their carers, but it has not addressed another set of relationships that may be pertinent to the experience of care. These relationships are those that may develop between people with dementia and other older people without dementia resident in the same care facility. Meacher (1972) concluded that these relationships varied from hostility, through indifference to sympathy. Wilkins and Hughes (1987), in their study of residential care from the 'consumers' point of view, claim that, 'A surprising degree of tolerance was shown by lucid people towards those who had become confused' (p. 175), a statement which, whilst it may reflect the overall analysis of their data, does not enter into the complexities of this tolerance. Golander and Raz (1996) provide more detail in their discussion of the construction of positive social identities and roles for people with dementia in an Israeli geriatric centre. They coined the term 'demented role' (an allusion to Parson's notion of the 'sick role') to describe the ways in which the behaviour of people with dementia (e.g. non-participation in social events, or non-adherence to social conventions) is constructed. Residents who did not have any cognitive impairment would describe dementia as being a 'release' from worries, particularly the distress of realising that they had become dependent and frail.

The study by Golander and Raz (1996) is fascinating in the way in which it describes the response of 'normal' residents to those with dementia, and for the questions it raises about the dynamics of relationships between residents. This moves us some way from the simplistic 'evaluation of outcomes' found in some studies, an endeavour that seems to have been singularly unsuccessful. Given the wide range of factors that may have a part to play in care, it seems unlikely that such studies can distinguish between them, and the strategy of comparing segregated and non-segregated units does little to overcome this problem, given the potential similarities across types of provision, and differences within types of provision. For practitioners working with people with dementia, research may more usefully focus on the processes of care, to make carers more aware of the dynamics of the relationships between people with dementia and those without, and how these can mediate the neurobiochemistry of cognitive impairment.

It is with the object of encouraging such research that this chapter has been written, and it is hoped that experts in dementia care will find it useful and thought-provoking. Although the study discussed below did not have an explicit focus on dementia care, the data it generated may help to inform debates on care for older people with dementia.

THE STUDY

The study was designed to follow a group of older people through the process of moving into a care home, in order to understand and articulate their experiences and views. In order to ensure, as far as possible, that the concerns and ideas of the older people in the study were given precedence over those of researchers, the study had a relatively unstructured qualitative approach and centred on sustained interaction with older people over a lengthy period.

The research schedule comprised a sequence of interviews with older people which followed them through the process of moving into care homes, beginning with interviews before the move, and three subsequent to it, ending when the research participant had been in the care home approximately 6 months (Table 8.1). The emphasis of the interviews was on developing life histories and personal narratives of residents, in order to produce data to illuminate these processes, and to place them in the context of previous life experiences. This approach, as Humphrey (1993) has stated, uses the notion of 'social career' to analyse life experiences and changes in lifestyle, and avoids the dangers of treating research participants as 'ahistorical', in other words that their meaningful experiences are confined to the duration of the study, and that the experiences observed in the study have no link with prior experiences. The interviews were augmented by two other exercises in both the first and last sessions. In the first exercise participants were to choose an image of their home (or the care home if it was the last interview) which to them summed up their experience there, a view that they felt would be a good souvenir of that place. In the second exercise participants were asked to draw a map of their relationships with friends or family, discussing who was close to them. With both of these exercises, the analysis centred not so much on the photographs or maps as data in themselves, but on the discussion that they stimulated, which was recorded as part of the interview.

A second strand to the study consisted of focus group meetings with staff from the homes involved in the research. These occasions were used to present to the staff some of the ideas generated by the interviews, and to invite their comments. As an aim of the study was to establish how the staff as a group saw their work, collecting people together to discuss these issues seemed appropriate. Group interviews show how groups interact and share ideas, whereas individual interviews only give individual perspectives. Kitzinger (1994) describes the advantages of forming focus groups like these where people are known to one another. She notes that

Table 8.1	*Sequence of interviews*
Interview	Focus
A	Pre-admission interviews using life history methodology Network maps and photographs
B and C	Early post-admission interviews – experiences of moving and strategies for coping. Interviews conducted in first 2 weeks after admission and at 6–8 weeks after admission, when the trial period of residence ends and a decision has to be made by the resident about whether to stay
D	Final post-admission interviews – summary of adjustment, evaluation of home-making and relationship-forming Network maps and photographs

such groups represent to some extent the naturally occurring context of everyday discussion of issues. She therefore proposes that such groups and the analysis of the interaction between participants provide an insight into language and the construction of ideas that is normally only available through participant observation techniques.

The early staff group meetings began when the resident study was well established, and some of the data from this were used to guide the staff discussion. These topics included the staff's perceptions of the ways in which residents settled in and the development of relationships. The later focus groups took place when the resident study had been completed, and possible changes in practice were presented to the staff groups for their comments.

The study sample

The study identified prospective residents awaiting places in nursing and residential homes for older people. Because of the logistic problems involved in this process, the decision was made to restrict the study to one local authority area, and to identify a number of homes within this. This strategy meant that the research team had to liaise with only one team of social workers, and a small number of home managers. The local authority area chosen was one containing two small towns and a number of small villages, originally built around coal mines. The population is extremely stable, and reflects the whole range of social groups.

In order to access a range of clients with different care needs, and homes with differing levels of staff input into patient care, the sample of six homes was selected from the residential care sector, the nursing home sector and the dual-registered sector (Table 8.2). The homes were all of a similar size, with 30–40 residents; those run by the local authority were in buildings that were less than 30 years old, whilst the privately run homes were in converted large houses. The homes were selected from lists supplied by local inspectors who were asked to identify places where the care was, in their opinion, of a high standard and where staff would be able to contribute to discussions about moving into care homes based on their awareness of this process. It was felt that in order to explore the ways in which older people could be supported through this process, placing the study in environments where it was likely that some such attempts had already been made would facilitate conversations about strategies and issues. This selection technique could be criticised as leading to an unrepresentative sample, but with only six homes in the study the goal of being 'representative' was not pursued, and the study's strategy came closer to ideas of 'theoretical sampling' as promoted by Glaser and Strauss (1967), where settings and participants are chosen for the potential they have to develop theoretical understanding of the issues or phenomena being studied.

Table 8.2	Homes recruited to the study	
Provision	Management	No. of participants recruited
Residential home	Private	6
Residential home	Local authority	6
Dual-registered	Private	10
Nursing home	Private	6
Nursing home	Private	6
Residential home	Local authority	7

Potential research participants were selected from the waiting lists for these homes, and were contacted prior to arrival via their local authority care managers or, in the case of self-funding residents, through the home managers. The target sample size was 30 residents (five from each home), but as attrition rates were likely to be high given the age and frailty of the sample, 41 participants were recruited to the study, and from this group five withdrew and one participant died.

Of all prospective residents, those who were able to understand the purpose of the interview and who could converse without serious difficulty were invited to participate. The notion of 'serious difficulty' was based on a pragmatic definition of ability to contribute to the study. In order to talk to people about the experience of moving to a new home, we needed to include people who were oriented to time, place and person. This degree of orientation also afforded some degree of assurance that the consent that they gave to participation in the study was sound and informed – see Reed and Payton (1996a) for a more detailed discussion. This means that the study did not involve people with significant degrees of dementia, although some of our participants did display some cognitive problems, and some were 'officially' diagnosed as having dementia at a later date. These official diagnoses were usually made when home managers or care managers called in specialist services to assess people whose behaviour was causing concern. The researchers were not party to these assessments, and often only found out about them in the course of casual conversations with staff. This means that there was no way of systematically checking the diagnoses of those who participated in the study or their fellow residents, and for this reason they could only be described as 'confused', based on participants' evaluations, rather than a more precise diagnostic term. The admission policy of the homes did not exclude people with dementia, but they did not provide any degree of specialised care for people with cognitive problems.

The intention was to conduct two focus groups with staff at each home in the study, but this was not always possible owing to the unavailability of staff. Ten focus groups were conducted, however, with all grades of staff invited to participate. The groups involved between three and six members of staff; only one group included a manager, the others being composed of carers whose training, where it existed, was based on National Vocational Qualifications.

Data analysis

As interviews were transcribed they were entered into a qualitative data analysis package (NUDIST) and coded. The initial coding framework was simply based on the topics discussed in the interviews, i.e. units of analysis were coded according to whether they discussed one or more topics. Some of these topics were derived from the interview agenda, but using the package it was possible to identify topics that were introduced by the participants, and were to some extent unexpected or not anticipated by the interviewers, such as relationships with other residents. Such introductions suggest that the interviews, while focused, did not exclude or prevent the concerns and interests of participants from being voiced, and that the researchers' prejudices and concerns did not completely overshadow the concerns and views of participants.

In examining what people said about these areas it was possible to develop theoretical categories that crossed over topics, such as 'settling in' processes which involved environmental and interpersonal dimensions. It was also possible, using codes to identify participants, to track the development of these themes throughout the interview sequence, and to identify processes over time. By using the same analytic framework for the focus group data it was also possible to compare remarks by residents and staff about the same aspects of life in care homes.

The analysis was wide-ranging, covering all of the topics that people had talked about. From this, the data presented in this chapter focus on those areas most pertinent to the issue of living with fellow residents who are confused: firstly, the importance of relationships with other residents – see Golander and Raz (1996) and Reed and Payton (1996b) for a fuller discussion – and secondly the complexities of relationships with residents who are confused.

RESULTS

Relationships with other residents

One of the most important concerns of the residents was the area of relationships with other residents. Whilst staff remained as benevolent but shadowy figures in many conversations, interactions with other residents were much more vividly described. Many of these descriptions concerned the support and help that residents offered each other, ranging from opportunities to participate in social activities to practical information about how to negotiate the routines of the home. Sometimes, however, relationships with other residents could be stressful or acrimonious, with conflicts and disagreements between residents. Whether positive or negative, however, these relationships were a major topic of conversation in interviews.

This importance can be explained partly on pragmatic grounds – as residents spend only brief periods with staff or visitors, and much longer periods in lounges or dining rooms with their fellow residents, it is logical that the relationships that occupy most of their time should dominate the conversation. At a more theoretical level, however, these relationships may also be important in the way that they maintain a sense of self in residents. By engaging in social interaction they present themselves as social beings, with personal histories and identities, and social activity becomes a medium for maintaining continuity with the self before the move, and of establishing a social self within the community of the care home (Reed and Payton, 1996b).

Relationships with confused residents

Some themes emerging from these data call into question the desirability of people with different problems living together, both for those who are not confused, and for those who are. These themes involve a range of responses and feelings which participants articulated, and indicate a degree of ambivalence about living with confused people.

In the interviews quoted in the following text, 'P' denotes 'participant' and 'R' 'researcher'.

Sadness

The central theme that was apparent was a sense of sadness, especially if people knew the confused person before and there was a comparison made between past and present. One woman, for example, described seeing someone that she knew when he came into the lounge for a musical evening at the home:

P: He lived in C—, he had a job singing. And we had a Salvation Army band, singers last night, and he came down in the wheelchair but he didn't know anybody, poor soul. I know him from me Sunday School days. I was married in the church that he went to.

R: Oh right, so was it nice to see a familiar face?

P: Oh, yes, it was. But there again. I suppose it was nice but it wasn't familiar to him. To me, he didn't know it was me.

R: Right, is that a bit sad?

P: It is, it is very sad. I mean I can go around now and meet people. I can go 'Oh, hello', but he didn't make an answer, no request, or answer, last night.

Another woman described the behaviour of someone who had lived in the same sheltered accommodation facility as herself, emphasising the differences in her acquaintance's behaviour between then and now:

P: And one poor soul, well she gets out, you see. She wants to be on the wander all of the time, she was never like that. She used to come to Jubilee Court and play dominoes with us. She knows you one minute then the next minute, like.

R: That must be upsetting to see.

P: Well, it does upset you, like.

Sometimes the sadness of confused people 'depressed' others, but often this seemed to be partly caused by the fears that this gave rise to for their own future, or in the way that confused people made visible and explicit concerns or feelings that they kept hidden. One participant, for example, when asked about his own feelings, referred immediately to the expressions of feeling emanating from confused residents, and in addition speculated on the possibility of himself becoming confused:

R: Mmm ... but this place, does it feel like home?

P: No, it doesn't to a lot of the old people that are here. They cry and they come and say, 'I want to go home,' when they meet you in the corridors and that. There's a few very, very funny, poor old souls. Worse than me because their brains have gone as well. Mine are going.

R: I don't think so.

P: But not quite yet.

For some participants the fear of becoming confused was ever present, evoked by the sight of confused residents – regardless of their behaviour, their mere presence was a reminder of the possible fate in store for others. One participant, when talking about other residents, reflected on this:

P: Oh yes, they are all nice, but there are some poor things, half asleep and I think my goodness, if I got like that, I would think why didn't

God take me before. I mean, why didn't he take me when I had this funny turn and let some of the younger ones live. It's not fair.

Keeping a distance

The possibility of future dementia was expressly denied by some who were at pains to emphasise that there was a great deal of difference between themselves and those who were confused, that these people were not like them. Defining the differences in their conversations with the interviewers was intended to establish them as not being confused. For example, one participant was very concerned that the interviewer would think that she was confused:

P: There's a lot who are confused, you know, they're daft. I hope you don't think I am, mind. I might be in here, but I've still got my wits about me.

Others, however, simply expressed distress at being with people who were confused because of the social isolation that they felt:

P: I've cried for hours, hinny, but I will get over it, won't I? These people down here are not what I thought they were, hinny. You know I thought I was coming into a home where there was people like myself.

This was also evident in comments people made about not being able to have conversations with confused people. Relationships with other residents were important as a means of establishing social identity, as discussed earlier, and this could not happen with people who were confused. The comments were, however, often non-judgmental, as though people could not be blamed for their confusion. One participant, for example, was careful to emphasise the 'niceness' of confused fellow residents:

R: What about the other people in here, did you say there's some nice people that you can talk to?

P: There is. There's some that you can talk to, but of course there's quite a lot that's the other way, that, that, er, they're all quite ... at the bottom of them they're all nice people, but of course you can't sometimes get a sensible conversation with them.

Another resident was keen to absolve confused residents of any 'blame' for their condition:

P: Because, well, there is three, three I have never spoken to.

R: Why is that?

P: Well, they are not, cannot get no sense out of them, you know what I mean.

R: Oh, are they a bit confused?

P: It's not their fault, you know.

Another resident suggested that confused fellow residents were not only blameless, but were actively fighting their condition:

P: So, anyway, and then after that, nice little bit chat to the six people that were at my table, five people that were at my table, I got on very nicely chatting with them. It was surprising how from little bits of conversation they were alright but the other people in the other dining room were a little bit ... er, well, they were there because their minds were going, and that's sad and that's what. They were all doing their best, don't let me be critical.

When pointing out differences between themselves and confused fellow residents, participants were engaged in establishing their own, non-confused identity. In the examples above these distancing statements were accompanied by riders which also absolved confused residents of any blame or responsibility for their condition, raising the possibility that participants may have been anticipating their own possible decline, and absolving themselves as well.

Caring

An extension of this permissive and sympathetic stance was demonstrated in descriptions that some residents gave of the ways in which they 'cared' for fellow residents who were confused. Again, the action of caring makes explicit the non-dependent role of the carer, and is a way of emphasising difference. This was particularly the case for participants who had formerly been nurses, as talking about the way they cared for others also evoked their previous occupation and status. One woman, for example, who had worked in a hospital described herself as drawing on this previous experience, and not only pointed out the differences between herself and her confused room-mate, but also between herself and her non-confused, non-qualified fellow residents:

P: And she's very unruly, in fact I don't think she should be in here, it's not just me she's annoying, it's the ones next door, you see, they can't get any sleep. Well, last night they were knocking on the wall, but there's no need to knock on the wall because I could do nothing about it and she was running about at half-past three this morning, half asleep. It's just the condition she's in you see … with working at [the hospital] when I realised what she was and there's nothing … they live among themselves, them at [the hospital], if they make a noise it doesn't annoy them at all, you see, but I think the ones next door's getting a bit sick of it.

Participants who had not had nursing experience also differentiated between their own enlightened approach and that of others. One participant explained the need for tolerance in the following way:

R: What about some of the residents who are confused?

P: Well, you have just got to talk and decide whether or not, you know, and try and put them in the picture and one thing and another, that's what I do. It's no good shouting, one or two of them have to be shouted at like, he is very, very, impatient, so they do get annoyed with him at times, they think that's the way they [should] use him, but I don't, I'm sitting talking to him, me.

In many of the descriptions of 'caring' approaches there were some phrases which were quite explicitly parental, and which presented confused residents as being child-like. One woman, for example, talked about her room-mate as if she were a little girl:

P: We talk as they talk, you see, if she talks that way, I just talk to her back and tell her she's pretty and things like that. If you see her dressed in anything, you know. Sometimes she's naughty and she shouts, but we had a good night last night, she never moved last night until about half-past five.

The consequences of this parentalism are, of course, potentially demeaning for people who are confused, in the way that it belittles their actions and makes what they say seem like the inconsequential chatter of a child. For the resident who adopts the parental role, however, there can be many benefits in terms of their own self-image. While much caring seems to be done from genuinely altruistic motives, like many acts of charity, there is an implicit payback for the giver in terms of enhanced status and esteem. One participant, who had 'adopted' a confused fellow-resident, was quite open about this:

P: Well, I've really taken to her, you know, she's a canny little thing, no harm in her, and she just looks so lost. I look after her, you know, see she eats and everything. Well, it gives me something to do, you know, makes me feel useful. And I often think, well, you should be grateful you're not like that.

Benevolence then, could have elements of infantilisation in it, and for some of the people who were 'adopted' by non-confused residents, life might well have been better if their adopter had left them alone instead of constantly supervising and directing their activities. Caring approaches were, however, largely altruistic, and afforded a substantial degree of tolerance and sympathy for those who were confused.

Hostility

Sometimes, however, residents expressed hostility, especially if there had been incidents of conflict or intrusion. The behaviour of some confused people sometimes flouted social conventions, and for those who were trying to negotiate the new social world of the care home, this could be extremely disconcerting and they could react angrily. One participant, for example, related the story of a social gaffe he had unwittingly committed:

R: Is it quite difficult to get to know people, then?

P: Well, well, I thought this woman was talking to us today and I just tapped her on the shoulder – 'Ooh', she says, 'don't touch me, don't punch me.' I thought, oh well, shut up.

R: And was she talking to you?

P: No, I thought she was, but she maybe just mumbling on to herself and I thought, oh, was she wanting something, you know. I didn't mean any harm, there was no need for her to shout like that. Well, bugger her.

Sometimes, however, it was a confused person who committed a social sin, such as coming into another person's room uninvited or interfering with their belongings. One participant talked about his mother's experience with a confused resident (both mother and son were residents in the home), and while disclaiming any anger on his own part, expressed some determination to protect his mother:

P: Aye, well, do you know what happened, last time she went into me mother's room, five o'clock in the morning, asked me mother if she'd had her breakfast yet, it was five o'clock in the morning. Well, she goes to everybody's room, she goes to everybody's room.

R: You just put up with that?

P: Aye, I just put up with it. Just doesn't bother me, man.

R: Mind, it is a strange thing to happen.

P: I mean to say if she does it again, I'll have her. I'll stop her, though.

Another resident was more forthright about his views of a confused resident who kept coming into his room:

R: So did she come in?

P: Yes, man, I tell you she's always in here, messing about. I told her 'get to hell, you stupid woman'.

R: So did she go away?

P: Aye, but she'll be back, but I've got me stick, that'll learn her, if she feels that.

Experience of exclusion

Not having access to the participants' medical notes, the interviewers often did not know whether the residents who participated in the study had been diagnosed as having Alzheimer's disease or any other form of dementia. However, a number of the people interviewed seemed to be experiencing some short-term memory problems, and their orientation seemed tenuous at times. These people provided some accounts of the experience of being confused in a home where there are non-confused residents. These accounts are few, but they do indicate that for some confused residents, their experience is largely one of exclusion. One woman who was later diagnosed as having Alzheimer's disease told us of her feelings about her confusion in an interview shortly after she had moved into a home:

R: Do you get a bit confused sometimes?

P: Oh! definitely. Definitely. I'm away with the mixer sometimes. [laughter] I am.

R: I suppose we all are at times.

P: Oh! thank you. [R and P laughter]

R: But you're finding it a problem feeling confused?

P: Terrible, I feel as I don't want to live, I'll tell you that much.

One of the reasons that this person felt that she did not want to live was loneliness. She felt that no-one wanted to talk to her, and that all overtures she made were rebuffed:

R: Oh, right, so have you not managed to get chatting with the other people who live here?

P: I never bothered; mind, I'm not going to say I could, because I can't.

R: You can't, why is that?

P: They just don't want you.

R: Do they not?

P: No, they want their own friends. They don't want somebody like me.

R: How do you mean?

P: Well, they don't want someone mixed up.

This participant had serious problems in mixing with other residents, not only because she felt unable to function competently and break down the barriers that other residents had put up, but also because her responses to this rejection compounded the problem. She became angry and emotionally labile which further embarrassed other residents. The staff came to see her as a trouble-maker, and when she approached other residents they would intervene, offering to take her away if she was 'bothering them'. This happened on one occasion when one of the researchers had visited her and was sitting with her in the lounge. A member of staff came up and apologised to the researcher for the participant's behaviour, commenting that 'she's always bothering people'. The staff member took some convincing that the researcher did want to talk to the participant.

Staff responses

The staff response detailed above seemed to stem from a concern that non-confused residents would be bothered by those who were confused, but in the discussions with staff in focus groups this seemed to be a somewhat unusual response. Many of the staff, when discussing residents, seemed to be quite comfortable in approaching care with the least able as the template or norm on which their actions were based. In one focus group, for example, we asked a question about residents' relationships with each other, and received this answer:

> We've got to remember a lot of them are confused, and you know you can say something and somebody only has to walk through that door and they'll look and when they look back to you it's gone [the memory of what has been said].

The anxiety that participants demonstrated about being seen as confused may come from many things, but seems likely to be exacerbated by staff attitudes like this. Staff frequently commented that most people were confused, or that they did not make distinctions between residents in the interests of egalitarianism: 'You have to treat them all the same, so that you're fair'. In other staff discussions, where distinctions were made, staff felt that confused people were treated unfairly, and they castigated residents for their intolerance. It seemed that non-confused residents would not be supported in disputes, as the sympathies of the staff were with the 'less fortunate'. In one group, a member of staff described the dynamics as she saw them:

> Well, they're very fickle, you know, you've got to watch them. They'll be all over them one day, you know, cutting up their food and doing their hair. The next day, they'll be bored, they don't want to know. And you'll see the demented ones just standing there, lost. It breaks your heart, it's cruel.

Such an approach, whilst it may have the merits of siding with 'the underdog', does not betray much sensitivity to the position of the non-confused residents, whose treatment of confused fellows may well reflect their sense of eroded identity, a sense created partly through the staff ethos of 'treating everybody the same'.

Where staff had developed strategies for managing conflict between confused and non-confused residents, these seemed to be based on unofficial forms of segregation, by placing residents in different lounges during the day, or sleeping areas at night. This, however, seemed to be also a strategy for observing and supervising confused residents. The lounges they sat in or the bedrooms that they slept in were close to the staff offices, or in self-contained areas where staff could be stationed. As covert and unobtrusive management strategies they were a dismal failure (in every home in the study residents could tell us where the 'confused lounge' was) and whilst they may have reduced conflict between groups of residents because there was less contact between them, these strategies did little to explore the feelings of residents about living together under one roof.

DISCUSSION

The data from this study, whilst limited, raise some interesting questions about the non-specialised care home as a place for both confused and non-confused people to live together. The view that this has a normalising effect on confused people is challenged by the mechanisms for exclusion and control used by other residents. Confused residents may be excluded from 'normal' social activities, and only allowed to participate in limited roles developed for them by others, for example the role of the helpless, child-like recipient of care. This does not seem to be a therapeutic environment for confused people, and indeed may be very limiting for them. For people who are not confused, living with those who are creates other dangers, mainly that their mental functioning may be called into question, and they will be seen as confused like their fellow residents. Their response to the presence of confused fellow residents may take the form of benevolent caring, parentalism or hostility, but all of these responses can be seen as mechanisms for maintaining distance and difference between themselves and others. If these mechanisms are also seen as a strategy for maintaining personal identity then they would seem to be inevitable, especially as staff recognition of identity is limited.

A circular pattern can be identified, which, albeit crudely, does demonstrate some of the processes revealed in this study. Non-confused residents are made anxious by the presence of those who are confused, and in their anxiety to distance themselves from those who are confused, use strategies that the staff disapprove of as being unfair. In their determination to be fair and to support those who are confused, staff condemn rather than try to understand the behaviour of the non-confused, and explicitly make no difference between the groups, thus increasing the anxiety of the non-confused residents.

This seems to be paving the way for some sort of segregationist policy, advocating that confused and non-confused people should be cared for in different facilities. This policy does have some merits for those who are confused, in that they can receive skilled, specialist care in an environment that does not exclude or infantilise them. For those who are not confused, a source of irritation is removed, and their identity as competent people is not challenged. There are, however, problems with this policy, not least for those who are on the borderline between the two groups. For those who are in the early stages of dementia, or who are anxious in case they will develop dementia in the future, the 'moving on' of those with cognitive problems can be both disruptive and distressing. Moving to a new environment is stressful at the best of times, but if one is feeling frail and disoriented then the impact is likely to be greater. Similarly, for those who worry about future dementia, the idea that their security of residence depends on maintaining cognitive ability is a frightening one: dementia then carries two sets of dangers, firstly that it will involve some sort of suffering, and secondly that it will mean being removed to some special facility, which is unlikely to be familiar or known.

These are reasons for leaving the care of people with mild or early dementia in the mainstream system for care of older people, and the lack of evidence that specialised facilities have clear therapeutic benefit adds weight to the argument. There are, however, a number of implications for such 'mixed care' which arise from the dynamics of the relationships between residents, and which carers would do well to be aware of. Firstly, there is the potential for distress that the presence of people with dementia may cause in those without cognitive impairment. People with dementia may provoke feelings of sadness, hostility or fear, and responses that are less than caring. Even when the responses are sympathetic, excessive infantilisation of those with dementia can be countertherapeutic. Understanding the dynamics behind these responses, however, can help staff to intervene constructively and avoid compounding problems. Understanding the perceived need to make a distinction between 'us' and 'them', as Kitwood (1993) describes it, focuses attention on the needs of those without dementia to have their personhood respected and their sense of self supported. Simply treating everyone the same, in some strange version of fairness, is not likely to be helpful, and may even reinforce anxiety and hostility. Treating people with dementia less preferably is one possible (and possibly quite common) way for staff to differentiate between residents, but this is counterproductive, not only in its impact on the quality of life for those with dementia, but also in the way that it reinforces ideas of dementia as being something to be afraid of. The consequences may be seen by those without dementia as an automatic reduction in care and respect.

In conclusion, then, I can only appeal, as so many have done before, for those caring for all older people to respect and protect their personhood and sense of self. More particularly, however, I suggest that a failure to understand the dynamics of relationships between residents with and without dementia is not only likely to lead to non-therapeutic practice, but is also a manifestation and reinforcement of the 'ageist' view that expectations of all older people should be low, and that they are all the same. It is simply making the distinction between 'us' and 'them' in a different way – not between those with and those without dementia, but between older people and younger people.

Acknowledgments

This study was funded by the Department of Health with the award of a Postdoctoral Research Fellowship to Jan Reed. The research staff on the project were Jane Macmillan and Dr Valerie Roskell Payton.

REFERENCES

Burgner, T. (1996) *The Regulation and Inspection of Social Services*. London: Department of Health Welsh Office.
Davison, N. & Reed, J. (1995) One foot on the escalator: elderly people in sheltered accommodation. In: Heyman, B. (ed.) *Researching User Perspectives on Community Health Care*. London: Chapman & Hall.
Douglas, M. (1991) *Purity and Danger*. London: Routledge.
Eley, R. & Middleton, L. (1983) Square pegs, round holes. The appropriateness of providing care for old people in residential settings. *Health Trends* **15**, 68–70.

Glaser, B.G. & Strauss, A.L. (1967) *The Discovery of Grounded Theory: Strategies for Qualitative Research*. Chicago: Aldine Press.

Golander, H. & Raz, A.E. (1996) The mask of dementia: images of demented residents in a nursing ward. *Ageing and Society* **16**, 269–285.

Humphrey, R. (1993) Life stories and social careers: ageing and social life in an ex-mining town. *Sociology* **27**, 166–178.

Kitwood, T. (1990) The dialectics of dementia: with particular reference to Alzheimer's disease. *Ageing and Society* **10**, 177–195.

Kitwood, T. (1993) Towards a theory of dementia care: the interpersonal process. *Ageing and Society* **13**, 51–67.

Kitzinger, J. (1994) Qualitative research. Introducing focus groups. *British Medical Journal* **311**, 299–302.

Meacher, M. (1972) *Taken for a Ride: Special Residential Homes for Confused Old People. A Study of Separatism in Social Policy*. London: Longman.

Ohta, R.J. & Ohta, B.M. (1988) Special units for Alzheimer's disease patients: a critical look. *Gerontologist* **28**, 803–808.

Preston-Thomas, H. (1901) Report in 13th Annual Report of the Local Government Board, p. 122–123. London.

Reed, J. & Payton, V.R. (1996a) Past the age of consent? A discussion of some ethical issues arising in a study involving older people. *Health Care in Later Life* **1**, 51–62.

Reed, J. & Payton, V.R. (1996b) *Working to Create Continuity: Older People Managing the Move to the Care Home Setting*. Report No. 76. Centre for Health Services Research, University of Newcastle.

Royal Commission on the Law relating to Mental Illness and Mental Deficiency (1957) Report. Cmnd 169. London: HMSO.

Sabat, S.R. & Harré, R. (1992) The construction and deconstruction of self in Alzheimer's disease. *Ageing and Society* **12**, 443–461.

US Congress Office of Technology Assessment (1992) *Special Care Units for People with Alzheimer's and other Dementias: Consumer Education, Research, Regulatory and Reimbursement Issues*. OTA-H-543. Washington: US Government Printing Office.

Webber, P.A. Breuer, W. & Lindeman, D.A. (1995) Alzheimer's special care units vs integrated nursing homes: a comparison of resident outcomes. *Journal of Clinical Geropsychology* **1**, 189–205.

Wilkins, D. & Hughes, B. (1987) Residential care of elderly people: the consumers' views. *Ageing and Society* **7**, 175–201.

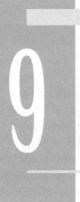

The family caring experiences of married women in dementia care

Christine E. Carter

KEY ISSUES

- Research addressing married women's experiences of caring for a husband with dementia is characterised by a lack of attention to their complex support needs

- This chapter illustrates particular disadvantages experienced by female spouses: limited support services were justified through discrimination based on the carers' marital status

- The caring experience is characterised by loss and change; carers became isolated, and marital relationships changed as their partner became their dependant

- Psychological pressure was experienced by women caring for a husband with dementia, through both the caring experience and the illness itself

- Complex social and psychological factors influenced women's decisions to care for their husband with dementia, thereby confounding simplistic theorising

INTRODUCTION

This chapter presents the results of a qualitative study that explored the experiences of married women providing full-time care for their husbands with dementia. This small-scale study conducted in the north of Britain involved interviewing women about their experiences of caring. A grounded theory approach was adopted in order to explore the complexity of this experience. The chapter begins with a summary of related research, examining the role of married women within family care. The methodology adopted is described, followed by the results of the study. The results are discussed with the aid of a case study and the conclusions focus on support issues. Finally, recommendations for practice and research are considered.

There appears to be a broadly based consensus in Britain that care in the community is good, care at home is better and care by the family is best (Webb and Tossell, 1991). Both within government policy and society, the unspecified link that ties the notion of 'community' to that of 'care' is women (Bornat et al, 1993). Despite the romantic image of family care, it can entail considerable disadvantages for both sides of the caring relationship, especially for married women who care for a husband who has senile dementia. However, a national survey confirmed that this social relationship provides the setting for most caring relationships (Green, 1988). The marital relationship within caring appears to create a complexity which presents problems for researchers (Twigg, 1989). The enormous social and psychological pressures on women to care for their husband, if required, appear to cloud any theorising regarding the uniqueness of this relationship, when their partner becomes their dependant (Parker, 1990a).

COMMUNITY CARE AND THE NOTION OF THE FAMILY CARER

The community is now established as the optimum environment in which to deliver health care and – more equivocally – as the most cost-effective form of care (Barret, 1992). 'Community' has been inextricably linked to 'care' in that they are perceived to link together naturally, and in turn 'care' has been inextricably linked to the notion of family. Debate continues as to whether this means care *by* the community or care *in* the community. It has been argued that the family can be represented as a truly human and supreme form of community care (Webb and Tossell, 1991). However, it is generally agreed that care in the community actually means care by women (Finch and Mason, 1990; Hammell, 1992; Lee, 1993). Although of the 6.8 million carers in Britain, 2.9 million are men, women still shoulder the major burden of family care (Parker and Lawton, 1994). Men are more likely to give financial assistance than be involved in physical and emotional tasks (Parker, 1990b; Suitor and Pillemer 1993). The 'family carer' therefore becomes synonymous with the 'female carer' – that is, the wife, the mother or the daughter.

Family care within marriage

Central to the effective implementation of community care policy are the kinship obligations amongst family networks. Analysis of family care has revealed a hierarchy of caring. Women are put under specific emotional and psychological pressure to care which is compounded by normative societal expectations and where the cost of not caring is guilt (Qureshi and Walker, 1989). This hierarchy of care has been viewed as a method of negotiation, in which women's role in the maintenance of family relationships is central. Finch and Mason (1990) have termed this as 'kin keeping'. These authors agree that the hierarchy of obligation is most definitive in the case of spouse carers. When caring for one's husband, the pressure from social bonds of duty are further compounded by emotional feelings of love and affection. The shift created when 'caring about' becomes 'caring for' has been termed a 'labour of love' (Graham, 1983). The former is to do with feelings for another person, the latter is related to carrying out tasks for another person. Most probably a true dichotomy does not occur, but rather both terms coexist within the caring experience, although this complexity is rarely acknowledged by health professionals.

Spouse carers have not received the same attention from researchers as other carers. This is possibly the result of assumptions held about the unitary nature of marriage and marital relationships. However, Parker (1990b) provides some insights into the specific relationship problems women experience when caring for their husbands. She highlights the loss of a relationship between equals that makes caring for a spouse so difficult. Hammell (1992) describes the social expectations of women's role in the provision of care. These expectations have not only reinforced women's role in the provision of care but have also traditionally maintained that role within the private sphere (Larrabee, 1993). This has resulted in limited care options being available to women who care: for example, caring for one's husband is either undertaken at home or within an institution, the latter being an unthinkable option for many women (Hammell, 1992). Rather than relinquishing their role as a wife, many women choose to care for their husbands at home through a combination of love, duty and obligation.

Although spouses may be happy to care reciprocally for each other, society generally assumes that this is an implicit part of the marriage contract. In so doing community services often underestimate or ignore the support needs of women caring for a husband with dementia. The decision to care for a partner who has dementia may also be influenced by a need to create a sense of control and normality over an increasingly chaotic situation. Dementia can create behavioural problems such as poor concentration, wandering and disorientation. However, one of the most distressing problems for a wife can occur when her husband's memory impairment results in sexual disinhibition, for example when her partner has forgotten appropriate intimate behaviour (Mace, 1990). Witnessing one's partner's change in personality, mood and behaviour exacerbates feelings, and relationships naturally become more intense (Wright, 1993).

Theories of women within family care

Historically, women's roles within familial care were first considered by Marx who focused on the private domain, examining how women reproduce and maintain health within the familial context (Haralambos, 1991). The 1980s onwards witnessed an upsurge in feminist literature which has explored, through role socialisation theories, the social divisions in which caring occurs. These theories were developed in conjunction with a growing feminist critique of community care. Finch and Groves (1980) criticised community care as intensifying inequalities already experienced by women. They believed that more women were caregivers owing to the gender role expectations of society. According to Scheyett (1990), the strength of these social pressures and the cultural assumption of women's 'natural' role as caregivers results in many women overidentifying with the caregiving role. Feminist literature has established caring as central to the experience of women and a form of oppression within Western culture, a culture that demands that women care but does not acknowledge the value of caregiving tasks (Ungerson, 1987; Dalley, 1988; Scheyett, 1990; Baldwin and Twigg, 1991).

Central to these studies is an emphasis on the socioeconomic costs borne by women carers. However, a growing number of feminist researchers have also examined the psychological aspects of the caring relationship. Carol Gilligan's theory on moral reasoning (Gilligan, 1982) is directly related to Jean Piaget's work on psychological development. Gilligan observed that women's sense of morality is mediated through the wish not to hurt others by fulfilling an altruistic need to care. The different explanations of the reasons why women choose to care were united in an essay by Hillary Graham. Graham (1983) points out that psychologists look to the affective components of caring and its peculiar attachment within femininity, whilst social policy analysts consider the function of family care within capitalism and patriarchy. Graham concludes that 'caring defines both the identity and the activity of women' (Graham, 1983). However, the situation is more complex than that initially described by Graham. Ungerson (1987) describes how for women, caring within the family often involves a complex process of duty, role and obligation whilst fulfilling a female identity. This process is further complicated by the situation of women caring for their husbands. The social norms and values attached to the marital relationship determine that a female spouse has an unquestioned responsibility to care for her husband. This becomes translated into her unquestioned ability to care, regardless of the situation or level of dependency or need.

Support networks of the female spouse carer

The complexity of the caring experience in relation to female spouse carers and support networks has been inadequately studied. The 1985 General Household Survey of Britain (Green, 1988) provided valuable data on support services utilised by carers. However, this survey is characterised by a traditional focus on dependants rather than carers and a lack of consideration for the emotional aspects of support. Particular problems stem from the normative ties of obligations surrounding a wife's role in caring for her husband, which as previously stated appears to be unquestionable within society. This results in the care and support needs of the carer not being addressed, as it is believed that the care they provide should be unconditional (Twigg, 1989). The strength and ties these obligations hold within marriage complicate the caring relationship further, by creating complex interpersonal dynamics. These dynamics appear to affect carers' expectations and levels of support (Collins et al, 1994). In reality this means that of all carers, female spouse carers receive the lowest levels of support. Evidence from the General Household Survey (1985) shows that the probability of an unmarried male carer receiving practical support is nearly two-thirds higher than that of a female carer who is married (Parker and Lawton, 1994).

Married women who take on the caring role may have to take on responsibility for many aspects of running a household that have been unfamiliar to them. Pre-existing roles are challenged, where before there may have been a very traditional division of labour in their marriages (Land, 1991). Older women may well be unfamiliar with household repairs, maintenance and financial affairs, creating an obvious need for practical support (Wright, 1993). This reversal of roles also involves a change in the balance of power within the relationship, accompanied by emotional stress, guilt and loss, creating further psychological support needs. However, these issues are often ignored and do not receive the consideration they deserve by health-care professionals.

The General Household Survey (1985) enquired about practical forms of support. However, interestingly, a study of spouse carers reveals how carers had a greater need for social activity rather than for practical interventions as a form of support (Parker, 1990a). Not only was social isolation the biggest burden for female spouse carers, but it also appeared to suppress their ability to express the need for support. The difficulties in distinguishing between caring tasks and obligations has been examined by Twigg and Atkin (1994). They observed that female spouses are not perceived as carers. This highlights the disparity in expectations placed on male and female spouses, characterised by a lack of theorising surrounding female spouse carers and their relationship with support services. The consequence of this is that insufficient attention is paid to their support needs.

THE STUDY

The research methodology

The study described here developed in response to my clinical observations while working as a community psychiatric nurse with older people who had dementia and their carers. Assumptions about levels of support were made by well-meaning health professionals, myself included. However, it became apparent through my contact with women caring for a husband with dementia that the levels of support offered did not address some of their specific needs. The aim of this study was therefore to elicit and explore the emotional context of caring, in relation to female spouses and support. Grounded theory is suitable for studying the social phenomenon of caring, and the multidimensional and complex nature of the caring experience quickly became apparent. Consequently such a broad aim was perhaps ambitious for the intended scale of the research. Any generalisations made from the study are made on the basis of the validity of inductive logic, rather than the representativeness of the sample.

The sample

Defining the sample

Identifying who carers are can be difficult. They are notoriously hard to find, as the nature of family caring is that it is done behind closed doors. Approaching statutory services was not as productive as one would imagine, because large numbers of carers never bring themselves to the attention of their local social service departments (Ungerson, 1987). Taking this into consideration, a sample selection criterion of belonging to a carers' support group was adopted as the best and easiest way of identifying carers for the study. However, this criterion naturally created a bias; one may regard the carers as being well-informed about services, and attendance at a support group for carers implies that they are already identifying with the caring role.

Locating the sample

Access was negotiated to 'Crossroads', a voluntary organisation for carers which ran a support group. Negotiations were made to attend the support group in person in order to avoid the problems of relying on postal consent, for example low response rates (Wright, 1986). Despite initial concerns about confidentiality, the project manager of Crossroads gave me permission to attend a support group. This provided an invaluable insight into the current issues and problems facing carers, and interview topics were therefore focused accordingly.

Obtaining the sample

A covering letter and consent form were distributed to all the female members of the support group. Stamped addressed envelopes were offered to avoid the pressure of an immediate response. Of the eight women attending the group, five signed the consent forms immediately and one replied by post. Respondents were given a full explanation of what was involved in the study: the interviews would be tape-recorded, last approximately 30–45 minutes, and would be undertaken at their convenience. All the respondents were happy to discuss the research and felt that it would be valuable. Feedback about the study was disseminated in a discussion with the carers and a report was circulated within the support group.

Of the six respondents, five were eventually interviewed. One carer's husband died and it was felt to be inappropriate to interview her. All the women in the sample were aged between 55 years and 70 years, and there was a wide range of social and caring circumstances. The mean length of time caring was 9 years, with a range of 6–18 years. All the dependants suffered from a dementing illness, the criterion adopted for this being a diagnosis from either their general practitioner or consultant which confirmed the presence of a dementia.

Data collection and analysis

Data collection

Data collection involved in-depth, semistructured interviews which were conducted in the informant's home, with the carer only. Open-ended questions were used as prompts and the interview was then directed by the informant's responses. Any distractions were minimised in order to increase receptivity. However, this was difficult to achieve when the dependant was in the same environment, hindering open discussion. After sensitive explanation with the carers, who were extremely amenable, arrangements were therefore made for the dependant to be at a day centre, in another room or with a relative when the interview occurred. Strict time limits of 30–45 minutes avoided interviews becoming exhausting for both parties. During the first interview questions started at a superficial level, but these increased in depth during subsequent interviews as relationships within the data were identified. Saturation was achieved when new data did not provide additional insights and at that point data collection was complete.

Data analysis using grounded theory

The process of data analysis involved open coding and axial coding. In open coding the social processes were broken down in order to examine, compare, conceptualise and categorise data. Data were categorised by identifying key words within the text which provided an understanding of the social processes within caring and therefore contributed to the emergence of codes. The frequency of key words within the transcripts qualified these emerging codes. Axial coding allowed data to be reassembled in new ways by making connections between categories through a 'coding paradigm'. However, addressing the categories in terms of the paradigm model as described by Strauss and Corbin (1990) was unsuccessful. The process of axial coding proved a difficult concept to grasp, and many ways of handling the data were tried before developing a method which was workable. The interrelationships of the data proved to be the main problem.

The small sample size and the complexity of the data resulted in categories overlapping under the axial coding headings. This meant that categories were not distinct and could be viewed as a limitation within the study, as the categories must be regarded as underdeveloped analytically. However, the paradigm features of axial coding were still considered to be useful. These were adapted in an attempt to link the categories analytically. Instead of a central category becoming the phenomenon within the paradigm, the 'caring experience' itself became the phenomenon. This allowed the development of a theoretical understanding of the social experience of female spouse carers and their levels of support.

RESULTS

In view of the qualitative nature of the data, the emergent categories are supported by extracts from interviews, giving a fuller understanding of each category and its grounding within the data. Analysis of the data revealed six categories which emerged as significant within the caring experience of female spouses:

- Pathways into care
- Medical services
- Support avenues
- Prerequisites of support
- Relationship change
- Lifestyle loss.

The caring experience of female spouses

Pathways into caring

This category describes the factors that influenced and determined the women's decisions to care for their husbands. Medical advice was a key factor in decisions to care for a husband at home: 'The doctor said "I think you could nicely take him home and we'll get you lots of support".'

Social roles and relationship bonds were also significant. Statements were characterised by positive feelings, as well as a sense of duty: 'Well, I mean we had been married forty years and we had always been close, I was his wife, it was my place'. This woman had been caring for her husband for 4 years and the most important factor in her decision to care was their length of time together. This emerged as a common pathway into caring for all the women interviewed.

Medical services

This category demonstrates an involvement between the women and the medical services (made up of health professionals) through and on behalf of their husbands. It involved processes of control and negotiation when their husbands entered the medical services and became a 'patient'. Carers and doctors exercised varying degrees of authority in relation to care for the dependant, whether through their role as legal partner, or as a professional practitioner with a duty to care. This was invariably fraught with conflict and created a sense of instability within the caring situation, which was characterised by both negative and positive experiences and appeared to be a common situation shared by all the women.

> The doctor come and he said, 'You seen the state your man's in, we'll send him away,' and I said, 'No, you're not.' 'We propose to transfer him from here to [the hospital] to a geriatric ward.' I said, 'What! He's not going there.' The doctor said, 'No? So what do you propose, then?' I said, 'He's coming home.' He said, 'Who else is there at home?' I said, 'Nobody.' He said, 'Well, you can't do it by yourself.' I said, 'Why not?' and he said, 'Well, for a start he's got a permanent body catheter in.' Well, I'd never had any contact with anybody like that and I didn't know what was involved, nobody explained it to me, but I still said, 'Oh no, he's coming home'!

The medical services defined dependance and many women felt unable to question or challenge doctor's statements in the manner shown by the previous quote.

Support networks

This category describes the support avenues that were available to carers, covering statutory and non-statutory services, friends and relatives, and also the home environment and aids to caring. Nursing interventions were particularly important, involving face-to-face contact with services and practical support. However, a disparity was noted between the types of support required and the support offered. All the support networks appeared to be geared to providing practical support, with little attention being paid to psychological support. Where the carer perceived that psychological support was provided, it seemed to be as a by-product of a practical intervention:

> We had the male nurse all last week and when he comes he stays nearly an hour – enough time to talk about problems and listen – but the others are just in and out.

Support networks involved control, and support could be withdrawn without consulting the carer:

> When he first came out of [hospital] we had a bath nurse once a week for six weeks, then she came one morning and said, 'Well, I won't be back, you've been crossed off the list'.

Options of support were often limited, and when extra support was required long-term care was invariably the only alternative option to community-based services:

> The doctors said, 'Look, he's getting worse and nobody would blame you if you wanted to put him into care.' The option was mine.

Interventions were sometimes in conflict with what the carer was trying to achieve. In one case the woman had originally rejected medical advice by choosing to care for her husband at home and because of this she felt that community services resented giving her support:

> Well, I got two nurses in every week, but mind you the nurses weren't altogether happy, two of them said to our doctor that they considered that he ought to be in hospital.

Prerequisites of support

This category refers to the levels of support received, and what determines those levels. There appeared to be two factors determining levels of support: one related to professional assumptions made about the levels of support required, and the other related directly to the carer and included her role, knowledge, ability, financial security and where she lived geographically. These determinants were therefore unique to each carer; for example, caring abilities were determined by how assertive carers were in requesting guidance, their capacity to adopt coping strategies and their knowledge of the services available. Economic factors also directly determined levels of support received. One woman was caring for her elderly father-in-law as well as her husband who had dementia, and yet this did not appear to be taken into account by social services:

> Well, they said that it's because [of] us living with his dad, his dad got a bit extra money because he was a miner and with his chest, having emphysema, so they turned round and said we could afford the stair-lift, but I don't know how they expect us to pay.

Professional assumptions about the carer's role as a wife were apparently crucial in determining the level of support which was perceived to be necessary by health-care professionals, for example:

> I said to the doctor, 'Where's the help, it hasn't come from anywhere'. We weren't getting any, and he said, 'But you have a home help, you know, and you are his wife'.

Relationship changes

Marriage emerged as a central theme within this category and was characterised by change and loss. The women's marital relationships inevitably changed as a result of caring for their partners and this was coupled with the devastating effects of dementia:

> Well, this sort of thing does alter it, we couldn't have any sort of physical contact: I mean we sleep in the same bed, but all that part of my marriage went when he became ill.

However, the women did describe a sense of closeness with their partner, identifying feelings that were different from the emotional bonds of husband and wife:

> I didn't feel love, I felt this tremendous kindness, it wasn't love like you have at the beginning like husband and wife.

Within this category roles changed as the spouse gradually became 'the carer' and the husband became 'the dependant'. In some ways this appeared to allow both partners an ability to retain some control over their situation. However, ultimately the tasks of caring for a husband with dementia altered that relationship irrevocably, resulting in the modification of roles and often characterised by a sense of loss:

> It's just become a habit, it's routine now, everything has changed between us. I have to do everything for him, all the personal things.

One woman took early retirement at 40 years of age to care for her husband, and is still caring for him 20 years later. She described how they had been catapulted into an 'old' relationship before their time, losing 20 years of their marriage:

> It's like having a child again but much worse, you get feedback from a child, much more feedback. No, it isn't marriage any more.

Lifestyle loss

Lifestyle loss refers to an experience shared by all the women. This category may be divided into external losses such as employment and family, and internal losses such as identity and freedom. Lifestyle loss was experienced to varying degrees; for example, loss of employment was invariably immediate, while other losses, such as loss of a sense of identity, were more gradual. As women adopted the caring role, internal and external losses were linked, for example socioeconomic losses through unemployment were coupled with a loss of identity:

> I've lost such a lot, plus that fact that at Christmas I would have retired on a very, very good salary, I've lost that. I was a teacher of mentally handicapped children.

Internal factors such as 'identity' and 'freedom' refer to how the women viewed themselves and how much time they had to make decisions in their lives, for example:

> I mean, you can't sort of just say, well I'm going to do this today or that today, you know; I mean my whole life is spent here.

> I'm more a carer than a person, your self goes, it just dies. I mean, there's some times that it's very easy to not wash your face because you're not going anywhere.

Health was also lost or certainly suffered while caring and specific problems resulting from the dementia (such as incontinence) resulted in carers not getting adequate sleep:

> If I could only have maybe two nights a week of good sleep, you know, you see because every night, the middle of the night I have to get him out for the toilet.

This 70-year-old woman had just moved to a purpose-built bungalow; for the previous 6 months she had slept on a settee after moving her husband's bed downstairs to be near the bathroom.

The analytical story

The categories described above display a process which may be conceptualised through non-progressive movement, that is, when 'change occurs in response to changing conditions' (Strauss and Corbin, 1990). The categories are therefore more easily explained through a series of interrelationships using the features of axial coding as headings. This is represented by a logic diagram and forms an analytical story (Fig. 9.1) (LoBiondo-Wood, 1994).

Figure 9.1 depicts how pathways into caring determine and shape the caring experiences of married women. This experience involves a process whereby the carers and professionals interact to determine and establish levels of support. Ultimately the women's caring experiences appeared to be characterised by loss within their lifestyle and change within their marital relationship.

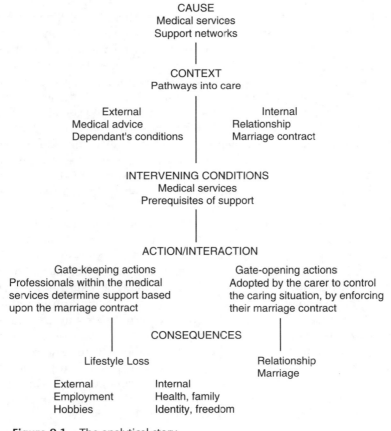

Figure 9.1 The analytical story.

Understanding the analytical story

The categories describe a process rather than a static 'caring experience'. Providing an explanation of these findings by simply discussing categories sequentially would therefore prove to be inadequate. To give a clearer understanding of this research study and the way categories relate to each other, an analytical story in the form of a case study has been compiled from within the sample. This demonstrates the detail and variations within the emergent categories and their contribution to the caring experience. Names and references to personal details have been changed to ensure anonymity. Hakim (1987) describes a case study as the social research equivalent of a microscope. Case studies, by their very nature, are open to selection bias; however, by giving descriptions of the main properties within each category, this has been partially reduced.

Case study: Mrs Brown Mrs Brown first had to consider caring for her husband when the medical services diagnosed Alzheimer's disease. Initially Mrs Brown did not seek any further explanation, as she felt relieved that her husband did not have dementia and further explanation was not offered by the medical services. When it became clear that Mrs Brown's husband was becoming increasingly confused she went back to the medical services. It was only then that she realised that Alzheimer's disease was a form of dementia. The medical services's prognosis that her husband was deteriorating rapidly constituted a pathway into care, as she realised he would need full-time nursing attention. Initially, respite care in a geriatric ward with a view to long-term care was offered as a support network.

However, Mrs Brown was unhappy with this advice and challenged the medical services, citing the length of their marital relationship as a reason why she did not want to be parted from him. These signify internal pathways into care, involving emotional bonds and ties embedded within marriage. Mrs Brown also stated that it was her duty as his wife to look after him, and that she could not bear the thought of him being in a geriatric ward. The medical services agreed that her husband would be happier at home and promised to provide support. This characterised an external pathway into care. Mr Brown deteriorated physically; a social worker was assigned to the case, and agreed that Mrs Brown needed home care to help bathe and dress him. However, the medical services refused to provide a bath nurse because Mrs Brown lived in the wrong geographical area, reflecting a disparity in services depending on location, although she was allocated a home help. This was helpful, but Mrs Brown felt very guilty at times that she could not cope with her own husband. As her husband's condition deteriorated and he became increasingly confused, Mrs Brown became isolated within her home. She could not leave him safely in the house when she went out shopping, but to take him meant enduring the stares of other people as Mr Brown often shouted in public or became very emotional. However, through Mrs Brown's social worker, and her own past experience working as a nursing auxiliary, she was aware that there were support networks available which provided sitting services. These factors constitute the prerequisites of support and intervening conditions, such as knowledge, experience and location. Together they produced an ongoing process of negotiation between Mrs Brown and the medical services, centring around gaining support networks.

Negotiations about support were characterised by a number of gate-keeping and gate-opening actions by Mrs Brown and the medical services. She felt that the support she had been promised by them had not materialised and she was still waiting for a nurse to help bathe her husband. When she approached the medical services about this, they felt that she did not require this sort of assistance because she was the dependant's wife and it would therefore be more appropriate if she assisted with his bathing needs. In this way the medical services acted as gate-keepers to support networks, emphasising her role as a wife to account for their rationing of support. It was only at a crisis stage, when Mrs Brown could no longer cope and considered putting her husband into care, that she began to receive more practical support. When the medical services made decisions about what was best for her husband, Mrs Brown used her role as his wife to reinforce her rights to have a say in this situation. Through gate-opening actions she was able to negotiate some control within the caring experience, in terms of determining the kind of practical support that would best suit her husband's needs.

While caring for her husband Mrs Brown felt that their relationship changed irrevocably. The change in her husband's personality and memory meant that at times he did not recognise her and she felt that he was not the person she had once known. Mrs Brown stated that she loved her husband and affirmed that caring for him was an unquestioned part of their marriage contract; however, at the same time she felt that they no longer shared a marriage in any emotional sense, and was deeply saddened by this. Although not consciously changing her role, Mrs Brown was aware that her husband had become child-like and she had become more of a mother or nurse, but felt that this transition made things easier to cope with.

Mrs Brown felt angry with the situation she was in, not the caring experience itself which she had never regretted, but the lack of a full explanation of what she was undertaking and the lifestyle losses incurred. Leaving her job so suddenly to care for her husband meant missing out on certain benefits and pension rights. Employment may be regarded as an external loss, but internal losses also occurred. Mrs Brown felt that she had lost her identity as an individual and believed that she was viewed instead as a 'carer', a title which she rejected as impersonal. She often felt frustrated and although receiving practical support, felt emotionally stressed and missed company. Regardless of these experiences Mrs Brown never regretted caring for her husband, asserting that it was her place to do so. However, she believed that it could have been made easier, and that if the situations were reversed he would not have cared for her.

DISCUSSION

Caring

A substantial amount of sociological and in particular feminist writing argues for caring to become valued as 'non-market work' (Evans and Ungerson, 1983; Dalley, 1988; Scheyett, 1990; Baldwin and Twigg, 1991). However, it has also been argued that this would strip caring of its emotional bonds (Lewis and Meredith, 1988). This is an important consideration where caring involves looking after a husband with dementia, as the maintenance of emotional bonds is vital in enabling carers to cope with their situation. The women in this study refused or disliked to see caring as 'work', thus demonstrating that caring is much more than an 'activity', and as such signifies a relationship. Maintaining a marital relationship was partially achieved by rejecting the term 'carer' and reinforcing the term 'wife' – for example, 'We are still husband and wife, whatever happens'. It will therefore be interesting to see how much benefit the Carers (Recognition and Services) Act (1995) holds for this particular group of carers in Britain, where recognising their role as a wife is more important than their role as a 'carer'.

The results of the study illustrate how the nature of the caring relationship is centred around the dynamics within marriage. The social roles of marriage are combined with the emotional bonds of the relationship itself. Together, women used these concepts to explain how they 'cared for' their husbands, because they 'cared about' them, thus supporting Graham's conceptualisation of caring as a 'labour of love' (Graham, 1983). Women supported role socialisation theories, adopted by feminists, and described their pathways into caring in terms of, 'It was my place', and, 'I was his wife – you have to depend on your wife'. Managing intimate and practical tasks were also explained in this way: 'Well, I just got on with it, I had to do it, me being his wife'. These statements were always preceded with expressions of emotion and bonding:

> I love him, I wouldn't do what I have if I didn't. We are very close, even the nurses commented on it.

Emotional expressions were used by the women to qualify and cope with a difficult situation, but these were not reciprocated by their partner. Dementia may create feelings of anger, mistrust and fear in a partner, resulting in the alteration of emotional bonds such as affection. It is this change in a relationship between equals that makes caring for spouses so complicated. Parker (1990a) terms this as the change from 'equal partner' to 'pseudo-child', reflected in the study through the loss of the physical and emotional features of marriage. However, the women remained committed to their relationship in the belief that they shared an alliance with their husbands. This partnership developed from a sense of unity and time together as a couple and is supported by Wright (1993), who described this as a 'committed dependent relationship'. This relationship appeared to enhance the women's ability to cope with the caring experience. However, it is difficult to ascertain how much this sense of partnership was shared by their husbands, and this was not investigated further within this study. Perhaps not surprisingly, this ambiguity was not highlighted by the women and did not seem to be a consideration; for example:

> Of course he can't tell me how he feels any more, but we know each other so well, I know better than the nurses what he means.

The women were obviously devoted to caring for their husbands, but this is a more difficult emotional task than has traditionally been acknowledged. The term 'going it alone' has been used to illustrate how carers rationalise and cope with their situation (Thompson et al, 1993), and the women in the study used terms such as 'Well, I just get on with it', and 'I have nobody to talk to'. This highlighted the lack of opportunity to socialise and receive supportive feedback, areas that were identified by the women as sources of stress. However, many didn't expect any form of emotional assistance from support networks, and the emotional support they received mainly came from neighbours or friends.

Support

The assumptions made in society about the nature of marriage result in a lack of appropriate support being available to female spouse carers

(Parker, 1990a; Hammell, 1992). Clark and Haldane (1990) identify 'mutual care and nurture' as one of several tasks within the marriage contract. These properties appear to be exploited by professionals within the medical services. It is unclear whether support was deliberately withheld on a basis of these assumptions. Rather, it is more likely that these actions reflect the 'ambiguity' Twigg (1989) identified surrounding female spouse carers in relation to support networks. Caring is a task only visible when it is not being done, and as such it is simply regarded as a natural part of marriage which is, therefore, open to exploitation. This is exacerbated by society's understanding of dementing illness, which is characterised by fear and stigma. The private domains of caring and marriage, coupled with the personal nature of dementia, result in professionals apparently speculating about rather than objectively assessing the support needs of this group of carers. This factor, combined with the social expectations of marriage, mean that support requirements often become trivialised. The difficulties associated with caring for a husband with dementia appear to be misunderstood by health-care professionals.

Parker (1990a) highlights the belief that within marriage caring is in some way seen as easier and less stressful than within other relationships. These assumptions are not only sexist but also ageist. There appears to be a perception that older men and women accept cross-sex caring tasks more easily and have few inhibitions in relation to personal tasks such as bathing and toileting. Parker (1990a) goes on to state how these assumptions are replicated in service provision. This is typified in the study by the way in which the medical services used a series of 'gate-keeping' actions to determine support levels. Limits on support services were justified through comments such as, 'Well, you are his wife'; this was the response to one woman's query as to why she had not received adequate support since the discharge of her husband from hospital. Another example is the withdrawal of a bath nurse from a couple because the help was perceived to be unnecessary, although the carer felt embarrassed when washing her husband and stated that he had been a very proud man and felt it would have been kinder to have a nurse bathing him.

Hammell (1992) describes the characteristics of marriage as 'love, duty and obligation'. Interestingly, these characteristics, on which many of the assumptions made by the medical services are based, were also adopted by the carer in a series of 'gate-opening' actions. Wright (1993) states that caregivers have more power to influence outcomes than they may realise and certainly the rights and obligations contained within the marriage vows were used by the women to assert their rights as spouses. Comments such as, 'Well, I'm his wife' and 'He was mine' were used to negotiate control within the medical services. This occurred where husbands required outside nursing intervention or long-term hospitalisation was considered. This allowed wives to manage their husband's care, but also reflected their commitment to the relationship with their husband as a partnership:

> We have always been together, I said to the doctor, I want him home with me, he is my husband!

However, by asserting these rights the existing preconceptions held by the medical services about the roles of women caring for a spouse were reinforced. Therefore a vicious circle of negotiating support and control developed between carer and professional. These interactions do not reflect the non-judgmental approach community care claims to advocate.

CONCLUSION

The complexity of the issues raised in the course of these interviews meant that identifying one event characteristic of the caring experience was not achievable. As a group, married women who care for a partner with dementia face a double burden. They are denied social support because of society's assumptions of marriage, and lose the emotional support within their married relationship as they witness their 'partner becoming their patient' (Parker, 1990a). However, the women also displayed a great deal of courage and personal commitment based on a sense of unity shared with their husbands. Until this complex experience is acknowledged by professionals within health and social services, wives who care for their husbands will continue to be viewed as a readily available resource, free at the point of delivery.

The results of this study identify factors that contribute and determine the caring experience and have implications for both policy and practice. Therefore these conclusions are summarised through their broader policy contexts, followed by recommendations for practice.

Community care policy and support

The study illustrates how definitions of support remain ambiguous within both the social and health services. This has resulted in a lack of psychological support being available to female spouse carers. Statutory services appear to believe that this group do not require extra psychological support. They assume that this support is available to them within their married relationship. This belief allows them to justify limiting or controlling support levels on the basis of the duties and obligations inherent within the marriage contract. Community care policy holds misconceptions about the tasks wives who care must undertake, and therefore statutory services appear to exploit the married relationship.

Caring for a dependent husband is a full-time activity, requiring attention 24 hours a day. Most of the women undoubtedly derived a great deal of satisfaction from the care they provided. However, the prolonged caring relationship they described also had negative psychological effects, such as stress, as caring became an increasingly isolating activity. Support services do exist and are provided by the local authority social services, but the availability of these services varies from region to region.

Future research

Caring for a husband with dementia involves the carer having to make huge sacrifices in terms of time, energy and money. At a practical level these sacrifices are similar to those of other caring groups. However, at a more personal level these 'carers' suffered a specific loss, the loss of their partner's identity as a husband. This blurring in roles changed their marital relationship irrevocably.

The immense sacrifices women make emotionally and psychologically in caring for a husband with dementia have not been considered in enough detail within this study. Motivations and personal satisfactions were not included owing to the sensitive nature of such questions, but these represent important areas for future research. Psychological theories remain important, adding further understanding of the caring experience. The distinct lack of emotional support means that psychology's contribution may become particularly valuable.

Caring for a husband with dementia is a unique individual experience which requires further qualitative research. Future longitudinal studies could provide a more complete picture of the changes within this experience. Questions have been raised surrounding support, marital roles and community care issues, all of which could be studied more thoroughly. Feminist theories alone fail to explain adequately women's desires to care, thus in recent years attempts have been made to utilise psychology to answer these questions. However, further integrated research uniting the disciplines of psychology and sociology is required. Psychological studies will contribute to understanding the interpersonal dynamics between husbands with dementia and their wives. Combined, these studies would lead to more effective understanding of the caring experience.

Future practice

Within the UK statutory services, clearer policy definitions of what constitutes support are required, taking the psychological dimension into consideration. A psychological understanding of carers' emotional needs may generate more support groups and networks. Practitioners such as nurses and social workers may then become more aware of the social isolation and emotional difficulties spouse carers experience. This would enable care managers to improve their assessment of individual needs, and community nurses could more accurately provide for those needs.

The development of support groups and networks should be locally based, within the carers' community, thereby increasing collaborative working between social services and carers' groups. This is a central requirement within community care policy. More assessments should be undertaken in the home environment rather than in hospital, and should include the carer's needs as well as the dependant's. This issue has been partly addressed by the Carers (Recognition and Services) Act (1995).

This study's qualitative nature may sensitise health-care practitioners to the specific needs faced by female spouse carers and question existing assumptions held by practitioners within community care. However, this must be reinforced with policy research of community care. This is essential in order to challenge the discriminatory practices of statutory services towards spouse carers.

Monitoring community care is essential to ensure that appropriate services are provided, such as psychological support. However, Wistow (1995) found that only 6% of monitoring activity of community care was aimed at carers. Until this imbalance is redressed it would appear that wives who care for husbands with dementia will continue to be viewed as a resource. Recognition of what it means to provide a 'labour of love' (Graham, 1983) is required by policy-makers and practitioners. Reliance on the marriage vow, 'in sickness and in health', is no longer an adequate response to community care.

REFERENCES

Baldwin, S. & Twigg, J. (1991) Women and community care – reflections on a debate. In: Maclean, M. & Groves, D. (eds) *Women's Issues in Social Policy*. London: Routledge & Kegan Paul.

Barret, D. (1992) Older people's experiences of community care. *Social Policy and Administration* **26**, 220–225.

Bornat, J., Pereira, C., Pilgram, D. & Williams, F. (1993) *Community Care – A Reader*. London: McMillian/Open University.

Carers (Recognition and Services) Act (1995) London: HMSO.

Clark, D. & Haldane, D. (1990) *Wedlocked*? Oxford: Polity Press.

Collins, C., Stommel, M., Wang, S. & Given, C.W. (1994) Caregiving transitions; changes in depression among family caregivers of relatives with dementia. *Nursing Research* **43**, 220–225.

Dalley, G. (1988) *Ideologies of Caring: Rethinking Community and Collectivism*. London: Macmillian.

Evans, M. & Ungerson, C. (1983) *Sexual Divisions, Patterns and Processes*. London: Tavistock.

Finch, J. & Groves, D. (1980) Community care and the family, a case for equal opportunities? *Journal of Social Policy* **9**, 487–511.

Finch, J. & Mason, J. (1990) Filial obligations and kin support for elderly people. *Ageing and Society* **10**, 151–178.

General Household Survey (1985) London: HMSO.

Gilligan, C. (1982) *In a Different Voice: Psychological Theory and Woman's Development.* Cambridge: Harvard University Press.

Graham, H. (1983) Caring: a labour of love. In: Finch, J. & Groves, D. (eds) *A Labour Of Love; Women Work and Caring.* London: Routledge & Kegan Paul.

Green, H. (1988) *Informal Carers: General Household Survey 1985.* London: HMSO.

Hakim, C. (1987) *Research Design; Strategies and Choices in the Design of Social Research.* London: Allen & Unwin.

Hammell, K.R.W. (1992) The caring wife: the experience of caring for a severely disabled husband in the community. *Disability, Handicap and Society* 7, 349–362.

Haralambos, M. (1991) *Sociology, Themes and Perspectives.* London: HarperCollins.

Land, H. (1991) Time to care. In: Maclean, M. & Groves, D. (eds) *Women's Issues in Social Policy.* London: Routledge & Kegan Paul.

Larrabee, M. (1993) *Gender and Moral Development, A Challenge for Feminist Theory.* London: Routledge/Chapman & Hall.

Lee, G. (1993) Gender differences in parent carer; demographic factors and same gender preferences. *Journal of Gerontology* 4, S9–S16.

Lewis, J. & Meredith, B. (1988) *Daughters Who Care; Daughters Caring For Mothers At Home.* London: Routledge.

LoBiondo-Wood, J. (1994) *Nursing Research Methods: Critical Appraisal and Utilisation,* 3rd edn. St Louis: Mosby.

Mace, N. (1990) *Dementia Care, Patient, Family and Community.* Baltimore: Johns Hopkins University Press.

Parker, G. (1990a) Spouse carers; whose quality of life? In: Balwin, S., Godfrey, C. & Propper, C. (eds) *Quality of Life; Perspectives and Policies.* London: Routledge.

Parker, G. (1990b) Whose care? Whose costs? Whose benefit? A critical research on case management and informal care. *Ageing and Society* 10, 459–467.

Parker, G. & Lawton, D. (1994) *Different Types of Care, Different Types of Carer; Evidence from the General Household Survey.* London: HMSO.

Qureshi, H. & Walker, A. (1989) *The Caring Relationship: Elderly People and their Families.* London: Macmillan.

Scheyett, A. (1990) The oppression of caring; women caregivers of relatives with mental illness. *Affilia* 5, 32–48.

Strauss, A. & Corbin, J. (1990) *Basics of Qualitative Research; Grounded Theory Procedures and Techniques.* Newbury Park: Sage.

Suitor, J. & Pillemer, K. (1993) Support and interpersonal stress in the social networks of married daughters caring for parents with dementia. *Journal of Gerontology* 48, 51–58.

Thompson, E., Futterman, A., Gallagher, D. Rose, J. & Lovett, S. (1993) Social support and caregiving burden in family caregivers of frail elders. *Journal of Gerontology* 48 S245–S254.

Twigg, J. (1989) Models of carers; how do social care agencies conceptualise their relationship with informal carers? *Journal of Social Policy* 18, 53–66.

Twigg, J. & Atkin, K. (1994) *Carers Perceived; Policy and Practice in Informal Care.* Buckingham: Open University Press.

Ungerson, C. (1987) *Policy is Personal; Sex, Gender and Informal Care.* London: Tavistock.

Webb, R. & Tossell, D. (1991) *Social Issues For Carers: A Community Care Perspective.* London: Edward Arnold.

Wistow, G. (1995) The waiting game. *Community Care* 2, 26–27.

Wright, F.D. (1986) *Left To Care Alone.* Aldershot: Gower.

Wright, L.K. (1993) *Alzheimer's Disease and Marriage.* Newbury Park: Sage.

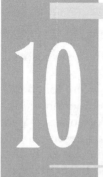

The long goodbye: the experience of loss in husbands who care for a wife with dementia

Liz Matthew

KEY ISSUES

- Husbands of women with dementia experience emotional trauma associated with the loss of their wife to dementia

- Husbands experience a wide variety of emotions such as feelings of isolation, anger and stress when caring for their wife

- Most of the husbands in the study had 'moved on' from their experience of coming to terms with the loss of their wife to dementia

- Loss counselling may well be a useful psychosocial intervention with husbands caring for a wife with dementia

- Loss associated with caring for a close relative with dementia should be understood in terms of present loss rather than anticipated grief

INTRODUCTION

In recent studies on caring for people with dementia, there has been a particular interest in the mental and emotional strain experienced by relatives who take on the role of primary family carer (Adams, 1997). Having worked as a community psychiatric nurse (CPN) dealing with older people and their family carers for a number of years, during which time I had frequent contact with people with dementia, I became aware that my work as a CPN focused more on giving practical support and advice to carers rather than helping the carers deal with the emotional and psychological trauma that they may have been experiencing throughout the course of their spouse's dementia. As Adams (1996) noted in a study on the work of CPNs, the type of emotional help offered to carers is 'supportive' and does not address to any great depth the psychosocial issues relating to providing care.

The period during which relatives provide care is often long and arduous, yet carers are often given little help to address the emotional traumas they experience, such as loss and grief that are often associated with losing a relative to dementia. Indeed, Pauline Taylor describes her experience of caring for her husband with dementia as a 'living bereavement' (Taylor, 1987). Various studies have examined the experience of loss in relatives caring for people with dementia (Austrom and Gendrie, 1990; Liken and Collins, 1993; Miesen, 1997; Sweeting and Gilhooly, 1997). Collins et al (1993) describe the experience of loss and grief as it appears prior to and following the death of a relative with dementia; six themes identified in their study are loss of the person and relationship; loss of hope; pre-death grief; expectancy of death; post-death relief; and caregiving reflections. In a study of caring for a relative with dementia, Loos and Boyd (1997) identified various areas of loss associated with the loss of social and recreational interaction, loss of control over life event, loss of wellbeing and loss of occupation. They argue that those caring for people with dementia incur a diminution of self in which they are subsumed by the needs of the person with dementia. This ties in well with the development of the concept of 'dual dying' developed by Jones and Martinson (1992), in which the primary family carer as well as the person with dementia effectively loses their life as the result of dementia.

This led to the development of the study described in this chapter, which examines the loss experienced by husbands whose wives have dementia. A further aim of the study was to examine how closely the carer's experience of loss mirrored the loss and grief experienced by people who had been bereaved. Having seen the positive effects of bereavement counselling in my work, I was interested in developing psychosocial interventions that could be employed by health-care professionals to benefit carers of people with dementia within an overall framework of partnership.

In the study, I decided to address the issue of loss with a particular type of carer: men giving care to a wife with dementia. This was partly because the majority of my work in bereavement counselling has been with men, but also because much of the work on family care has related to female carers only. As various writers have pointed out, male carers have a different experience of providing care, for example men have been found to be more able to manage the provision of care to a family member, to set limits and delegate where necessary (Colerick and George, 1986). Parsons (1997), in a study of men providing care to a relative with dementia, identified eight interrelated themes: enduring; vigilance; a sense of loss; aloneness and loneliness; taking away; searching to discover; the need to discover; the need for assistance and reciprocity. I therefore thought it would be worth while to examine the experience of men losing a wife to dementia.

THE STUDY
Method

Data were collected in the form of open-ended interviews with husbands caring for wives with dementia at home. The interviews took place in the family home and consisted of an informal, open-ended discussion. The aim of the interview was to obtain the carer's ideas about caring for a wife with dementia. The data was tape-recorded and excerpts that were particularly illuminating were transcribed. These were placed into categories relating to insights into the carer's emotional experience of providing care for the person with dementia. Fourteen categories were developed from the data. It was also considered worth while to develop carer biographies, which presented an overall view of the carer.

Carer biographies

Carer 1 – Mr A

Mr A is in his 70s and has known his wife for nearly 60 years. Mr A used to work at a printers but has had a variety of jobs over the years. He developed epilepsy when he was young and subsequently found it difficult to obtain regular work. He was recruited into the army, but was soon discharged on health grounds. Although times were hard for Mr A and his wife, he nevertheless described them as having a happy marriage. Mr A has suffered generally from bad health due to his epilepsy. Each week Mr A took his wife to the hairdressers and then to the pub, and treated her to flowers and sweets every Saturday. They have four children, two of whom now live abroad. A daughter keeps in touch with them regularly, despite the fact that she lives many miles away in the south of England. They also have a son who is a local market trader.

Carer 2 – Mr B

Mr B is in his early 80s and has been caring for his wife for 13 years. They met each other over 60 years ago. Mr B worked for a company as a driver/chauffeur. Early in their marriage, he also started his own business in scrap paper which he has now passed on to his son.

Mr B talked positively about his wife; however, he spoke about her in terms of the tasks she performed rather than about the personal qualities she possessed. His description of her was generally in terms of her ability as a housekeeper. Mr B considered these qualities of his wife were the key to his happiness. When he later talked of his relationships with other women, the idea of being looked after seemed to be of primary importance. Mr B's relationship with his children has deteriorated in recent years; he was clearly bitter about this in the interview. During the interview Mr B frequently stopped talking about his wife, and gave detailed descriptions of his relationship with his former employers and his children. In the interview it was notable that Mr B frequently used the word 'I', talking about himself and his relationship with 'his family'. However, he talked warmly about his wife, though usually in the past tense, and presented problems that had arisen as being his fault.

Carer 3 – Mr C

Mr C is in his early 70s and had lived in India for most of his working life. He was employed as a manager of a tea plantation. He married his English-born wife in India about 50 years ago and brought up his two children. Returning to England, he worked for a time with his wife managing a historic building on behalf of the National Trust. On retirement, he moved to his present location to be near his daughter and enjoys close links with both his children

In the interview, it was clear that Mr C is a very articulate and methodical man. His lively personality made the interview very colourful and descriptive. When his wife's illness was diagnosed he responded by careful planning. He displayed little knowledge of informal and formal support and how they may be obtained, having lived abroad for most of his life, but he has now enough help and support to allow himself to take on a part-time job. He is very appreciative of the help offered and positive about what has been received, whether it is help from the consultant psychiatrist or from his next-door neighbour.

Carer 4 – Mr D

Mr D has been married for 57 years and is 83 years old. He has been caring for his wife for about 4 years. He was married in the early stages of World War II, but was then separated from his wife until it ended. His sister's husband was killed in the closing days of the war and his father died shortly afterwards. Consequently he took it upon himself to look after and support their widows, but this led to disagreements with his wife. Gradually the problem was resolved and Mr D settled down to a happy marriage. He worked in an office for nearly all his life, and that is where he met his wife. He has a son, a company executive, whom he sees rarely, and a daughter of whom he is obviously very proud. A close family link is maintained with the daughter, and his three grandchildren visit regularly.

Carer 5 – Mr E

Mr E is 75 years old and lives with his wife, who has been diagnosed with dementia. They live on the same council estate as Mr A, though they do not know each other. Mr E has worked in a variety of manual occupations throughout his life, and had to take early retirement through illness. He has limited contact with other people and most of his friends are people whom he had known at work. Mr E has one son who sometimes comes to help him. In the interview Mr E disclosed little about his own personal background.

Carer 6 – Mr F

Mr F is 62 years old and has been caring for his wife for 8 years. He married late in life and his wife had been married twice before. She has a son from a previous marriage who is currently living abroad. Mr F was a commercial artist running his own business. He and his wife, who was a teacher, worked abroad in Cyprus and Scandinavia, living what he calls the 'lotus-eating life'. On his return to England, becoming disenchanted with the bureaucracy of the system of working, he set up his own studio and worked for himself. He gradually slipped into retirement as his role of being a carer increased. He has had a female companion for some time and she is also involved in caring for his wife, in addition to her job as a care assistant in a nursing home. In the village where he lives there is some disapproval of this relationship.

Categories developed

Category 1: Husbands' perceptions of their wives as they were prior to the onset of dementia

A considerable amount of what the husbands said in the interviews related to how they viewed their wife in the past. All but one of the husbands interviewed went to great lengths describing how wonderful their wife had been. At first sight, it may be that these descriptions were associated with their experience of losing someone to dementia, since people often see someone they have lost through 'rose-coloured spectacles'. On closer examination, however, these descriptions may be placed into context, as they make a comparison between the wife they once had and the wife they have today. This explains to some extent the preoccupation that the husbands had with regard to hygiene and tidiness, which were often contrasted to their wife's current condition.

These descriptions by the husbands are also important because they demonstrate they have actually accepted the loss of the person to dementia. All the husbands interviewed in the study expressed clearly the view that they had lost someone they valued:

[She was] so good, can't fault her in any respect. Morals, good housekeeper, clean, honest, good saver, everything under the sun.

Mr B

[My wife] was a lovely person … always immaculate and impeccably dressed and her hygiene was second to none.

Mr C

Category 2: Husbands' denial that wife has dementia

The descriptions the husbands provided suggest that the denial they expressed may be understood as a means of protecting the identity of their wife as a rational person. This was facilitated by the symptoms of the dementia, which may develop slowly.

It was noticeable that denial was less pronounced in husbands to whom information was readily available. Some of the husbands found that ignoring their wife was a useful method of minimising problems. For example, Mr A commented:

I lived normally and ignored [what the general practitioner had said] … but my daughter had noted it.

While Mr A was not aware of the symptoms of dementia or its implications, he is being protective of his wife.

She was talking to me last night, saying [in the past] I would not listen to her.

Mr A

Mr C, on the other hand, is aware but does not want to accept the situation. Gilhooly (1984) found this not uncommon and attributed this partly to the stigma of mental illness and consequent reluctance to ask about it or seek help. However, there is no evidence to suggest that this was the case with Mr C.

Category 3: Understanding dementia and recognising its implications

Although the dementia had been diagnosed some time previously, there was a general view that the explanation given by the medical profession had not been thorough enough for the husbands to realise the progressive effects of the disorder. This can be seen in the following comments:

I've been in touch with the Dementia Association, etc. – I have been in touch with all the people it's humanly possible to get in touch with, but at the time [of diagnosis] ... I did not [understand the implications]. To me it was completely new.

Mr A

The doctor said, 'I don't know but I think she may have something like Alzheimer's disease.' I'd never heard of dementia. I didn't know what dementia was.

Mr C

Although there were variations in the progression of the dementia, most of the wives at the time of the interview were in the latter stages of dementia. Moreover, most of the husbands recognised that their wife's condition was deteriorating.

In the near future ... however long, in a month, in a year, she will not know me ... I realise that the day is coming and I don't think it will be very long [before she needs to go into formal care].

Mr A

I know that one day I won't be able to do it [care].

Mr C

Lack of knowledge is common in carers, as Gilhooly (1984) noted:

Although supporters [carers] ... appeared reluctant in many cases to speak to the [general practitioner] about the dementing old person's behaviour, this does not mean that they did not want information or advice. Supporters expected the GP to volunteer information which, it seems, at least from my study, they rarely do. (p. 118)

It may be seen that the husbands interviewed did not know what to expect as their wife's dementia progressed.

Category 4: Husbands' guilt

The main area of guilt for the husbands related to the times when they thought they were being asked to abandon – or thought they had already abandoned – their wife. As one carer said, '[my daughter] actually made an appointment with my GP and I said, "I'm not going behind her back".' Another husband commented, 'We had arguments about her driving ... Now I know more about her illness, I realise that was irresponsible – that makes me feel pretty bad.'

Resolving this guilt was probably one of the most difficult problems for the husbands to address. As Wilkin (1979) acknowledges, family carers are often in a 'no-win situation' regarding providing satisfactory care for family members with dementia: carers who support the relative at home are seen as overprotective; if they continue as normal, they are accused of ignoring the problem; and carers who seek to place the relative in residential care are accused of neglect.

Category 5: Husbands' anger

A number of the husbands interviewed expressed strong feelings of anger. For example:

> I do get angry. You can't do anything else. I don't go to extremes, just nasty. I'm not angry for myself, just worried what she will do if anything happens to me.

> *Mr E*

Anger and guilt have been associated with the experience of loss (Parkes, 1996). In the interviews, the husbands expressed two types of anger: anger towards 'the system', and anger towards particular people.

Category 6: Stress

It was clear from the carers who were interviewed that they all experienced considerable stress when caring for their wives:

> They said, 'You're suffering from a lot of stress', and I said, 'I am – I've no social life anymore' ... The stress is always there, but I just cope all the time.

> *Mr C*

All the husbands at some point in the interview talked about the difficulties they encountered dealing with day-to-day activities. These difficulties were not referred to directly but rather were discussed in terms of the relief they experienced at receiving support such as respite care. Sandford (1975) identified various problems that family carers find difficult to tolerate, such as sleep disturbance, faecal incontinence, night wandering, shouting and micturition. The husbands interviewed did not consider these behaviours to be particularly stressful, although they all mentioned them at some point in the interview. The problems they did mention were more associated with risk and dangerous behaviour, or strange and bizarre behaviour. In the study, guilt associated with not being able to care was a likely cause of stress to the husbands.

Category 7: Husbands' perceptions of their own health

Of all the husbands interviewed, only Mr A recognised his health as being a problem: he had suffered from epilepsy, and said that his health was not good. The others interviewed made comments such as, 'At my age you can't complain' (Mr B). However, most of the men were undergoing some form of medical treatment, but they often put this down to their age, believing that illness was only to be expected at their time of life. Mr F emphasised that any minor health problems he had incurred were not related to his wife's illness. Generally speaking, the husbands interviewed appeared to be in good health.

Category 8: Isolation

Negative feelings were expressed by the husbands relating to the physical separation that had occurred as the result of admission to hospital. These feelings were often spoken about in terms of isolation:

> Next to sickness is loneliness and don't I know it, I've cried. I can look across to the lights of the hospital [when his wife is there] … and say a little prayer. Now that sounds funny for a man, but sometimes I cry.
>
> *Mr B*

> It's a blessing if someone calls in because I can talk and get an answer.
>
> *Mr D*

It was interesting to note that the husbands continued to talk to their wives, even though they had dementia:

> I really can make her laugh. It may be something simple, but I can still recognise a sparkle there.
>
> *Mr F*

Moreover, a number of the husbands said that they felt 'cut off'

> I used to enjoy playing the church organ, going to choral concerts. I've had to stop everything, but I accept it.
>
> *Mr C*

Sometimes friends stopped visiting:

> Two of her close friends … just washed their hands of her … and they meet me in the street and say, 'How's –? It is a shame'. They don't say, 'I'll drop round and see her'.
>
> *Mr B*

The isolation the husbands reported took two forms: separation from their wife, and also separation from other people. In this sense, isolation was a double loss. The difficulties the husbands experienced in communicating with their wives were largely due to the lack of response, although there was some reason to believe that the husbands still talked to their wives. The loss of the companionship their partners provided was exacerbated by isolation elsewhere, that is, their rejection by family and friends. What is interesting here are the attempts to fill this 'empty space'.

Category 9: Feelings of helplessness

A few of the husbands expressed feelings of helplessness:

> It's an illness, and that's all there is to it. I've had many illnesses in my time and there's nothing you can do about it. I accept her for what she is now.
>
> *Mr A*

The focus of this helplessness was directed towards coping with their wife's condition. There was no firm evidence from the interviews that the husbands felt helpless at the prospect of continuing their own lives. Three of the husbands were particularly active in moving on, so this negative element seemed to have been either overcome or averted in some of the husbands interviewed.

Category 10: Accepting the situation

All the husbands interviewed had accepted their situation, however with varying degrees of resolve.

> It's a job to be done. Get on with it. It helps keep her on course. It's a job I've got to do.
>
> *Mr D*

> It's not a relationship now – I have to look after her. That's the way it is.
>
> *Mr E*

This acceptance is linked closely with the 'helplessness' identified above. In this case, acceptance relates to the role of carer. All the husbands interviewed recognised that the caring had to be done. From the language used by the husbands, in most cases providing care seems to have been undertaken somewhat reluctantly. However, associated with this reluctance there was often a strong sense of duty which was particularly noticeable. None of the husbands talked about giving up, and indeed, most fought to continue caring. It may be argued that this sense of duty is related to the behaviour described by Barusch and Spaid (1989) who suggest that today's older man tends to be stoic, complaining little 'regardless of the extent of their emotional discomfort'.

Category 11: Support from the family

The support provided by other members of the family was frequently referred to in the interviews:

> He went to London to make his fortune ... he's in advertising, a real whiz kid ... Caring's not in his book – it's dirty. [When he first heard] he said, 'I'll send her to Harley Street, get it sorted out'. I said, 'You can't, it's irrevocable', and then of course he washed his hands of her.
>
> *Mr F*

> My granddaughters passed my door to visit their mother who lived around the corner, and I never knew. [When they were finally persuaded to call] I was washing [my wife]; 'Aren't you marvellous,' they said, 'I could never do that' – and then they went!
>
> *Mr B*

> I told everybody in the street [about her condition]; I wasn't ashamed of it, I didn't try to hide it. They've all been lovely about it. She'd suddenly call on them [telling them a strange man was in the house]. They'd make her a cup of tea and within twenty minutes she'd be back. They were terribly nice.
>
> *Mr C*

There is little in the literature which looks at the willingness of children to rally round in caring. Gilhooly (1984), for example, suggests that support is often not forthcoming and when it is, it usually comes from a woman – this was in keeping with this study.

It is also worth noting that there may be other reasons for non-involvement with care. Isaacs et al (1972) found that in cases where old people had not received care from available relatives, there had usually been a long history of conflict or rejections of help and love by the dependant.

Category 12: Support from formal agencies

Some of the husbands were very appreciative of the help they had received. Mr B spoke highly of the general practitioners and consultants whom he had met and their eagerness to help him. Mr C went further, extending his appreciation to the nurses and the voluntary sector sitting service. It is also clear that sometimes the consultant was instrumental in persuading a relative to accept the offer of respite care:

> [The consultant] was the final push that made me decide [to use respite care].'
>
> *Mr A*

However, there are also examples where the support of the consultant was lacking:

> The consultant said, 'Sorry' and shook my hand. I asked the receptionist if I had another appointment. She said, 'No'. I felt so alone.
>
> *Mr A*

All the husbands interviewed had a formal support network. Clearly they did not wish to give up their caring responsibilities, but at the same time they were openly appreciative of the care their wife was receiving; Mr C and Mr F in particular emphasised the value of the relative support group.

The value of relative support groups is supported by other research findings. Levin et al (1989) found that services were utilised disproportionately by men, but recognised this may relate to current services being more oriented to male needs, specifically domestic help.

Category 13: Coping strategies (dependant)

All the husbands in the study had developed strategies of being able to deal with their situation. They were keenly independent and did not wish to relinquish care until it was absolutely necessary:

> I wouldn't let her go in. I absolutely would not let her go in. I argued with the doctor for an hour.
>
> *Mr A*

> I'm not ready – not yet. She's still got a home here.
>
> *Mr F*

They were also generally upset about the deterioration of their partner both physically and mentally:

> She was witty, intelligent, but now she's gone completely.
>
> *Mr F*

There is strong evidence from the husbands interviewed that all the men were reluctant for their wives to leave the home environment for care. The implications for this with regards to bereavement counselling would suggest a problem in 'letting go' by providing a constant reminder of the dependency of the wife.

Category 14: Coping strategies (self)

Providing care to a wife with dementia had made all the husbands interviewed take stock of their lives, and in spite of their surrounding difficulties, most of them realised that life had to go on:

> It's no use jumping under a bus, putting your head under a cushion. Quite right! Life has to go on.

Mr B

Some of the husbands realised things that were of value in their life which helped them continue to provide care:

> The thing that makes life worthwhile, and helps me retain my sanity, is my part-time job.

Mr C

Some of the husbands had succeeded in filling, or starting to fill, the 'empty space' created by their increasing detachment from their wives. This was certainly the case with Mr B and Mr F, both of whom had established relationships with other women. This clearly helped them to cope, but was not necessarily accepted by other people. This raises the question of what is the appropriate balance between emotional detachment and involvement of the husband towards a wife with dementia. There is no easy answer to this question and it is probably best to suggest that it is a matter of personal judgment, in the context of a network of supportive relationships that the carer needs to make.

DEMENTIA AND BEREAVEMENT: A COMPARISON

The main aim of this study was to examine the loss that husbands of wives with dementia encountered. However, other studies have highlighted the effect of loss in a wide range of situations such as the loss of a house through removal and the loss of a limb through amputation (Parkes, 1996). A frequent loss that people encounter is the loss of a close relative through death. This raises the question: what are the similarities and dissimilarities between losing a relative to dementia and losing a relative to death, i.e. bereavement?

Denial

Numerous studies reveal that people who have lost someone they love experience feelings of denial and numbness (Parkes, 1996). The interviews revealed that the numbness and shock that has often been associated with bereavement did not occur to the same extent in the husbands who had lost their wife to dementia. This, of course, does not lessen their difficulties, but rather acknowledges the nature of the loss. There are various reasons why the husbands in the study might not have experienced numbness and shock, and these may lie in the differences between the two forms of loss. For example, when someone dies it happens at a particular point in time and the effect of the loss may therefore be much more intense. Secondly, there is no ambiguity when someone dies: the person is physically and mentally absent. However, when someone has been lost to dementia, there is an ambiguity: the person is physically present but mentally absent. As Boss (1988) points out, 'ambiguous loss' is particularly distressing for families containing people with dementia. And so, the experience of loss is drawn out over a prolonged period of time.

In the interviews, certain statements by the husbands could be understood as instances of denial. However, this denial seemed to be related to protecting their wives. Denial on the part of the husbands was encouraged by the slow and insidious nature of dementia as well as by the perception that the wives did not recognise its presence themselves. Denial was less noticeable in husbands who had access to information about dementia and the services that were available. Moreover denial, particularly in the early stages of dementia, may be a way in which the husbands coped.

Emotional pain

Studies of people who have been bereaved indicate that they experience considerable emotional pain (Parkes, 1996). The husbands in the study expressed distress about the loss of their wife to dementia. This distress was often described in terms of 'feeling lost' and 'helplessness'. On occasions the husbands admitted to 'crying'. However, this was the exception rather than the rule, and in the accounts the husbands gave there was little talk of physical symptoms associated with their emotional pain. This rather stoic position of the husbands may be due to their internalisation of a stereotypical view of men within Western society which inhibits them from expressing their emotional distress.

It may be that various aspects of the carer's life provide painful reminders of a time when the wife did not have dementia, such as visiting familiar places, and living in the same surroundings as those before the illness. This was not something that was mentioned by the husbands, but it was clear that often social contacts had been severed and that this had caused a considerable amount of anger in the husbands interviewed.

Acceptance

The acceptance stage of the process of loss was particularly significant in this study. In the interviews, it was apparent that the husbands interviewed had not become physically and psychologically detached from the person with dementia, indeed there was still some vestige of 'partnership' between themselves and their wives. It was also clear that the husbands who were interviewed had progressed to a 'moving on' stage which enabled them to take up tasks such as housework that they would never have done prior to the onset of their wife's dementia. In some ways, the husbands were limited by social norms, but in others they had already developed. This corresponds well with the idea of Jones and Martinson (1992), who suggest that people caring for relatives with dementia experience a 'dual dying'.

COUNSELLING CARERS

Various writers have recognised the value of providing support to people who are experiencing the emotional effects of losing a close family member to dementia (Garner, 1997). Adams (1997) applies various principles of counselling people who have been bereaved that may also be successful with husbands who have lost a wife to dementia. These principles could be used to underpin the practice of a wide range of health-care practitioners, including CPNs.

1. **Admit the loss.** Counselling should be directed towards helping husbands recognise their loss. Accordingly, the practitioner may encourage the husband to talk about what his wife was like before she had dementia. The carer should be encouraged to talk about the qualities and attributes which his wife had lost through the development of dementia as a means of helping him adjust to the loss.
2. **Identify and ventilate feelings**. The practitioner should encourage the carer to talk about the variety of feelings such as anxiety, anger, guilt and helplessness that he is experiencing.
3. **Exploration**. The practitioner should help the carer explore the implications of losing their relative to dementia. One way might be to help the carer go through some problem-solving exercise, by asking such questions as, 'What will be the problems now that

your [husband, wife, mother] is demented?' 'How can these problems be solved?'

4. **Discourage emotional withdrawal**. The practitioner should encourage the carer to maintain old and develop new friendships. This may be difficult because of the restraints that giving care places on the carer. However, it is important that the carer maintains a supportive social network and resists the temptation to become emotionally withdrawn.

5. **Allow time for grief**. Carers should be allowed time to go through the work they must accomplish to get through their feelings of loss about what has happened to their demented relative. Worden (1991) usefully describes this process as 'grief work'.

6. **Interpret normal behaviour**. Following the loss of a relative to dementia, carers may have a sense that they, too, are 'going mad'. The practitioner should take every opportunity to reassure carers that what they are going through is a normal experience. Odd and funny things that happen to the carer may need interpreting back to let the carer know that it is fine to feel and act that way.

7. **Allow time for individual differences**. Everybody reacts differently to losing someone to dementia. This may be difficult for other family members to come to terms with. The practitioner therefore may need to reassure the rest of the family that the way in which a particular family member is reacting is normal.

8. **Provide continued support**. The practitioner needs to provide support for the carer and therefore will need to keep in contact with the carer, as it may well be that feelings of loss may return. The feelings may be particularly acute in the carer at significant times such as birthdays and wedding anniversaries.

9. **Examine defences**. The practitioner should help carers examine their defences. These will be exaggerated during the period of loss. Some of the defences will help carers adapt to their situation; however, other defence mechanisms will not be adaptive, such as excess alcohol consumption.

CONCLUSION

The findings of this study suggest that it may well be useful to develop loss counselling as a means of helping people caring for a family member with dementia. Whilst there are differences between the phenomena of bereavement and losing someone to dementia, there is enough evidence from the interviews to suggest that it would be worth while to explore the possibility of using techniques that have been employed in other areas of loss with husbands who are providing care to a spouse with dementia. However, it should be pointed out that it would be worth extending and developing the study described here to include a greater number of husbands as a means of making some sort of generalisation about the phenomena. The knowledge gained from such a study could then be used to develop educational approaches that would enable health-care professionals to employ such techniques in practice. At this stage, it would be appropriate to develop a means of evaluating the effectiveness of the approach through a controlled trial.

One issue that has to a certain extent been circumvented in this present study is whether the loss that was experienced by the husbands in the study arose as a result of losing a close relative to dementia or whether it was actually anticipated grief. This is a thorny question and one that is difficult to answer. Jones and Martinson (1992) argue that what the carers in their study experienced was 'not anticipatory grief, but acute grief related to immediate and permanent loss of a relative's human abilities and personhood while still living' (p. 175), and state that the concept of 'dual dying' is a better way of understanding the phenomenon. Garner (1997) agrees, and suggests that whilst carers experience elements of anticipatory grief, the emphasis in the case of dementia is the present loss, not the loss that will occur. Moreover, she points out that in cases of dementia, there is no confidant(e) for the partner for the anticipatory elements of loss, for example, to negotiate the anticipation of loss. In this way, the resolution of the personal relationship between the partner and the patient is denied or is a solitary task.

REFERENCES

Adams, T. (1996) A descriptive study of the work of community psychiatric nurses with elderly demented people. *Journal of Advanced Nursing* **23**, 1177–1184.

Adams, T. (1997) Dementia. In: Norman, I. & Redfern, S. (eds) *Mental Health Care for Elderly People*. London: Churchill Livingstone.

Austrom, M. & Gendrie, H. (1990) Death of the personality: the grief responses of Alzheimer's family caregivers. *American Journal of Alzheimer's Care and Related Disorders Research* **5** (2), 16–27.

Barusch, A. & Spaid, W. (1989) Gender differences in caregiving: why do wives report greater burden? *Gerontologist* **29** (5), 667–676.

Boss, P. (1988) *Family Stress Management*. London: Sage.

Colerick, E. & George, L. (1986) Predictors of institutionalisation among patient patients with Alzheimer's disease. *Journal of American Geriatrics Society* **7**, 483–489.

Collins, C., Liken, M., King, S. et al (1993) Loss and grief among family caregivers of relatives with dementia. *Qualitative Health Research* **2**, 236–253.

Garner, J. (1997) Dementia: an intimate death. *British Journal of Medical Psychology* **70**, 177–184.

Gilhooly, M.L.M. (1984) The impact of care giving on care-givers. *British Journal of Medical Psychology*, **57**, 35–44.

Isaacs, B., Livingstone, M. & Neville, Y. (1972) *Survival of the unfittest: a study of geriatric patients in Glasgow*. London: Routledge & Kegan Paul.

Jones, P.S. & Martinson, I.M. (1992) The experience of bereavement in care givers of family members with Alzheimer's disease. *Image: Journal of Nursing Scholarship* **24** (3), 172–176.

Levin, E., Sinclair, I., & Gorbach, P. (1989) *Families, Services and Confusion in Old Age*. Aldershot: Gower.

Liken, M.A. & Collins, C.E. (1993) Grieving: facilitating the process for dementia caregivers. *Psychosocial Nursing* **31** (1), 21–24.

Loos, P. & Boyd, A. (1997) Caregivers of persons with Alzheimer's disease: some neglected implications of the experience of personal loss and grief. *Death Studies* **21**, 501–514.

Miesen, B.M.L. (1997) Awareness in dementia patients and family grieving: a practical perspective. In: Miesen, B.M.L. & Jones, G.M.M. (eds) *Care-giving in Dementia*, Vol. 1, London: Routledge.

Parkes, C.M. (1996) *Bereavement: Studies of Grief in Adult Life*, 3rd edn. London: Routledge.

Parsons, K. (1997) The male experience of caregiving for a family member with Alzheimer's disease. *Qualitative Health Research* **7** (3), 391–407.

Sandford, J.R.A. (1975) Tolerance of debility in elderly dependants by supporters at home. *British Medical Journal* **3**, 471–473.

Sweeting, H. & Gilhooly, M.L.M. (1997) Dementia and the phenomenon of social death. *Sociology of Health and Illness* **19** (1), 93–117.

Taylor, P. (1987) A living bereavement. *Nursing Times* **30**, 27–30.

Wilkin, D. (1979) *Caring for Mentally Handicapped Children*. London: Croom Helm.

Worden, J.W. (1991) *Grief Counselling and Grief Therapy: A Handbook for the Mental Health Practitioner*, 2nd Edn. London: Routledge.

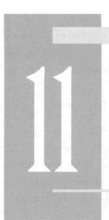

11

The early experience of Alzheimer's disease: implications for partnership and practice

John Keady, Jane Gilliard

KEY ISSUES

- The projected course and clinical criteria for establishing mild dementia remain to be defined

- Grounded theory is a methodological approach which makes its greatest contribution in areas where little research has been conducted

- In Alzheimer's disease there is a 'preclinical' phase which may last up to 7 years before symptoms can be diagnosed

- Coping with the onset and transition into Alzheimer's disease is a secretive process coupled with a heightened state of anxiety

- People with the early experience of dementia cope one day at a time

INTRODUCTION

This chapter is based on 15 interviews conducted with people with an awareness of their Alzheimer's disease and a willingness to discuss its impact. As such the research design immediately fell headlong into the murky waters of identifying and accessing a theoretical sample, ensuring the subject's informed consent to interview and gaining ethical approval to implement the research design. Controlling fully such sensitive considerations may well explain why so few qualitative, quantitative or survey studies exist that interpret the early experience of dementia and/or describe its subjective impact upon the individual concerned; for a discussion of this topic, see Keady (1996).

Writing at the beginning of the 1980s on the stressful nature of caring at home for a person with dementia, Zarit et al (1980) started a social research agenda that was to occupy the rest of the decade. A cursory glance through the social science literature on dementia care from this time reveals a plethora of research studies utilising a variety of research designs aimed at understanding this caregiving experience (Zarit et al, 1980; Greene et al, 1982; Gilhooly, 1984; Gilleard et al, 1984; Chenowerth and Spencer, 1986; George and Gwyther, 1986; Morris et al, 1988; Levin et al, 1989; Pearlin et al, 1990; Kuhlman et al, 1991; Vitaliano et al, 1991; Mace et al, 1992; Knight et al, 1993; Downs, 1994; Aneshensel et al, 1995; Woods, 1995). Consequently, people with dementia largely became seen as incidental subjects and passive recipients in the process of their dementia. This marginalisation of people with dementia was present in environments such as residential and nursing homes, where professional frameworks for assessment traditionally centred upon identifying, interpreting and overcoming 'problematic' behaviour such as 'wandering' and 'incontinence' (e.g. Stokes and Goudie, 1990; Blackburn, 1993), although the development of dementia care mapping (Kitwood, 1992) appears to be improving the situation. Moreover, the brief assessment schedules used to screen for the existence of dementia, e.g. the Mini-Mental State Examination (MMSE) (Folstein et al, 1975), are constructed on the basis of identifying cognitive loss and assigning scores to measure such incapacity. Rarely have people with dementia been seen as partners in the process of their dementia with support available for the empowerment of their own decision-making. Interestingly, in their thoughts on empowerment, Bell and McGregor (1995) state that the only generalisation they feel comfortable in making about people with dementia is that the condition primarily affects two areas – memory and communication – and that 'we' (presumably professional care staff) must always look at the person and not the diagnosis. Bell and McGregor (1995) also suggest that people with dementia 'naturally adjust to the changes that occur to themselves and their lives' (p. 14). But how true is this statement? Coping with the onset and transition into Alzheimer's disease is anything but a natural process. Our interviews showed this transition to be secretive in nature and coupled to a heightened state of anxiety; only later, do patterns of acceptance emerge, and even then, the degree of understanding differs from one individual to another.

However, the winds of change are blowing. Recent research and practice trends are attempting to uncover the 'personhood' of people with dementia (Kitwood and Bredin, 1992; Kitwood and Benson, 1995; Kitwood, 1997) – although in these studies the descriptions appear locked within advanced dementia – and are augmented by the recent needs-led shift in the direction of community care legislation and assessment procedures (Department of Health, 1990). This chapter aims to add to this understanding, in four steps: first, by selectively reviewing the literature on the early experience of dementia, with a particular emphasis on Alzheimer's disease, from a medical, social, policy and practice context, with an emphasis on the 'preclinical' phase of Alzheimer's disease; second, by describing the research aims and ethical considerations involved in the design of two separate but interrelated grounded theory studies conducted by the authors. The interviews involved exploring the early experience of dementia, and the sample presented here involves 15 people with diagnosed (very mild) Alzheimer's disease recruited from one memory disorders clinic in England. The interviews were conducted between 1994 and 1996 and were divided into study 1 (conducted by JK during 1994–5) and study 2 (conducted by JG during 1995–6), with both data sets being combined and analysis shared. Thirdly analysis of these interviews provides insight into individual transition into Alzheimer's disease and disclosure of its impact, through the strategies of 'taking stock' and 'sharing the load'. Finally, the practice implications of these strategies are explored, together with ideas for developing partnerships around an axis of people with dementia, families, community involvement and professional support.

THE EARLY EXPERIENCE OF DEMENTIA
Assessment and clinical considerations

The acquisition of cognitive impairment and dementia in both old and young age has been significantly correlated with a reduction in life expectancy (Eagles et al, 1990), with Magnússon and Helgason (1993) placing an upper age limit of 75 years on this positive correlation. Whilst it has been known for some time in Huntington's chorea (Folstein, 1989), there is emerging evidence of the genetic inheritance of dementia, particularly amongst younger people with Alzheimer's disease (Newens et al, 1993; Post, 1994; Li et al, 1995). The need to define precisely what is meant by 'cognitive impairment and dementia' is therefore crucial if support, services and new pharmacological treatments are to be offered at an earlier point in its trajectory.

The need for standard diagnostic criteria in dementia has been recognised since the early 1970s. The fourth edition of the *Diagnostic and Statistical Manual of Mental Disorders* (DSM-IV) (American Psychiatric Association, 1994) and the World Health Organization's ICD-10 classification of mental and behavioural disorders (WHO, 1993) both divide the syndrome of dementia into three distinct stages – mild, moderate and severe. For an early diagnosis of dementia to be made, therefore, it is essential that the individual is assessed as soon as possible during the mild stage, although, as we shall see later, this is easier said than done. The ICD-10 diagnostic criteria define mild dementia as having the following properties (WHO, 1993):

> *The decline in cognitive abilities causes impaired performance in daily living, but not to a degree that makes the individual dependent on others.*
> *Complicated daily tasks or recreational activities cannot be undertaken.*
> *(p. 30)*

However, the medical profession itself appear at odds over the relative merits of a standard definition, as 'complicated daily tasks' such as driving can still be undertaken relatively competently by people with very mild Alzheimer's disease (Hunt et al, 1993). Arguably, the diverse signs and symptoms attributable to the vast range of the dementias (Lishman, 1981) have led to clinical dissatisfaction with such overarching definitions. In turn this has led to the development of seemingly more sensitive and personalised rating scales to grade the severity and impact of dementia. Examples of these rating scales include the Global Deterioration Scale (GDS) (Reisberg et al, 1982) and the Clinical Dementia Rating (CDR) (Hughes et al, 1982), with both scales being frequently cited as admission criteria and sample identification in medical and psychological research. In content the CDR expanded upon the three stages of dementia described in DSM-IV and ICD-10, to view dementia on a scored continuum ranging from healthy (0) to questionable dementia (0.5), mild dementia (1), moderate dementia (2) and severe dementia (3). The score and criteria for inclusion were applied to six domains covering memory; orientation, judgment and problem-solving; community affairs; homes and hobbies; and personal care. For instance, people with questionable dementia – CDR 0.5 – under the memory domain were seen as experiencing mild consistent forgetfulness, partial recollection of events and 'benign' forgetfulness whilst under the orientation domain were seen as being fully oriented.

There is an apparent validity in staging the progression of dementia and anecdotal evidence suggests that these transitions are certainly recognisable to cares (Chenowerth and Spencer, 1986; Wilson, 1989a,b; La Rue et al, 1993). On the one hand, a persuasive argument could be tendered for staging dementia in this way as it can actually help carers to shape their day-to-day decision-making, as well as indicate what the future has in store (Barnes et al, 1981; Fortinsky and Hathaway, 1990; Keady and Nolan, 1995a). On the other hand, there remains an insensitivity in forcing people with dementia into predetermined criteria, when clinical judgment over what constitutes mild dementia is so uncertain (Burvill, 1993) and where the inclusion criteria may still be evolving – for instance in the recent 'discovery' and reporting of Lewy body dementia (McKeith et al, 1995). This point is also reinforced by Rubin et al (1989) who suggests that the CDR 0.5 stage of 'questionable cognitive impairment' actually represents very mild Alzheimer's disease. Bell and

McGregor (1995), in agreement with Carr and Marshall (1993), view the stage theories of dementia and clinical rating scales as 'problematic', with Bell and McGregor (1995) going as far as seeing the composition of such stages as 'positively dangerous' (p. 14). However, we would suggest that a balance needs to be struck between these opposing viewpoints and, perhaps, the real test of the validity of clinical staging is to be made by people with dementia themselves; a study that remains to be conducted.

For assessment and case identification of the early experience of dementia to improve, a better understanding of the disorder's onset and progression is essential. To investigate this phenomenon Flicker et al (1991) compared 32 elderly people who had clinically identified mild cognitive impairment with a group of 32 'normal' subjects matched for age and education. In this study the mildly impaired subjects were found to perform more poorly on tests of recent memory, remote memory, language function, concept formation and visuospatial praxis. In specifying these findings to Alzheimer's disease, Almkvist and Bäckman (1993) suggest that this represented a sequential model of neuropsychological decline. They observed that Alzheimer's disease starts by slowly progressive impairment of long-term episodic memory related to the medial temporal regions (Delieu and Keady, 1996 a,b) which 'occurs about 5 years before the first (clinical) examination' (Almkvist and Bäckman, 1993, p. 761). From a sociological standpoint the passage of time from very early symptom onset to its need for clinical assessment may well explain the uncertainty and personal struggle that people with Alzheimer's disease experience, whilst also accounting for the amount of time available to instigate compensatory cognitive and behavioural coping strategies.

In their informative study Almkvist and Bäckman (1993) further suggested that this time delay amounts to a 'preclinical' phase of Alzheimer's disease and that, overall, the onset of decline in Alzheimer's disease occurs first in episodic memory, then in psychomotor speed, semantic memory and visuospatial functions, and, eventually, in primary memory (Weingartner et al, 1993; Sliwinski et al, 1996). Expressive language disorders were also seen to occur early in Alzheimer's disease, and Almkvist and Bäckman (1993) suggested that case identification would be improved via sensitively designed tests for measuring subtle changes in episodic memory. In adopting a longitudinal study design Linn et al (1995) also supported the finding that changes in memory were amongst the earliest signs of Alzheimer's disease, but implied that these subtle changes could be identified up to 7 years before a 'confident' clinical diagnosis could be made – a 'preclinical' phase of Alzheimer's disease a full 2 years longer than that described by Almkvist and Bäckman (1993). Linn et al (1995) also found that in Alzheimer's disease measures of verbal learning and memory (paired associates, logical memory-percentages retained) and immediate auditory attention span (digit span) may be amongst the most sensitive to the early changes in cognitive functioning.

Traces of this finding were also seen in an individual case study undertaken by Morris and Fulling (1988) who assessed an 82-year-old cognitively healthy man until very mild Alzheimer's disease was diagnosed some 3 years later. The subject had a high level of education, and one of their study's key findings was that intellectual performance in highly selected older adults can be expected to 'hold' over time, and that brief cognitive scales for detecting the early signs of dementia may not have the necessary refinement and sensitivity to locate these changes, a finding consistent with others in the field (Galasko et al, 1990; Beardsall and Huppert, 1991). Morris and Fulling (1988) also identified the need for 'an observant collateral source' (i.e. a close relative or friend) to aid accurate case identification. This finding was noted earlier by Henderson and Hupport (1984), who suggested that reliance on self-reports by informant interview about cognitive performance is 'one of the most reliable methods of case identification' (p. 10).

The tapestry of potential signs and symptoms of mild dementia becomes ever more threadbare when other clinical conditions emerge and conspire to create a similar presentation. Keady (1996), in a review of the literature on the experience of dementia, found that confirming an early diagnosis of dementia is an extremely complex act which involves the exclusion of other symptomatology, including benign senile forgetfulness, age-associated memory impairment, depressive pseudo-dementia and other underlying physical causes such as normal pressure hydrocephalus, cerebral tumour and drug toxicity (Byrne, 1994). Coupled with concern over the ability of general practitioners to diagnose mild dementia in primary care settings (O'Connor et al, 1988; Cooper et al, 1992) and the inability of brief cognitive screening tools to comprehensively identify the early signs of dementia, it is, perhaps, not surprising that the prevalence rate of mild dementia varies considerably. For instance, Henderson and Hupport (1984) estimated that the prevalence of mild dementia in the community could range from 2.6% to 52.7%. At present there are around 650 000 people with dementia living in the UK, of whom half a million are thought to have Alzheimer's disease (ADS, 1995), and if the latter prevalence figure was applied to this total it would result in over 340 000 people with mild dementia living in the UK, the vast majority being older people living in their own home.

One way of providing an early diagnosis, and thereby increasing the reliability of prevalence rates, involves the role of memory clinics. Memory clinics themselves were first introduced in the UK in 1983 for the purpose of early diagnosis, and whilst they perform a vital function, they have come under increasing criticism for being too concerned with diagnostic research and for not providing enough support to meet the long-term needs of people with dementia and their families (Wright and Lindesay, 1995; Gilliard and Gwilliam, 1996). Undoubtedly, this position will come under further scrutiny as the prescription of donepezil hydrochloride, the first pharmacological treatment specifically for Alzheimer's disease at the mild to moderate stage, becomes more widely available (Harvey and Fairey, 1997).

Policy and practice: right from the start?

The focus of a recent Alzheimer's Disease Society (ADS) report was the need for services and the diagnosis to be 'right from the start' (ADS, 1995); in short, the earlier the better, as this confirmation allows people with dementia and their families time to prepare for their respective futures. However, this subtle shift in emphasis from a reactive to a proactive response in the identification of dementia (ADS, 1995; SSI/DoH, 1996, 1997) raises some complex questions for service providers and policy makers. Arguably, most research attention and service provision is targeted at people in the more advanced stages of dementia where services can be visible and support for the carer recognisable. Practical approaches to assessment and intervention with people in the mild stage of dementia have received only minimal attention, and where reports do exist a mixed message is heard. For instance, separate studies by Pollitt et al (1989) and O'Connor et al, (1991) dispute the importance of early intervention and its impact on family care. Indeed, the study by Pollitt et al, (1989) questions the usefulness and justification for intervention which, at this early point in the process of dementia, they contend was not recognised 'as a problem' by those living with its impact, and hence could afford to be overlooked. In contrast, other studies, notably those by Chenowerth and Spencer (1986), Bowers (1987, 1988), Motenko (1989), Clarke and Watson (1991) and Williams et al, (1995), highlighted the culmination of stressors placed upon carers at this transitional time and their pronounced uncertainty over what was happening. From these latter studies an early diagnosis was seen as pivotal to resolving this uncertainty, and there was an initial urgency to place changing and unusual behaviour within an illness, and thereby a medical, context.

This uncertainty leads to an uncomfortable question: just what is the current practice of informing people with dementia of their diagnosis? Rice and Warner (1994), in conducting one of the most authoritative surveys on the subject, only succeeded in adding more fuel to the fire of uncertainty. Rice and Warner (1994) reported on a UK survey of consultants in old age psychiatry ($n = 259$, response rate 79%) about their practice of informing people with dementia about their diagnosis and prognosis. Little uniformity was found in the responses, although carers were almost invariably told the diagnosis, which is similar to the practice in memory clinics. (Gilliard and Gwilliam, 1996), thus shifting the ultimate burden of responsibility. As Rice and Warner (1994) stated, the results for mild dementia 'demonstrate the wide variation in practice', with people in this diagnostic category being more likely to be told their diagnosis. The dividing line on 'to tell or not to tell' appeared to be one of human conscience coupled to the severity of the dementia. Moreover, even when the diagnosis was shared, the prognosis was rarely communicated. This lack of communication and partnership with people with dementia was rationalised through its status as an underresearched and underdebated area of medical ethics. Rice and Warner (1994) are, quite rightly, highly critical of this standpoint and concluded firmly that:

> *Patients have a right to know about their condition. Our view is that people*
> *with mild dementia should be given enough information for them to*
> *understand the diagnosis and prognosis. Carers should not be given*
> *information that cannot also be imparted to patients. (p. 470)*

For this to occur there will need to be an emphasis on training in breaking bad news (Buckman, 1984; McLauchlan, 1990; Davis, 1991; Rice and Warner, 1994) and an infrastructure to support people with dementia, and their families and support networks (including employers where appropriate), through the diagnosis. There is emerging evidence that such a view is gaining support, although, from a carer's perspective, considerable uncertainty remains over telling the person with dementia the diagnosis for fear of making that person depressed (Maguire et al, 1996). Black (1995) in an article for the Alzheimer's Disease International newsletter provided a balanced account of the rights and wrongs of people with Alzheimer's disease being told their diagnosis. In this article people with mild dementia were made to be a case where withholding the diagnosis and prognosis was seen as 'unfair and unethical'. Like the psychiatrists in the study by Rice and Warner (1994), Black (1995) drew a dividing line on 'to tell or not to tell' the diagnosis along the severity of the impairment. Whilst the language is 'patient-centred' and not 'people-centred', Black (1995) cogently draws out the central arguments for disclosing the diagnosis of dementia (Box 11.1).

Respect for the individual's intrinsic right to know the truth was evident in the writings of a carer named Lynne Bell. Within the pages of the ADS newsletter, Bell (1995) outlined the responsibility of living with her mother's diagnosis of Alzheimer's disease, and declared that, after much soul-searching, she found that sharing the diagnosis was 'the right thing to do.' As Bell (1995) sensitively described, after many shared tears her mother's response to being informed of the diagnosis was that 'they would have to do the best we can' (p. 5). This openness meant that the full meaning of Alzheimer's disease could then be shared and jointly used to understand and manage the experience of forgetfulness. Moreover, the

Box 11.1 The pros and cons of informing people with dementia of their diagnosis.

For:
Maximises individual autonomy
Affords opportunity to seek the best possible information and choose or reject treatment, even if experimental or unconventional
Accommodates need to formulate specific advance directives, and for complete financial and personal planning and identification of surrogates
Respects the individual's intrinsic right to know the truth
Offers opportunity for individuals to express themselves, resolve conflicts and make known last wishes before the opportunity is forever lost
Acknowledges patient's preference based on past knowledge.

Against:
Diagnosis of Alzheimer's disease cannot be assigned with prefect accuracy and prognosis is imprecise
Therapeutic options are limited – may lead to hopelessness and compromise quality of life
The patient may not have the ability to understand the diagnosis
Avoids severe depression or catastrophic reaction, or unnecessary functional decline or suicide attempts
Acknowledges patients preferences based on past knowledge.

From Black (1995).

burden of responsibility and knowledge of deceit could also be released and channelled into more purposeful activity.

Individual considerations

In 1989 the publication of a book entitled *My Journey Into Alzheimer's Disease* (Davis, 1989) drew attention to the voice and awareness of people with dementia. Underpinned by his Christian faith, the Reverend Davis articulated his transition and adjustment to the onset of Alzheimer's disease and the fear and uncertainty that accompanied his journey (pp. 21–82). Another younger person with dementia living in the USA, McGowin (1993), also provided a lucid account of being 'dragged' into Alzheimer's disease. McGowin movingly described the emotional, physical and social turmoil that this process inflicted upon her life and that of her family; in particular the denial experienced by her husband, their overriding sense of fear and the matter-of-fact way in which the diagnosis was initially communicated to her. It is interesting that professional interventions are mentioned only rarely in both these books, and when they are, it is usually with feelings of frustration and hostility. More specifically, both individuals expressed their distress at:

- The time it took to establish a diagnosis
- Being kept in the dark over the outcome of assessment investigations
- The lack of dedicated support services, especially support groups to facilitate discussion
- The inadequate supply of information
- Lack of support for memory training.

From a research perspective, Froggatt (1988) produced an interesting and well-received chapter for an Open University publication and study course on mental health problems in old age which focused on self-awareness in early dementia. Whilst the research methodology and sample size were not made explicit in her study, the research design involved interviews and observation of people with the early experience of dementia. The aim of this study was to explore how people with dementia perceived themselves and how they could be helped to retain a sense of identity. In this study the early experience of dementia was seen as a complex interplay of social, psychological and biological factors with memory failure quickly resulting in social isolation. The social construction of memory failure was seen as an episodic mixture of forgetfulness over recent events, absentmindedness and internal preoccupation with thoughts and daydreams. Much to her credit, Froggatt (1988) also looked at the 'retained social skills repertoire', such as the person's ability to continue to express politeness, be friendly to strangers and put on a good presentation of self. Memory failure itself was found to be masked by confabulation, and the professional skill of creating and maintaining trust was seen as crucial in gaining entry into this world. In a similar vein, McCormick et al (1994) found that people with Alzheimer's disease complained of symptoms clearly related to cognitive impairment early in the course of their illness, but underreported those symptoms. The study also found that people with probable Alzheimer's disease also experienced a range of other illnesses (similar to a 'normal' older population) such as gastrointestinal symptoms, joint pain, rash and cough.

Other attempts at interpreting the experience of dementia have been described in a range of process models (Willoughby and Keating, 1991; Kobayashi et al, 1993; Taraborrelli, 1993; Collins et al, 1994; Harvath, 1994; Clarke, 1995), although only a few have used the experience of people with dementia as part of the generated model (Keady and Nolan, 1994, 1995b; Wuest et al, 1994). Keady and Nolan (1994, 1995b) described the process of dementia as moving through nine stages. This process of dementia was seen to begin with a stage of *slipping* (1) and end in *death* (9). As the model was used to underpin the research interviews described below, an overview of its properties is given in Box 11.2.

In a separate and informative study, Gillies (1995) interviewed a convenience sample of 19 people with dementia drawn from a range of local service providers in the Dundee area of Scotland. Carers were also

Box 11.2 Nine stages of dementia

1. **Slipping**: the person gradually becomes aware of minor and seemingly trivial slips and lapses in memory and/or behaviour. These slips and lapses are initially ignored, but as they become more frequent can no longer be so easily dismissed. At this time emotion-focused coping behaviours such as 'discounting' and the 'normalising of events' are seen to be used to deny the significance of the symptoms. The stage shades into *suspecting*:
2. **Suspecting**: incidents occur with greater frequency or severity so that they can no longer be rationalised or ignored. The 'discounting' and 'normalising of events' become less successful coping strategies and the individual begins to suspect that something could be quite seriously amiss.
3. **Covering up**: the person makes a conscious and deliberate effort to compensate for these difficulties and actively hides them from family members, friends and colleagues. As the condition progresses and covering up becomes more difficult, the person begins to restrict activities in certain areas where competence is difficult to sustain. If they have not noticed before, it is at this point where the individual's partner or family may begin to notice changes in the level of cognitive and behavioural activities.
4. **Revealing**: in this stage individuals reveal their difficulties to the person closest to them. This may be as a result of a conscious decision, or as a result of being confronted with patterns of loss. At this point shared knowledge may still be kept within the immediate family and a formal confirmation of suspicions may be delayed.
5. **Confirming**: open acknowledgment of the problem is made and the process of diagnostic confirmation can begin.
6. **Maximising**: the person continues to adjust to the dementia by the use of adaptive coping techniques to compensate for cumulating losses.
7. **Disorganisation**: cognitive difficulties and associated behavioural problems become an increasingly dominant feature. There is diminishing decision-making ability and awareness of actions may become lost.
8. **Decline**: any semblance of a normal and overtly reciprocal relationship becomes clouded and uncertain. The instrumental demands of care become a more prominent feature of the caregiving relationship, together with increased dependency needs. At some point along this road decisions on the person's admission into continuing care may be taken by the carer.
9. **Death**: finally, the person with dementia is presented with the ultimate phase and transition, death.

recruited into the sample. In reporting her findings Gillies (1995) made the observation that carers were often reluctant to leave their relative during the interview, a situation consistent with our own study and that of Bowers (1987) when she described the cognitive mechanism of 'protective caregiving', i.e. protecting the self-image of the cared-for person, as the most stressful feature in caring at home for a person with dementia. Gillies (1995) also found that humour helped the carer cope with the situation and that the carer experienced degrees of emotional isolation from the person with dementia, for example during prolonged periods of silence. These experiences highlight the importance of establishing the subjective meanings attached to illness and care.

THE STUDY
Method

Chenitz and Swanson (1986) suggested that grounded theory 'makes its greatest contribution in areas in which little research has been done' (p. 7). As such, its methodological application to people with an awareness of their dementia would appear an appropriate choice. The aims of the study resulted from the need to refine and test stages 1–6 ('slipping' to 'maximising') of the nine-stage process model of dementia (Keady and Nolan, 1994, 1995b) and required contact with people with an awareness of their dementia. The research aims of study 1 (JK) were:

1. to explore the experience of dementia and personal coping behaviour
2. to explore when and how decisions are made to seek professional help
3. to explore stresses and coping behaviours of family supporters
4. to explore how resources are viewed by people with early dementia and their family supporters.

Study 2 (JG) was built upon the findings of study 1, in particular the person's awareness of the diagnosis and its prognosis, and shared its research aims. Overall, these aims were exploratory in nature, and people with the early experience of dementia and their family supporters were invited to be interviewed as soon as practicable after the symptoms were diagnosed as mild dementia using DSM-IV criteria – usually within about 6 months of initial contact with the memory clinic. The samples for both parts of the study were gained through contact with a respected memory clinic in England, and diagnostic and profile screening for the interviews was undertaken by the clinic's medical and psychology staff. In study 1, a total of 50 requests for interviews were screened and sent by the memory clinic over a 6-month period in 1994. The requests for interview were handed separately to the person with dementia and to the family supporter by the responsible clinic staff, with the offer of a joint interview if preferred. This approach resulted in 20 replies from 10 couples (nine married couples, and one daughter and her mother) which resulted in 11 family-centered interviews (one married couple were interviewed again later in the study), although it was made clear in the request to interview that it was the person with cognitive impairment who was to be the focus of the interview; further details of the sample composition and ethical considerations can be found elsewhere (Keady et al, 1995; Keady and

Nolan, 1995b,c; Clarke and Keady, 1996). Each interview was tape-recorded and conducted in the person's own home. Field notes were kept and all tapes were transcribed and analysed on the day of the interview. Ethical approval restricted the formal length of each interview to 45 minutes, although on eight occasions the family supporter and person with dementia asked if the researcher (JK) wanted to stay 'for a cup of tea' after the formal interview had concluded. This act of hospitality gave an additional opportunity for incidental data collection which was recorded in the field notes. Seven people in the sample had a diagnosis of (very mild) Alzheimer's disease, two had vascular dementia and one had frontal lobe dementia. One interviewee, who had been recently diagnosed with Alzheimer's disease, was found to be in a state of denial and the interview did not proceed. On all but one occasion, the family supporter of the person with dementia wanted to be present during the interview. Following the procedure of the memory clinic, the supporters only had been informed officially of the diagnosis, but on interview four people with the early experience of dementia stated that they had taken steps independently of their supporter to find out what was wrong, whilst four others had been informed by their spouse of the diagnosis.

In study 2 (JG) a similar research protocol was adopted, although all interviewees were aware of their diagnosis of dementia prior to interview, with this knowledge being known to the researcher. Nine people with diagnosed very mild Alzheimer's disease were recruited into this study (one person was interviewed twice). Study 2 commenced in mid 1995 and the spacing of the data collection involved one interview per month. Both studies followed a grounded theory design with the data subject to constant comparative analysis; this inductive technique allows themes and categories to emerge from the data (Glaser and Strauss, 1967; Glaser, 1978). From study 1 only the six transcripts and interviews with people with Alzheimer's disease (one additional interview being discounted) are included here to maintain specificity and qualitative rigour in reporting the research findings. This results in a full data set of 15 people with Alzheimer's disease (12 women and 3 men, age range 72–84 years and 67–86 years respectively) and their family supporters.

Each interview required a sensitive approach in which the development of trust was essential. The opening minutes of the interview were vitally important in allaying suspicion (as far as possible) and we found it of immense benefit that the interviews were conducted by researchers who had a clinical or social work background in working with people with dementia. Interviews usually commenced with the words: 'As you know, I am here to talk with you about your experience of living with memory loss – could you please tell me how it started?' Anecdotal evidence from our study suggests that people with dementia found the interviews a therapeutic experience and, after a process of trust had been established, were often amazed that someone was actually taking an interest in their situation.

Living with Alzheimer's disease: a transitional experience

Comparison and analysis of the interview data suggested that in Alzheimer's disease the individual enters a period of transition which involves adaptive coping behaviours. This transition was augmented by feelings of fear and anxiety in living under the shadows of constant uncertainty (Cohen, 1993). So far two strategies have emerged from the data which explain this process, and we have labelled these as *taking stock* and *sharing the load*. Both strategies are interdependent.

Taking stock

Taking stock comprises three tactics which we have named *closing down*, *regrouping* and *covering your tracks*. Taking stock is preceded by an awareness, and self-acknowledgment, that 'something is wrong'. Adapted from the work of Keady (1997), Box 11.3 draws together the physical, psychological and sensory sensations which people with Alzheimer's disease described as their first awareness of the onset of the disease. Upon experiencing one or a combination of these phenomena, no-one in the sample ascribed these 'slips and lapses' to the onset of Alzheimer's disease. Concentration difficulties were particularly perceived as a nuisance, a problem, the effects of growing older: 'I thought it was to be

---

Box 11.3   First signs and symptoms of Alzheimer's disease. This list is not intended to represent fully all reported first signs; some people reported an initial experience of a combination of these signs

Problem-solving difficulties
Being unable to concentrate for prolonged periods
Thought block
Inability to recall names quickly
Losing track of conversations
Feeling disassociated from reality
Becoming sad and depressed
Feeling unduly angry
Tearfulness
Feeling and becoming lost in familiar surroundings
Decline in coordination and control of speech and actions
Writing block
Heightened sense of taste and smell

expected', as one subject described it. Others believed that their feelings of depression or anger were extensions of lifelong personality traits; a reaction to their retirement, or the retirement of their spouse. However, whilst initially discounted, the signs were nevertheless monitored at an intuitive level and as they continued, or accumulated, people with Alzheimer's disease began to live through shifting degrees of uncertainty, gradually suspecting that something serious was happening to them. Significantly, these initial signs were also seen as an embarrassment and, potentially, as an admission of 'not being right'. This situation is typified by the following reactions:

> At the beginning it was so dark. I couldn't believe I was doing these things. I felt so stupid and didn't want to share it with anyone else. I had trouble getting the right word out and forgetting people's names. It was awful.

> The first time I noticed was when I used to do crosswords and gradually over the years the recalling of words become harder and harder until, well, they were quite difficult to do and I got a bit fed up with doing them then.

Another person in the study did not experience this early awareness because his problems had been masked by bereavement. As he stated during an interview.

> I'll tell you how it did start. I went to the doctor to get a signature so I could get the buses and he did that for me. After the doctor had signed it he stood up and he said, 'How many children did you have?' I said, 'Seven', and he said, 'Well, what are their seven names?' And I got five of them and I couldn't tell him the other two and that hurt me.

None of these early experiences was shared or openly communicated to others. Reaching the first tactic of 'closing down' was, itself, a protracted process involving many months of trying to explain away – to yourself – the impact of the signs identified in Box 11.3. Thus, in interpreting the early experience of dementia, it would appear that the original 'slipping' 'suspecting' and 'covering up' themes (see Box 11.1) had empirical validity, but only accounted superficially for the role and life transitions experienced by people with Alzheimer's disease. Indeed, it is the frequency, duration and concern posed by the signs outlined in Box 11.3 that become the marker to employing the tactic of 'closing down'.

Closing down The tactic of 'closing down' was employed by each person in the study; its primary purpose was twofold, allowing people with (undiagnosed) Alzheimer's disease time to adjust to their new-found reality, as well as space to reframe existing events. In effect, 'closing down' is a self-protective strategy aimed at maintaining the person's integrity and sense of 'who I am'. The tactic of 'closing down' was an intensely private experience and when people with Alzheimer's disease spoke retrospectively of using this tactic, it was expressed through feelings of fear, anxiety, bewilderment, puzzlement, uncertainty and loss. In sharing this tactic the body language of people with Alzheimer's disease also altered significantly and there was a great deal of comfort rubbing and clenching of fists or rubbing of hands. Eye contact also diminished rapidly, giving life to the described feelings of fear and anxiety. The act of 'closing down' was not shared, even in relationships that were obviously loving and close, and was expressed through the following set of coping strategies:

- Keeping my real fears and feelings secret
- Withdrawing from conversations
- Remaining in familiar surroundings
- Constantly repeating things to myself to aid memory and recall
- Engaging in mentally challenging activities such as puzzles and crosswords
- Having a good cry when no-one is around
- Keeping as active as possible by concentrating on familiar tasks
- Trying to avoid new situations as far as possible
- Relying on myself to find answers to the problems.

With the intensely private and secretive nature of these coping strategies, it is little wonder that people with (undiagnosed) Alzheimer's disease experienced depression and a lowering of mood (Verhey et al, 1993). The awareness and secrecy of these behaviours, coupled to a rapidly shrinking social world, without an explanation of what was happening, were a shattering blow to the individual. Moreover, the impact of employing such restrictive coping strategies was magnified enormously as their efficacy led to sources of conflict within a relationship, with spouses or adult children being confronted with 'new' behaviours which made little, if any, sense. These 'new' behaviours included the person suddenly starting to keep quiet during conversations; not following favourite television programmes; not wanting to go out of the home; restricting any driving activities to the local area; becoming argumentative for no obvious reason, and so on. These conflicts often led the carer to expressions of guilt and self-directed anger later in the caregiving trajectory once the full impact of Alzheimer's disease was out in the open.

The transition into 'closing down' also began a voyage of self-discovery in which strands of the individual's personality were being lost and mourned by their owner; indeed, we would describe it as a process of saying good-bye to parts of the self, and its functioning, that had previously been taken for granted. It is tempting to equate this phenomenon with the 'bargaining' stage of the Kübler-Ross (1970) five-stage model of death and dying, but the people in our sample were not dying in the accepted meaning of the word. Their philosophical bargaining with loss was more of a functional mechanism which allowed the person time to draw on other compensatory coping behaviours, rationalise their meaning and 'construct a new me' from within a shifting reality. We hypothesise that it is at this point where some people with (undiagnosed) Alzheimer's disease are unable to rationalise the feelings and experiences of loss, and plummet to the depths of helplessness and hopelessness; from here it is only a short cognitive step to suicidal ideation (Williams and Pollock, 1993). Indeed, as cognitive or genetic screening improves to detect the very early signs of Alzheimer's disease, it is likely that it will be at this point that turning suicidal ideation away from direct action (when possible) will become an increasing feature of dementia care practice, an example is given by Rohde et al, (1995). The following exchange between one of the authors (JG) and a person with Alzheimer's disease (M) attempts to illustrate this evolving process of loss and adaptation:

JG: You've told me about the 'old' Mary who used to go to work and run a household and look after the family, and now all these things are harder for you. Do you miss the 'old' Mary?

M: Yes.

JG: Do you grieve for her?

M: I don't think so, because I've got a lovely family and they're very good to me. No, I don't think so. I take life as it comes. If you do business, that has its problems as well. And now I've got my problems.

The dialogue reveals a personal acceptance of the impact of Alzheimer's disease, its process of rationalisation and the fact that the person has seemingly come to terms with its impact upon her life. Within the tactic of 'closing down' it is the eventual acceptance that things are not going to return to normal that triggers the next tactic of 'regrouping'.

Regrouping Regrouping is a time-limited tactic aimed at providing the person with the confidence and resilience to 'keep going'. Regrouping involves an acceptance of the purpose of 'closing down', and that the shifting reality cannot be returned to normal. In order to regroup, people with Alzheimer's disease drew on a diverse set of coping behaviours, including self-belief, and whilst it was not verbalised at the time, drew comfort from the familiarity of their surroundings and the support received from family and friends. From one set of field notes made at this time (JK), this process was described as 'reciprocity without visible exchange', but the exchange was evident in the compensatory feelings of comfort that familiar surroundings and people bring. Moreover, in supporting the tactic of 'regrouping', people with Alzheimer's disease stated that they talked to themselves a great deal, in effect giving themselves confidence to prepare for their future, whatever this might hold.

The function and meaning of engaging in self-dialogue was an interesting feature and one that warrants additional investigation. Keady and Nolan (1996) have termed this process 'tacit collusion', i.e. colluding with yourself to maintain a veneer of normality, and through tacit collusion people with Alzheimer's disease drew the inner strength to enter a more proactive yet stoically secretive tactic, of 'covering your tracks'.

Covering your tracks This is the final tactic of the 'taking stock' strategy and defines how long the person with (undiagnosed) Alzheimer's disease could, or wanted to, live out their condition without being found out. Covering your tracks also proved to be a tactic that was used jointly by the person with Alzheimer's disease and the supporter once the dementia was out in the open, but its consequences were to remain concealed within the family unit. However, in its initial form, 'covering your tracks' is employed to retain control over the individual's situation and proactively continue with the tacit collusion. The following coping strategies were described as being useful in controlling the progression of (undiagnosed) Alzheimer's disease:

- Keeping my fears and feelings secret
- Using lists and other memory aids
- Constantly repeating things to myself to help me remember
- Keeping any further memory loss to myself for as long as possible
- Fighting the memory loss and trying not to let it get the better of me
- Engaging in mentally challenging activities such as puzzles and crosswords
- Making up stories to fill in the gaps
- Trying to keep calm and relaxed at all times
- Taking things one day at a time.

There is some overlap in the range of coping strategies with the ones in 'closing down', such as engaging in mentally challenging activities, but it is the meaning and purpose of the strategy that has altered. For instance, engaging in mentally challenging activities was first used in 'closing down' as a self-administered test for determining the extent of memory failure. However, by the time it was used within the tactic of 'covering your tracks', its purpose was either to 'hold' the degree of cognitive loss, or in some instances to actively challenge it.

Thus 'covering your tracks' required adaptive and imaginative coping patterns, including writing down significant matters of concern such as important birthdays, ages of children, dates of anniversaries, directions to the local shop, where important keys are kept and what they are for, a pictorial representation of the value of money, and so on. These lists were usually secreted in places where the chances of their discovery were minimal; even so, there was an associated fear that discovery of such a list could reveal the depths of an individual's loss and perceived sense of failing. Interestingly, in carrying out this adaptive coping strategy, there were gender differences in places of concealment. For men, a common hiding-place for the lists was usually outside the house in places such as the garden shed or inside the car, whilst for women a handbag or a garment hanging in a wardrobe was frequently cited as a secret place. However, the purpose of the list was tacit self-collusion to perpetuate the veneer of normality and to preserve feelings of self-worth, identity and control.

The physical and emotional energy invested in this process should not be underestimated, and in our sample 'covering your tracks' was engaged in for periods stretching from months to years. Moreover, in some families, sources of conflict gradually diminished as the new behaviours began to be questioned less and less and became assimilated into daily living routines – it was 'Dad being difficult again', or as one family supporter stated:

> After a while I began to think what he [her husband] was doing wasn't a problem. He wasn't doing any harm, you know. I got frustrated at first not being able to go out as often as I would have liked, to get the shopping mainly, but I just thought he had gone off the idea of driving. That's what he told me anyway, and there are worse things in this life than not going out in the car, don't you think? I picked up some old interests of mine and life just went on.

How long 'covering your tracks' could be tolerated, and its surface meaning interpreted by others, was the hinge upon which the success and longevity of the tactic turned. Supporters unwittingly began to collude with the stories and behaviours of their partner, thus twisting their meaning and making a seemingly abnormal situation 'normal' again. Eventually, however, 'covering your tracks' became an increasingly fraught and difficult tactic to manage. In time, the people with Alzheimer's disease started to react to events and not to shape them, with others eventually beginning to notice the 'slips and lapses' and note their frequency. For the individual with dementia, long-held coping mechanisms aimed at concealment also began to break down and the cognitive skills were not sufficient to successfully reshape them. At this point 'covering your tracks' began to shade into the strategy 'sharing the load', as this quotation from a 71-year-old man with Alzheimer's disease attempts to illustrate:

You see, I couldn't carry on pretending anymore. I knew others knew, you could tell it in their eyes – they were watching me more, asking me questions, things I should have known but didn't. I felt I was on a roundabout and I couldn't get off. In the end I wanted them to know. It's a relief now.

Sharing the load

The strategy of 'sharing the load' is one of unburdening, and at this time a number of potential options and responses are available. For instance, family members may openly confront the person with Alzheimer's disease or, acting in a more subversive way, seek an independent confirmation for their partner's or their parent's unusual behaviour. This independent confirmation was sought either from other members of the family or from the general practitioner, although this path does not always run smoothly, with the supporters' concerns often in danger of being discounted with the signs being attributed to some other cause, such as normal ageing or depression (ADS, 1993; Keady and Nolan, 1995a). Alternatively, people with (undiagnosed) Alzheimer's disease may disclose their experiences and concealment activities to the person closest to them. However, no person in this study sought an independent explanation of changes in cognitive and emotional behaviour directly from a doctor or other member of the primary health care team. Steps to the diagnosis were taken by the supporter without the person's initial knowledge (in 4 cases) or, more commonly, jointly by the family member and the person with (undiagnosed) Alzheimer's disease (11 cases).

No matter how this stage of revealing is reached, for all individuals concerned this period of sharing was a cathartic experience. For instance, on four occasions reported during these interviews, when the subject was initially approached by the person with Alzheimer's disease, the family supporter denied firmly the existence of the exhibited signs and symptoms, suggesting instead that 'things would get better', or that the behaviour was simply 'due to their retirement'. This denial placed enormous additional pressure on the person experiencing Alzheimer's disease and often resulted in feelings of self-doubt and depression. Indeed, in most cases the way in which this process of informal confirmation was handled between the partners had a significant impact upon the future direction of care and the mutual seeking of a diagnosis. Obviously, in this part of the study, people with Alzheimer's disease and their family supporters were willing to discuss openly and share their thoughts, feelings and experiences. This open disclosure between partners may not be fully representative of the picture and this is a phenomenon where additional research inquiry is necessary. However, from our study data, a mutual acceptance of the existence of loss and adaptation moved the coping behaviours into a different domain, and people with Alzheimer's disease were able to feel a weight taken off their shoulders. At this time coping behaviours were expressed by the following thoughts and actions:

- Being thankful for the close support of family and others around me
- Relying on the support of the person closest to me
- Trying to keep calm and relaxed at all times
- Talking over my memory loss with people I trust.

However, it would be a mistake to believe that cognitive and behavioural concealment activities just vanished – they did not. Perhaps the most moving experience we encountered during the entire set of interviews was when people with Alzheimer's disease admitted to their supporter, at times to the latter's utter astonishment, that they were continuing to conceal further memory loss from them. As it emerged, the purpose of this concealment activity was to protect the supporter from evidence of further loss, thus covertly maintaining the tactic of 'covering your tracks'. For those who had passed to this point there was also a general feeling of satisfaction that no-one else knew, or had suspected, their earlier attempts at 'taking stock', in particular the deployment of the tactic of 'covering your tracks', – a reaction that we had not anticipated. In all likelihood this points towards people with Alzheimer's disease developing a sense of mastery over their situation, a mastery grounded in an intimate knowledge of adapting to cumulative and consistent losses. Within this experience lies an untapped pool of knowledge and, we would suggest, what is needed to reveal its properties is a professional mechanism and partnership able to dip into this reservoir of experience. The ensuing knowledge could then be used as a means of building upon past coping patterns in order to shape future events.

This professional partnership also extends to the task of sharing the diagnosis. This is a nettle which must be grasped, and 'sharing the load' is a responsibility we all must bear. From the study data, and bearing in mind the normal practice of the memory clinic only to disclose the diagnosis to the supporter, some relatives believed that informing the person with Alzheimer's disease of the diagnosis was their duty, and they preferred to do this at a time, and in a place, which suited them. This was explained by one carer (C) in the following exchange with JG:

C: I wanted it to be my job, and I told the doctor this. He said, 'I'll tell your wife', and I said, 'No, I'll tell her myself.' He said, 'How are you going to do that?' and I said, 'Time … I'm a great believer that life gives you little windows and it's just the ideal time.' I felt that at this terrible time it was my duty to explain to my wife in a way I knew she would accept it. She would have been shocked rigid if a stranger had told her.

JG: Was this difficult?

C: It was hard to tell her the exact thing. But when I told her I felt I had a terrific weight taken off my shoulders because the facade we'd been living for eight to ten months had gone. There was all this honesty now. We both felt that a cloud had gone off us and we felt entirely different.

For supporters in this study, provision of the diagnosis helped to place retrospective and present events in context. For people with Alzheimer's disease this process appeared to follow the same course. Armed with knowledge and information about their diagnosis, people with the onset of Alzheimer's disease no longer appeared frustrated when they forgot simple points, or dropped something which could otherwise be construed as being clumsy. They could explain it to their family and friends, and most importantly, to themselves. Providing the diagnosis also helped people with Alzheimer's disease to make sense of their evolving behaviours, actions and feelings. The people interviewed in this study had been ready to hear the truth, having worked through earlier feelings of shock and distress via the strategy and tactics identified in 'taking stock'. The diagnosis was, at times, a relief and a confirmation that 'they were not going mad'. For example, on being informed of his diagnosis, one subject – a devout Catholic – compared his Alzheimer's disease to the Devil, 'and I'm going to fight it'. To prepare himself for the fight he set himself mental and physical challenges underpinned by a motivation to win, thus engendering a sense of hope. On this same issue another woman in the study said, 'Well, it's there now and we can't change that, so I just have to make the best of it'. Sharing the load was not an admission of defeat, but a process whereby relationships and the meaning of illness could be reconstructed and rediscovered.

DEVELOPING PARTNERSHIPS: DISCUSSION POINTS

During one of our interviews, the person with Alzheimer's disease was asked to describe what it felt like to live with such a disease. He described it as if 'my head was full of little bubbles, like a glass of lemonade, and sometimes the bubbles all rise to the surface and my head clears. Then it slowly fills with bubbles again'. His wife would say that he had both good times and bad times. To us this man's experience of Alzheimer's disease described a general feeling of receptivity. However, 2 months later when the same man was asked if he could describe again how it feels to have Alzheimer's disease, he talked about his head 'feeling as if it's full like a bowling ball – heavy and solid – quite different from before'. The interpretation is that the clear times appeared to have been lost. He was asked if he could identify with the 'foggy feeling' another man had described at the onset of his Alzheimer's disease, but could not. This second man had said:

It's one thing I've been getting for quite a time now and that is a distant feeling that things are misting over and that I'm trying to remember. There's things coming through faintly that I'm trying to remember what they are. There was a patch of that and it's in a shroud of mist and I can't remember what it was I was trying to remember.

Without doubt, policy-makers and service providers will need to develop ways of responding more fully to this voice, the subjective meaning it creates for the individual and the impact it has upon family supporters and social networks. The depth and breadth of investment necessary to operationalise this act of partnership should not be underestimated, and there is an urgent need for more openness and honesty in working with people with Alzheimer's disease. A standpoint should be adopted whereby their voice and their experiences are the foundations for dementia care practice and service planning. From the study data, this call for partnership was heard most loudly in the following areas.

Developing a range of information needs

If service providers are going to offer people with cognitive loss an early assessment and diagnosis, and if that diagnosis is then to be shared, an understanding of the individual's experiences and information needs is crucial. But what information do people with the onset of Alzheimer's disease actually want? From the study this was often very difficult for people with Alzheimer's disease to articulate. Quite simply, if you do not know what information there is to have – if any – then you are unlikely to know what you want. One person with Alzheimer's disease was very clear that he wanted access to a central reference point as he felt he had been passed from 'pillar to post' during the time of his assessment and diagnosis. Other information needs emerged from people with Alzheimer's disease, and these were described as follows:

1. Technical information about what was happening to their brain so that they could try to make some sense out of the maze in which they were living.
2. Help to overcome feelings of anxiety during the diagnostic process: in particular, information on what to expect from the assessment procedure; the purpose of the memory and screening tests; how long each test would last, and the role of professional staff involved in the assessment procedure.
3. Reassurance about the cause of Alzheimer's disease, especially that it was not their fault.

4. Practical information about services and benefits to which they were entitled.
5. Advice about coping within the caring relationship. People with Alzheimer's disease expressed a great deal of concern about the burden they posed for their supporter.
6. Accessible information which may be provided in diverse forms, such as audio cassette, video cassette or large-print writing, which would allow for repeated access.

However, what we heard loudest and most clearly in the interviews was what people with Alzheimer's disease did *not* want. In particular, they did not want detailed information about the future. As one typical interviewee stated:

> I don't know anything about it. I don't want to know. I just take things day by day. The only thing I know about it is eventually I won't be able to do the things I could do before and I shall be in a chair or something. But I don't want to know.

Our feelings are that people with Alzheimer's disease know that the future is pretty bleak and they do not need this to be reinforced. They simply want to take one day at a time and we would suggest that practical support, information-giving strategies and approaches to partnership are constructed around this simple philosophy.

Creating separate and distinct services

During the interviews there was, at times, a degree of hostility expressed towards the supporter. The reason for this anger was distress that the supporters were receiving group support to which the people with Alzheimer's disease were not invited, although they knew that they were being discussed. Seven people in the sample also stated that they would like the opportunity to discuss and share their feelings with others living through similar experiences. Others wanted the opportunity to learn how to improve their memory performance. In our sample, no professional member of staff from either health or social service authorities visited the person with Alzheimer's disease at home. The absence of involvement from agencies outside the relationship meant that people with Alzheimer's disease themselves had no-one else to turn to. At times people with Alzheimer's disease wanted to keep additional losses to themselves, such as suddenly being confronted by additional lapses of memory, but, paradoxically, they also wanted to share this development with someone who would understand. It would appear, therefore, that there is a need for people with the early experience of dementia, no matter what the diagnosis, to have access to an independent confidante outside the family relationship where, if they so choose, they can confide such fears and patterns of coping. A step towards this partnership has begun in the formation of support groups specifically designed for people with the early experience of dementia (Jackson and Wonson, 1987; McAfee et al, 1989; Yale, 1989; Van-Wylen and Dykema-Lamse, 1990; Duff and Peach, 1994; Gatz, 1995; LaBarge and Trtanj, 1995; Gibson and Moniz-Cook, 1996), but the development and availability of these groups still remains an exception rather than a rule (Reilly, 1995).

Involvement in professional training

The early identification of dementia is crucial, and yet access to specialist services and centres, such as memory clinics, is dependent more upon geographical accident than on a coordinated and planned national strategy. Furthermore, in this study, no one person was able to align the initial symptoms (Box 11.3) to the onset of Alzheimer's disease. To increase public awareness about this onset it would seem appropriate for responsible authorities to engage in local health promotion and education campaigns. It is also crucial that the training of professional staff in dementia care practice generally, and the early experience of dementia specifically, is improved and that joint training programmes are initiated (Nolan and Keady, 1996a,b). Without the professions moving forward in a clear direction and with clear objectives – and we see identification and response to the early experience of dementia as one of these directions – the present service fragmentation and status quo will remain. This is one relic of the twentieth century it would be good to leave behind on entering the new millennium.

Acknowledgments

Grateful thanks to Professor G. Wilcock and staff at the BRACE Memory Clinic, Blackberry Hill Hospital, Bristol, for their time and help in assisting with the research design and for screening the interviewees. Thanks also to Mike Nolan, Professor of Gerontological Nursing, University of Sheffield, for his supervisory skills and facilitation of the research design and to the BASE Practice Research Unit (BPRU), University of Wales, Bangor for funding the Study 1 research interviews.

REFERENCES

Almkvist, O. & Bäckman, L. (1993) Progression in Alzheimer's disease: sequencing of neuropsychological decline. *International Journal of Geriatric Psychiatry* **8**, 755–763.

[ADS] Alzheimer's Disease Society (1993) *Deprivation and Dementia*. London: Alzheimer's Disease Society.

[ADS]Alzheimer's Disease Society (1995) *Right From the Start: Primary Health Care and Dementia*. London: Alzheimer's Disease Society.

American Psychiatric Association (1994) *DSM-IV: Diagnostic and Statistical Manual of Mental Disorders*, 4th edn. Washington: American Psychiatric Association.

Aneshensel, C.S., Pearlin, L.I., Mullan, J.T., Zarit, S.H. & Whitlatch, C.J. (1995) *Profiles in Caregiving: The Unexpected Career*. San Diego: Academic Press.

Barnes, R., Raskind, M., Scott, M. & Murphy, C. (1981) Problems of families caring for Alzheimer patients: use of support groups. *Journal of the American Geriatrics Society* 29, 80–85.

Beardsall, L. & Huppert, F.A. (1991) A comparison of clinical, psychometric and behavioural memory tests: findings from a community study of the early detection of dementia. *International Journal of Geriatric Psychiatry* 6, 295–306.

Bell, L. (1995) To tell or not to tell? *Alzheimer's Disease Society Newsletter* May, 5.

Bell, J. & McGregor, I. (1995) A challenge to stage theories of dementia. In: Kitwood, T. & Benson, S. (eds) *The New Culture of Dementia Care*, pp. 12–14. London: Hawker.

Black, J.S. (1995) Telling the truth: should persons with Alzheimer's disease be told their diagnosis? *ADI Global Perspective Newsletter* 6 (1), 10–11.

Blackburn, P. (1993) Freedom to wander. In: Johnson, J. & Slater, R. (eds) *Ageing and Later Life*, pp. 155–159. London: Sage.

Bowers, B.J. (1987) Inter-generational caregiving: adult caregivers and their ageing parents. *Advances in Nursing Science* 9 (2), 20–31.

Bowers, B.J. (1988) Family perceptions of care in a nursing home. *Gerontologist* 28 (3), 361–367.

Buckman, R. (1984) Breaking bad news: why is it so difficult? *British Medical Journal* 288, 1597–1599.

Burvill, P.W. (1993) A critique of current criteria for early dementia in epidemiological studies. *International Journal of Geriatric Psychiatry* 8, 553–559.

Byrne, E.J. (1994) *Confusional States in Older People*. London: Edward Arnold.

Carr, J.S. & Marshall, M. (1993) Innovations in long-stay care for people with dementia. *Reviews in Clinical Gerontology* 3 (2), 157–167.

Chenitz, W.C. & Swanson, J.M. (1986) Qualitative research using grounded theory. In: Chenitz, W.C. & Swanson, J.M. (eds) *From Practice To Grounded Theory: Qualitative Research in Nursing*, pp. 3–15. Menlo Park: Addison-Wesley.

Chenoweth, B. & Spencer, B. (1986) Dementia: the experience of family caregivers. *Gerontologist* 26 (3), 267–272

Clarke, C.L. (1995) Care of elderly people suffering from dementia and their co-resident informal carers. In: Heyman, B. (ed.) *Researching User Perspectives on Community Health Care*. London, Chapman & Hall. pp. 135–149.

Clarke, C.L. & Keady, J. (1996) Researching dementia care and family caregiving: extending ethical responsibilities. *Health Care in Later Life: An International Research Journal* 1 (2), 87–95.

Clarke, C. & Watson, D. (1991) Informal carers of the dementing elderly: a study of relationships. *Nursing Practice* 4 (4), 17–21.

Cohen, M.H. (1993) The unknown and the unknowable – managing sustained uncertainty. *Western Journal of Nursing Research* 15 (1), 77–96.

Collins, C.E., Given, B.A. & Given, C.W. (1994) Interventions with family caregivers of persons with Alzheimer's disease. *Nursing Clinics of North America* 29 (1), 195–207.

Cooper, B., Horst, B. & Schäufele, M. (1992) The ability of general practitioners to detect dementia and cognitive impairment in their elderly patients: a study in Mannheim. *International Journal of Geriatric Psychiatry* 7, 591–598.

Davis, R. (1989) *My Journey into Alzheimer's Disease*. Amersham on the Hill: Scripture Press.

Davis, H. (1991) Breaking bad news. *Practitioner* 235, 522–526.

Delieu, J. & Keady, J. (1996a) The biology of Alzheimer's disease: 1. *British Journal of Nursing* 5 (3), 162–168.

Delieu, J. & Keady, J. (1996b) The biology of Alzheimer's disease: 2. *British Journal of Nursing* 5 (4), 216–220.

Department of Health (1990) *NHS and Community Care Act*. London: HMSO.

Downs, M. (1994) *Dementia: A Literature Review for the Northern Ireland*. Dementia Policy Scrutiny. Stirling: Dementia Services Development Centre.

Duff, G. & Peach, E. (1994) *Mutual Support Groups: A Response to the Early and Often Forgotten Stage of Dementia.* Stirling: Dementia Services Development Centre.

Eagles, J.M., Beattie, J.A.G., Restall, D.B., Rawlinson, F., Hagen, S. & Ashcroft, G.W. (1990) Relation between cognitive impairment and early death in the elderly. *British Medical Journal* **300**, 239–240.

Flicker, C., Ferris, S.H. & Reisberg, B. (1991) Mild cognitive impairment in the elderly: predictors of dementia. *Neurology* **41**, 1006–1009.

Folstein, S.E. (1989) *Huntington's Disease: A Disorder of Families.* Baltimore: Johns Hopkins University Press.

Folstein, M.F., Folstein, S.E. & McHugh, P.R. (1975) Mini-Mental State: a practical guide for grading the cognitive state of patients for the clinician. *Journal of Psychiatric Research* **12**, 189–198.

Fortinsky, R.H. & Hathaway, T.J. (1990) Information and service needs amongst active and former family caregivers of persons with Alzheimer's disease. *Gerontologist* **30** (5), 604–609.

Froggatt, A. (1988) Self-awareness in early dementia. In: Gearing, B., Johnson, M. & Heller, T. (eds) *Mental Health Problems in Old Age: A Reader*, pp. 131–136. Buckingham: Open University Press.

Galasko, D., Klauber, M.R., Hofstetter, R., Salmon, D.P., Lasker, B. & Thal, L.J. (1990) The Mini-Mental State Examination in the early diagnosis of Alzheimer's disease. *Archives of Neurology* **47**, 49–52.

Gatz, I. (1995) Early stage Alzheimer's patients find comfort in their own support group. *ADI Global Perspective Newsletter* **6** (1), 6–7.

George, L.K. & Gwyther, L.P. (1986) Caregiver well-being: a multi-dimensional examination of family caregivers of demented adults. *Gerontologist* **26** (2), 253–259.

Gibson, G. & Moniz-Cook, E. (1996) It's good to talk – man to man. *Journal of Dementia Care* **4** (5), 20–22.

Gilhooly, M.L.M. (1984) The impact of caregiving on caregivers: factors associated with the psychological well-being of people supporting a dementia relative in the community. *British Journal of Medical Psychology* **56**, 165–171.

Gilleard, C.J., Gilleard, E., Gledhill, K. & Whittick, J. (1984) Caring for the elderly mentally infirm at home: a survey of the supporters. *Journal of Epidemiology and Community Health* **38**, 319–325.

Gilliard, J. & Gwilliam, C. (1996) Sharing the diagnosis: a survey of memory disorders clinics, their policies on informing people with dementia and their families, and the support they offer. *International Journal of Geriatric Psychiatry* **11** (11), 1001–1003.

Gillies, B. (1995) *The Subjective Experience of Dementia: A Qualitative Analysis of Interviews with Dementia Sufferers and their Carers and the Implications for Service Provision.* Stirling: Dementia Services Development Centre.

Glaser, B.G. (1978) *Theoretical Sensitivity.* Mill Valley: Sociology Press.

Glaser, B.G. & Strauss, A.L. (1967) *The Discovery of Grounded Theory: Strategies for Qualitative Research.* New York: Aldine.

Greene, J.G., Smith, R., Gardiner, M. & Timbury, G.C. (1982) Measuring behavioral disturbance of elderly demented patients in the community and its effects on relatives: a factor analytic study. *Age and Ageing* **11**, 121–126.

Harvath, T.A. (1994) Interpretation and management of dementia-related behaviour problems. *Clinical Nursing Research* **3** (1), 7–26.

Harvey, R. & Fairey, A. (1997) Drug treatments on the way. *Alzheimer's Disease Society Newsletter* March, 6.

Henderson, A.S. & Hupport, F.A. (1984) The problem of mild dementia. *Psychological Medicine* **14**, 5–11.

Hughes, C.P., Berg, L., Danziger, W.L., Coben, L.A. & Martin, R.L. (1982) A new clinical scale for the staging of dementia. *British Journal of Psychiatry* **140**, 566–572.

Hunt, L., Morris, J.C., Edwards, D. & Wilson, B.S. (1993) Driving performance in persons with mild senile dementia of the Alzheimer type. *Journal of the American Geriatrics Society* **41**, 747–753.

Jackson, D. & Wonson, S. (1987) Alzheimer's re-socialization: a group approach towards improved social awareness among Alzheimer's patients. *American Journal of Alzheimer's Care and Related Disorders and Research* **2** (5), 31–35.

Keady, J. (1996) The experience of dementia: a review of the literature and implications for nursing practice. *Journal of Clinical Nursing* (review section) **5** (5), 275–288.

Keady, J. (1997) Maintaining involvement: a meta concept to describe the dynamics of dementia. In: Marshall, M. (ed.) *State of the Art in Dementia Care*, pp. 25–31. London: Centre for Policy on Ageing.

Keady, J. & Nolan, M.R. (1994) Younger-onset dementia: developing a longitudinal model as the basis for a research agenda and as a guide to interventions with sufferers and carers. *Journal of Advanced Nursing* 19, 659–669.

Keady, J. & Nolan, M. (1995a) A stitch in time: facilitating proactive interventions with dementia caregivers: the role of community practitioners. *Journal of Psychiatric and Mental Health Nursing* 2 (1), 33–40.

Keady, J. & Nolan, M.R. (1995b) IMMEL 2: working to augment coping responses in early dementia. *British Journal of Nursing* 4 (7), 377–380.

Keady, J. & Nolan, M.R. (1995c) IMMEL: assessing coping responses in the early stages of dementia. *British Journal of Nursing* 4 (6), 309–314.

Keady, J. & Nolan, M. (1996) *Maintaining involvement; a meta concept to describe the dynamics of dementia.* Paper presented at the Royal College of Nursing Research Advisory Group Annual Conference, Newcastle upon Tyne, 31 March 1996.

Keady, J., Nolan, M.R. & Gilliard, J. (1995) Listen to the voices of experience. *Journal of Dementia Care* 3 (3), 15–17.

Kitwood, T. (1992) Quality assurance in dementia care. *Geriatric Medicine*, 22 (9), 34–38.

Kitwood, T. (1997) Person, dementia and dementia care. In: Hunter, S. (ed.) *Dementia: Challenges and New Directions*. London: Jessica Kingsley.

Kitwood, T. & Benson, S. (1995) *The New Culture of Dementia Care*. London: Hawker.

Kitwood, T. & Bredin, K. (1992) Towards a theory of dementia care: personhood and well-being. *Ageing and Society* 12, 269–287.

Knight, B.G., Lutzky, S.M. & Macofsky-Urban, F. (1993) A meta-analytic review of interventions for caregiver distress: recommendations for future research. *Gerontologist* 33 (2), 240–248.

Kobayashi, S., Masaki, H. & Noguchi, M. (1993) Developmental process: family caregivers of demented Japanese. *Journal of Gerontological Nursing* 19 (10), 7–12.

Kübler-Ross, E. (1970) *On Death and Dying*. London: Routledge.

Kuhlman, G.J., Wilson, H.S., Hutchinson, S.A. & Wallhagen, M. (1991) Alzheimer's disease and family caregiving: critical synthesis of the literature and research agenda. *Nursing Research* 40 (6), 331–337.

LaBarge, E. & Trtanj, F. (1995) A support group for people in the early stages of dementia of the Alzheimer type. *Journal of Applied Gerontology* 14 (3), 289–301.

La Rue, A., Watson, J. & Plotkin, D.A. (1993) First symptoms of dementia: a study of relatives' reports. *International Journal of Geriatric Psychiatry* 8, 239–245.

Levin, E., Sinclair, I. & Gorbach, P. (1989) *Families, Services and Confusion in Old Age*. Aldershot: Avebury.

Li, G., Silverman, J.M., Smith, C.J. et al (1995) Age at onset and familial risk in Alzheimer's disease. *American Journal of Psychiatry* 152 (3), 424–430.

Linn, R.T., Wolf, P.A., Bachman, D.L. et al (1995) The 'preclinical phase' of probable Alzheimer's disease: a 13-year prospective study of the Framingham cohort. *Archives of Neurology* 52, 485–490.

Lishman, W.A. (1981) *Organic Psychiatry*, 2nd edn. Oxford: Blackwell.

Mace, N.L., Rabins, P.V., Castleton, B.A., McEwen, E. & Meredith, B. (1992) *The 36-Hour Day: A Family Guide to Caring at Home for People with Alzheimer's Disease and Other Confusional Illnesses*. London: Hodder & Stoughton.

Magnússon, H. & Helgason, T. (1993) The course of mild dementia in a birth cohort. *International Journal of Geriatric Psychiatry* 8, 639–647.

Maguire, C.P., Kirby, M., Coen, R., Coakley, D., Lawlor, B.A. & O'Neill, D. (1996) Family members' attitudes toward telling the patient with Alzheimer's disease their diagnosis. *British Medical Journal* 313, 529–530.

McAfee, M.E., Ruh, P.A. & Bell, P. (1989) Including persons with early stage Alzheimer's disease in support groups and strategy planning. *American Journal of Alzheimer's Care and Related Disorders and Research* 4 (6), 18–22.

McCormick, W.C., Kukull, W.A., van Belle, G., Bowen, J.D., Teri, L. & Larson, E.B. (1994) Symptom pattern and comorbidity in the early stages of Alzheimer's disease. *Journal of the American Geriatrics Society* 42 (5), 517–521.

McGowin, D.F. (1993) *Living in the Labyrinth: A Personal Journey Through the Maze of Alzheimer's Disease*. Cambridge: Mainsail.

McKeith, I.G., Galasko, D., Wilcock, G.K. & Byrne, E.J. (1995) Lewy body dementia – diagnosis and treatment. *British Journal of Psychiatry* **167**, 709–717.

McLauchlan, C.A.J. (1990) Handling distressed relatives and breaking bad news. *British Medical Journal* **301**, 1145–1149.

Morris, J.C. & Fulling, K. (1988) Early Alzheimer's disease: diagnostic considerations. *Archives of Neurology* **45**, 345–349.

Morris, R.G., Morris, L.W. & Britton, P.G. (1988) Factors affecting the emotional well-being of the caregivers of dementia sufferers. *British Journal of Psychiatry* **153**, 147–156.

Motenko, A.K. (1989) The frustrations, gratifications and well-being of dementia caregivers. *Gerontologist* **29** (2), 166–172.

Newens, A.J., Forster, D.P., Kay, D.W.K., Kirkup, D.W.K., Bates, D. & Edwardson, J. (1993) Clinically diagnosed pre-senile dementia of the Alzheimer's type in the northern Health region: ascertainment, prevalence, incidence and survival. *Psychological Medicine* **23**, 631–644.

Nolan, M. & Keady, J. (1996a) Training together: a challenge for the future. *Journal of Dementia Care* **4** (5), 10–13.

Nolan, M. & Keady, J. (1996b) Training in long term care: the road to better quality. *Reviews in Clinical Gerontology* **6**, 333–342.

O'Connor, D.W., Pollitt, P.A., Hyde, J.B., Brook, C.P.B., Reiss, B.B. & Roth, M. (1988) Do general practitioners miss dementia in elderly patients? *British Medical Journal* **297**, 1107–1110.

O'Connor, D.W., Pollitt, P.A., Brook, C.P.B., Reiss, B.B. & Roth, M. (1991) Does early intervention reduce the number of elderly people with dementia admitted to institutions for long term care? *British Medical Journal* **302**, 871–874.

Pearlin, L.I., Mullan, J.T., Semple, S.J. & Scaff, M.M. (1990) Caregiving and the stress process: an overview of concepts and their measures. *Gerontologist* **30** (5), 583–594.

Pollitt, P.A., O'Connor, D.W. & Anderson, I. (1989) Mild dementia: perceptions and problems. *Ageing and Society* **9**, 261–275.

Post, S.G. (1994) Genetics, ethics and Alzheimer's disease. *Journal of the American Geriatric Society* **42** (7), 782–786.

Reilly, A. (1995) *Breaking through the conspiracy of silence for the empowerment of the person with dementia: the implications for a rethinking of the social work role* (unpublished MA dissertation). Cardiff: University of Wales.

Reisberg, B., Ferris, S.H., DeLeon, M.J. & Crook, T. (1982) The global deterioration scale for assessment of primary degenerative dementia. *American Journal of Psychiatry* **139**, 1136–1139.

Rice, K. & Warner, N. (1994) Breaking the bad news: what do psychiatrists tell patients with dementia about their illness? *International Journal of Geriatric Psychiatry* **9**, 467–471.

Rohde, K., Peskind, E.R. & Raskind, M.A. (1995) Suicide in two patients with Alzheimer's disease. *Journal of the American Geriatrics Society* **43**, 187–189.

Rubin, E.H., Morris, J.C., Grant, E.A. & Vendegna, T. (1989) Very mild senile dementia of the Alzheimer type: I. Clinical assessment. *Archives of Neurology* **46**, 379–382.

Sliwinski, M., Lipton, R.B., Buschke, H. & Stewart, W. (1996) The effects of preclinical dementia on estimates of normal cognitive functioning in aging. *Journal of Gerontology: Psychological Sciences* **51B** (4), 217–225.

[SSI/DOH] Social Services Inspectorate/Department of Health (1996) *Assessing Older People With Dementia In The Community: Practice Issues for Social and Health Services*. Wetherby: HMSO.

[SSI/DOH] Social Services Inspectorate/Department of Health (1997) *At Home With Dementia: Inspection of Services for Older People with Dementia in the Community*. Wetherby: HMSO.

Stokes, G. & Goudie, F. (1990) *Working with Dementia*. Bicester: Winslow.

Taraborrelli, P. (1993) Exemplar A: becoming a carer. In: Gilbert, N. (ed.) *Researching Social Life*, pp. 172–186 London: Sage.

Van-Wylen, M.D. & Dykema-Lamse, J. (1990) Feelings group for adult day care. *Gerontologist* **30**(4), 557–559.

Verhey, F.R.J., Rozendaal, N., Ponds, R.W.H.M. & Jolles, J. (1993) Dementia, awareness and depression. *International Journal of Geriatric Psychiatry* **8**, 851–856.

Vitaliano, P.P., Young, H.M. & Russo, J. (1991) Burden: a review of measures used among caregivers of individuals with dementia. *Gerontologist* **31**(1), 67–75.

Weingartner, H.J., Kawas, C., Rawlings, R. & Shapiro, M. (1993) Changes in semantic memory in early stage Alzheimer's disease patients. *Gerontologist* **33** (5), 637–643.

Williams, J.M.G. & Pollock, L.R. (1993) Factors mediating suicidal behaviour: their utility in primary and secondary prevention. *Journal of Mental Health* **2**, 3–26.

Williams, O., Keady, J. & Nolan, M.R. (1995) Younger-onset Alzheimer's disease: learning from the experience of one spouse carer. *Journal of Clinical Nursing* **4**(1), 31–36.

Willoughby, J. & Keating, N. (1991) Being in control: the process of caring for a relative with Alzheimer's disease. *Qualitative Health Research* **1**(1), 27–50.

Wilson, H.S. (1989a) Family caregivers: the experience of Alzheimer's disease. *Applied Nursing Research* **2** (1), 40–45.

Wilson, H.S. (1989b) Family caregiving for a relative with Alzheimer's dementia: coping with negative choices. *Nursing Research* **38**(2), 94–98.

Woods, B. (1995) Dementia care: progress and prospects. *Journal of Mental Health* **4**(2), 115–124.

World Health Organization (1993) *The ICD-10 Classification of Mental and Behavioural Disorders: Diagnostic Criteria for Research*. Geneva: WHO.

Wright, N. & Lindesay, J. (1995) A survey of memory clinics in the British Isles. *International Journal of Geriatric Psychiatry* **10**, 379–385.

Wuest, J., Ericson, P.K. & Stern, P.N. (1994) Becoming strangers: the changing family caregiving relationship in Alzheimer's disease. *Journal of Advanced Nursing*. **20**, 437–443.

Yale, R. (1989) Support groups for newly diagnosed Alzheimer's clients. *Clinical Gerontologist* **8**(3) 86–89.

Zarit, S.H., Reever, K. & Bach-Peterson, J. (1980) Relatives of the impaired elderly: correlates of feelings of burden. *Gerontologist* **20**(6), 649–655.

Zarit, S., Orr, N. & Zarit, M. (1985) *The Hidden Victims of Alzheimer's Disease*. New York University Press.

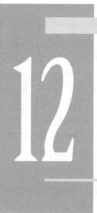

Young-onset dementia

Jill Walton

KEY ISSUES

- The prevalence of dementia is generally accepted as rising exponentially with age. The reported prevalence rises from 1.2 in 100 people aged 65–70 years to a staggering 50 in 100 people over the age of 85 years

- There is an urgent need to provide early and accurate diagnosis to people with young-onset dementia

- The issues of partnership in the provision of care are discussed with special relationship to the Multidisciplinary Young Onset Dementia Clinic and CANDID (Counselling and Diagnosis in Dementia), founded at the National Hospital for Neurology and Neurosurgery, Queen Square, London

- People with young-onset dementia have special problems and are in need of specialist services

INTRODUCTION

For the purposes of this chapter, 'younger people with dementia' are defined as people below the age of 65 years. There is much debate regarding the term that should be used to refer to dementia syndromes in this age group; again, for the purposes of this chapter, the term 'young-onset dementia' is used.

Whilst the majority of dementia syndromes are caused by sporadic disease, some are the result of inherited disease. Whether the cause is sporadic or genetic, the person with dementia requires high-quality care delivered in an appropriate setting. Dementia is a particularly harrowing and cruel disease at whatever age it occurs. Whilst acknowledging that many care needs are common to younger and older people suffering from dementia, this chapter seeks to highlight areas that require particular attention in relation to the younger sufferer.

EPIDEMIOLOGY

Dementia is described by Rossor (1992) as a clinical syndrome of progressive cognitive impairment with a variety of underlying pathological causes. Its prevalence was reported by Jorm et al (1987) to vary from 1.2 per 100 people aged 65–70 years to 50 per 100 people over the age of 85 years. Whilst Alzheimer's disease is generally accepted as the most common cause of dementia, there is considerable debate regarding the prevalence of other causes. Some researchers have reported studies in which Lewy body dementia has been shown as the next most common cause after Alzheimer's disease (Tobiansky, 1994). Other researchers suggest that in people below the age of 65 years, Alzheimer's disease may account for less than half of all cases of dementia (Harvey et al, 1996).

The epidemiological breakdown of prevalence statistics is to some degree an academic debate. For the majority of the people affected by young-onset dementia, an explanation of the symptoms they are experiencing and information with regard to prognosis are more important. Figure 12.1 shows the dementia syndromes most frequently

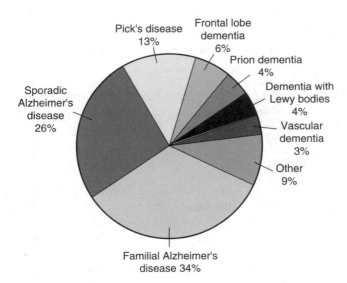

Figure 12.1 Breakdown of clients attending the specialist dementia clinic, by condition.

diagnosed at the specialist Multidisciplinary Young Onset Dementia Clinic at the National Hospital for Neurology and Neurosurgery, London.

Varieties of dementia affecting younger people

Alzheimer's disease

Alzheimer's disease is characterised by the formation of senile plaques and neurofibrillary tangles which are seen on neuropathological examination. Memory impairment, disorientation, impaired visuospatial abilities and motor skills, word-finding difficulties and dysphasia are among the 'core' symptoms of Alzheimer's disease.

Vascular dementia

The vascular dementias are a result of impairment of the blood supply to the brain. This may take many forms, including strokes, restriction of the blood supply due to narrowing of arteries, inflammation of blood vessels (vasculitis) and haemorrhage into the brain. The classical presentation is of sudden onset of cognitive impairment followed by a stepwise and fluctuating decline. The presence of vascular risk factors such as high blood pressure, smoking, raised blood cholesterol level and other vascular problems such as heart attacks and strokes often provides important clues to the diagnosis.

Dementia with Lewy bodies

Lewy body dementia may present in one of two ways: either as late-onset Parkinson's disease, followed months or years later by visual hallucinations, episodes of confusion, memory loss and then global dementia; or as cognitive or psychiatric symptoms followed by milder parkinsonian features later in the course of the disease. The main pointers to a diagnosis of dementia with Lewy bodies are fluctuating cognitive performance with episodes of confusion, persistent visual hallucinations or paranoid delusions, early gait disturbance, any combination of rigidity, bradykinesia, tremor and flexed posture, or temporoparietal dementia with inattention in a patient with Parkinson's disease.

Pick's disease

Pick's disease is an irreversible condition commencing usually between the ages of 40 and 65 years. Gradual dissolution of language (not just speech) is the only salient finding for 2 years and may continue for up to 14 years. Patients are aware of the deficit and usually are adept at communicating. As the condition progresses, so memory, attention, personality and behaviour are affected. The pathological findings are of Pick cells and Pick bodies in the cerebral cortex.

Frontal lobe degeneration

Frontal lobe degeneration usually starts in the frontal lobes, though the temporal lobes may also be affected. Symptoms include personality change, attentional deficit, obsessive behaviours, gluttony, lack of insight, sexual disinhibition, stereotypy and indiscriminate mouthing of objects. Memory deficits tend to occur later. The pathological findings are often a non-specific nerve cell loss without specific hallmarks, though occasionally features of Pick's disease are also found. Frontal lobe degeneration and Pick's disease are often grouped under the term 'frontotemporal dementia'.

Prion diseases

Prion diseases are a closely related group of neurodegenerative diseases known to occur in humans and animals. The transmissible agent can either be genetic or an abnormal form of the prion protein. Creutzfeldt–Jakob disease is one of the prion dementias, the new variant of which, though very rare, has a very young onset with sufferers often in their teens.

Corticobasal degeneration

Symptoms and signs of corticobasal degeneration include apraxia, rigidity, involuntary movements, dystonia, the 'alien limb' sign, dysarthria and a supranuclear disorder of the eye movement. Mental impairment occurs late. Progressive supranuclear palsy is a variant of this.

The majority of dementia syndromes are sporadic: they start unexpectedly and there is often no family history. However, some dementias such as Huntington's chorea are inherited in an autosomal fashion: this means that people with the affected gene will develop the illness if they live long enough. Children of sufferers have a 50% chance of inheriting the condition.

The number of people with young-onset dementia in the UK is thought to be about be 18 000 (Newens et al, 1993). However, the accuracy of any estimate of the prevalence is limited. Dementia must be diagnosed in order for it to feature in prevalence statistics. To be diagnosed it must be recognised, and the problem here is twofold: firstly, it depends upon people presenting to medical or social service professionals with a request for help, and secondly it depends on recognition by professionals of the problem and a correct diagnosis being established.

Prevalence figures for young-onset dementia are further complicated by cases in which dementia diagnosed when the person is (say) 68 years old may actually be the culmination of 4–5 years of progressive deterioration, so the diagnosis of young-onset disease will be missed. Similarly, misdiagnosis may also hide a significant number of sufferers from the statistics. It is therefore suggested that the true prevalence of dementia is much higher than statistics indicate.

DIAGNOSIS

Early and accurate diagnosis has been highlighted as particularly important in the care of younger people with dementia. Distress and anxiety caused by the symptoms of dementia, the effects of changed behaviours and risk factors associated with them, and the need for information which will enable both sufferer and carer to make appropriate legal, financial, occupational and welfare decisions are examples of reasons why an early and accurate diagnosis is so crucial (Quinn, 1996). Contrary to arguments that an early diagnosis serves mainly to label or stigmatise the sufferers as having a progressive, irreversible and essentially untreatable disease and thus makes their plight worse, early diagnosis and information are important in the care of younger people with dementia.

According to a report by the Alzheimer's Disease Society (ADS, 1995), many health authorities in the UK are failing to identify the numbers or the care needs of younger people with dementia in their area. Stories of carers fighting to have their relative's symptoms taken seriously, of misdiagnosis, and ultimately of a lack of appropriate services once the correct diagnosis has been established, are not uncommon. Cayton (1995) gives one example of a carer who spent 4 years trying to obtain redress for the wrongs done to her and her husband in terms of misdiagnosis, 'professional bungling' and neglect.

Often the onset of a dementia syndrome is insidious. Occasional episodes of unusual or uncharacteristic behaviour are ignored or put down to tiredness, stress at work or the pressures of a new job. Dementia is not an illness that people expect to suffer in their 40s or 50s and it may be several months or even years before the sufferer or a relative begins to suspect that there may be something more serious than tiredness or stress at the root of the problem. It is not uncommon for relatives and friends to look back once a diagnosis of dementia has been established, and reinterpret unusual, inappropriate and out-of-character incidents. It often takes a particular event such as going on holiday or moving house to make the early symptoms of dementia really apparent (Quinn, 1996).

Recognising that something may be seriously wrong and that further investigation is needed is often the starting point of a long and complicated journey towards diagnosis. Lack of insight into one's own problems is a feature common to many dementia syndromes. This can make it difficult for relatives to persuade the person with dementia that there is a need to visit a doctor. People under 60 years old are often still in highly active roles at work, within the home and socially. It requires great tact and sensitivity to suggest that they are having difficulties maintaining those roles. In most cases the general practitioner is the first port of call, and relatives frequently explain how they 'set up' an appointment for their relative under the auspices of a routine medical check, having previously briefed the doctor in private about their concerns.

The weeks and months leading up to the diagnosis of dementia can be particularly distressing for both sufferer and relative. Lloyd (1993) comments on the problems experienced by younger people with dementia and their carers in the time leading up to a diagnosis. Not only do delays in diagnosis add to the distress and burden, but misdiagnoses can further complicate the plight of those seeking to understand what is happening to them and their loved one. The process of eliminating any possible reversible or treatable causes for the symptoms does take time, but the finding of Lloyd (1993) that in some cases 8 years elapses between the onset of symptoms and diagnosis is alarming and highlights a cause for concern. Whilst depression and dementia can and do coexist, misdiagnosis of depression in people with dementia have been reported (Ryan, 1994). Whilst such misdiagnoses are eventually apparent, their effects are multifarious. Not least are the social and financial implications of misdiagnosis (discussed below).

The process of diagnosis usually begins with a visit to the general practitioner, who will take a history from the patient and relative, and conduct basic cognitive assessments, physical examinations and routine investigations such as blood tests. This is normally followed by referral to a specialist medical service. Sometimes, however, the relatives of younger people with dementia have to fight to have their situation referred to a specialist, particularly where the general practitioner is sceptical of the problem or has made a misdiagnosis.

Referral is usually to either a psychiatrist or a neurologist. The ideal would be for a specialist psychiatrist or neurologist with a particular understanding of young-onset dementia to be available in every health authority, but in a survey in 1995 by the Alzheimer's Disease Society, 72% of their branches reported that their health authority did not have an identifiable consultant with special responsibilities for diagnosis, assessment and referral of younger people (ADS, 1995).

PARTNERSHIPS IN CARE
The specialist Multidisciplinary Young Onset Dementia Clinic

As a response to the particular needs of people with young-onset dementia, the specialist Multidisciplinary Young Onset Dementia Clinic (Box 12.1) was set up at the National Hospital for Neurology and Neurosurgery in Queen Square, London. The clinic is an example of health-care provision where professional and academic knowledge has been used directly to influence professional practice in an attempt to offer a service providing early and accurate diagnosis of dementia in younger people. The progression of both patient and carer through the clinic is shown in the flow chart in figure 12.2. To enable the health-care professionals to obtain as clear a picture as possible from the appointment, the clinic requests that people are accompanied by a carer or relative. The appointment letter also explains that the various investigations may take several hours.

Every patient and carer routinely sees a neurologist and/or a psychiatrist. The relative or carer will be scheduled to see the nurse

---

Box 12.1   The specialist Multidisciplinary Young Onset Dementia Clinic

The specialist clinic was established in 1991 at The National Hospital for Neurology and Neurosurgery, Queen Square, London, operating on an outpatient basis once a month. It targets individuals with a possible diagnosis of young-onset dementia and their relatives or carers. Owing to increased need the clinic is now held three times a month, and deals with on average 5–6 new referrals and 8–10 follow-up appointments per clinic. At the clinic a wide range of professionals come together to provide diagnoses wherever possible of early or unusual dementias affecting people predominantly in the under-65 years age group. Neurologists, psychiatrists, neuropsychologists and nurses are involved with the remit, which extends to careful follow-up of this vulnerable patient population.

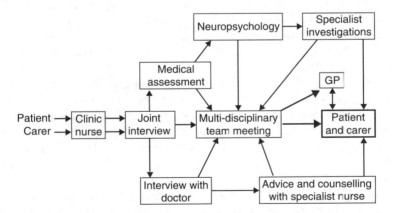

Figure 12.2   Movement of clients and carers through the specialist dementia clinic.

counsellor, usually while the patient is undergoing extensive neuropsychological testing. In addition to gaining a general medical and social history from the sufferer and the relative, various specialist investigations may also be undertaken. Some or all of the following may be required:

- *Magnetic resonance imaging (MRI)* allows brain tissue to be studied in minute detail with visualisation of structures deep inside the brain. As well as excluding certain intracerebral disorders, MRI may be able to indicate the amount of brain shrinkage in particular areas of the brain associated with Alzheimer's disease or Pick's disease.
- *Blood tests*: routine blood screening may be performed in order to eliminate some of the reversible causes of dementia for example thyroid disorders.
- *Electroencephalograms* record the electrical impulses inside the brain, and may be a useful aid to diagnosis of dementia.
- *Detailed family history* may reveal other family members who have suffered from dementia or a similar illness. In such cases the family tree would be carefully traced and investigated.
- *Neuropsychology*: cognitive function is assessed by testing comprehension, orientation, concentration, language and motor skills and the ability to retain and recall information. Specialist neuropsychological testing can discern very subtle changes in a person's performance in any one of these areas.
- *Lumbar puncture* allows examination of the cerebrospinal fluid.
- *Brain biopsy* is performed very occasionally, mainly to exclude treatable causes of dementia when circumstances dictate further confirmation is necessary.

It may not be possible to arrange for all the investigations to be performed on the day of the appointment. In some cases people are requested to return for a scan as an outpatient. In other instances they are admitted as an inpatient for a few days in order to undergo the relevant investigations. As much information as possible is gleaned as the patient and carer progress through the clinic.

The health-care professionals meet at the end of the clinic to discuss their findings and impressions. Diagnoses and appropriate management issues are considered from social, clinical and neuropsychological perspectives. A letter is written to the referring clinician explaining the conclusions reached. The patient may be requested to attend the clinic for follow-up appointments. It is sometimes appropriate to refer the patient to a local consultant for follow-up care.

Whilst early and accurate diagnosis is the overall function of the clinic, the specific role of the nurse counsellor within the clinic is to provide relatives or carers with a forum in which to express their concerns. The nurse counsellor also has an agenda of advice and information to share with the relative or carer, and this is based upon a knowledge and understanding of the particular problems associated with dementia in younger people.

PROBLEMS EXPERIENCED BY YOUNGER PEOPLE WITH DEMENTIA

Although most of the problems discussed here are applicable to all people with dementia and their carers regardless of age, there are additional implications when the person with dementia is of a younger age.

In the specialist clinic described above the nurse counsellor enters into an informal client-led discussion with the carer, who is invited to speak about any perceived problems. The discussion may cover a range of issues, depending upon the type and severity of the symptoms of the affected person. While listening to and accepting what is being said, throughout the discussion the nurse counsellor will endeavour to raise a number of points, based upon a working knowledge of young-onset dementia and some of the issues that typically need to be addressed.

Ethical issues

Like the diagnosis of cancer in the past, ethical dilemmas surround the issue of *if* and *how* the sufferer should be told of the diagnosis of dementia. The dilemmas are complex: sometimes sufferers have no insight into their problems which raises the question of how they can discuss the diagnosis. Sometimes the family carer specifically requests that the sufferer should not be informed of the diagnosis, believing this to be in the sufferer's best interest. In other instances the person with dementia directly requests an explanation of the diagnosis. Husband (1996) concludes that there is a great need for the training of health-care professionals with respect to whom to tell and how to tell. In a survey of UK psychiatrists, Rice and Warner (1995) found that the practice of giving information to carers is common, but that of giving information to people with dementia is not. Their survey also revealed that some doctors were 'economical with the truth' when discussing diagnoses with the patient, using terms such as 'memory problems' rather than presenting clear-cut facts about their diagnosis and prognosis. Helping people to understand that they have dementia and giving them the emotional and practical support they need is time-consuming and requires great skill. It must not be entered upon lightly (Husband, 1996). As the needs of younger people with dementia are pushed to the fore, these issues need to be properly addressed.

Accepting the diagnosis

Sometimes the diagnosis comes as a relief, as it provides an explanation of the symptoms and changes in behaviour. However, for the sufferers and their relatives, accepting the diagnosis of a progressive, degenerative disease for which there is no cure is a major challenge. Coming to terms with a terminal disease at any age requires an investment of mental and emotional energy. An unexpected diagnosis of dementia at a young age complicates the process of acceptance, because thought-processing and coping mechanisms are themselves affected by the illness.

Changes in relationships

A particular tragedy for younger people with dementia is that they are being robbed of their future. Many of their relationships are in relative infancy. Professional potential may not yet have been fully realised, ambitions not achieved, places of interest not visited. Spouse's, children's relatives' and friends' memories of the person with dementia will have to be drawn from a much shorter life span. It is often helpful for sufferers, carers, families and friends to get on and do many of the things they had hoped to do together before it is too late to appreciate them fully.

It is not uncommon for the parents of a young person with dementia to be still alive and to witness the progressive deterioration that Alzheimer's disease or Pick's disease has upon their child and the child's family. Feelings of guilt that their offspring should be experiencing such a devastating illness are commonly expressed. Parents may find the diagnosis of dementia in their offspring particularly difficult to accept. Not fully understanding the disease, they may attribute blame to the person's spouse or to pressure at work, as a means of trying to find an explanation.

Inevitably there will be many changes in the roles and relationships between people with dementia and their partners, children, siblings, parents, friends and colleagues. Sainty (1995) describes how the division of labour in marriage is radically altered by the changing level of dependence, deteriorating abilities and interest of the person with dementia. With young-onset dementia this shift towards a dependent relationship, with its inequalities in shared tasks and responsibilities, comes at a time when people would otherwise expect to have been independent and active. General companionship between husband and wife is affected by dementia, and people describe the loneliness of losing their partner to dementia long before they lose the person in death. With regard to the sexual relationship, lowered libido, tiredness or seeing sex as inappropriate may all reduce the amount of sexual intimacy between people with dementia and their partners. Sexual disinhibition or increased sexual demands on the part of the person with dementia also need to be recognised as factors that may affect the relationship. Partners often need permission to talk about these issues. Similarly, permission must also be given for carers to admit that their relationship with the person with dementia was not ideal or without its problems before the onset of the illness. One must not assume that every marriage or partnership is held together by love.

Young children and adolescents cannot be spared the challenge and trauma of accepting and understanding the diagnosis of dementia in their parent or a close relative. Learning to cope with inappropriate behaviour, accepting the loss of the father or mother they once knew and adjusting their world view and expectations accordingly are deeply traumatic transitions for a child to make. Being embarrassed to bring friends home, being frightened of their parent's aggression, having to lock the bedroom door at night because of a parent wandering, and having to adjust to reversed roles as they partake in their parent's care needs, are some examples of the issues children face. Children react differently to these experiences, and show their distress in different ways. Attention-seeking behaviour, nightmares, difficulty sleeping, hypochondria and changes in school performance may all be signs that a child is finding it difficult to cope and needs more support.

Children, like everyone else, need clear explanations in order to cope with the changing situation, and require reminders of why their parent is behaving in a strange way. They need to understand that no one is to blame for the illness. It is important that children in this situation are supported, and it may help them to have the opportunity to meet other children in a similar situation. Referrals to a child psychologist, counselling and genetic counselling can be offered where appropriate. There are cases of young adults still in therapy as a result of the difficulties associated with a parent having young-onset dementia.

Finances and employment

The long-term implications of Alzheimer's disease usually include a significant change in the financial circumstances of sufferers and carers alike. The substantial cost of care is well documented (Gray, 1993), and as dementia usually takes several years to run its course to death, it is at any age an expensive illness. Having to contribute towards the cost of day care, respite care or nursing care is obviously expensive, but other expenses include extra clothing and washing because of incontinence, having to buy different foods because of changed dietary preferences, and increased heating and lighting bills.

For the younger person with dementia, there may be several years of lost income, national insurance and pension contributions, and so the issue of employment and finances for younger people with dementia is particularly crucial. Unlike many of their older counterparts, younger people with dementia are usually still many years from completing their mortgage, have cars to run, concurrent standing orders to meet, children's education to fund and substantial household bills to pay.

Depending upon the course of events leading up to and after the diagnosis, younger people with dementia find themselves in a wide range of employment situations. Some continue to function at varying degrees of efficiency in their usual employment; some take early retirement because of the implications of their memory or behavioural problems at work. Others may be demoted, be made redundant or sacked, and thus find themselves unemployed. Those who are dismissed or who leave work often find that their pension rights are less than they would have been if they had obtained early retirement on health grounds from their employer. This problem is particularly acute because diagnoses of dementia often come too late, after the person has finished paid employment.

Each situation must be seen as unique to the people it involves. What is, however, common to all situations is the need for early and accurate diagnosis. In addition to the social difficulties that arise when there is no diagnosis or an inaccurate diagnosis, the financial complications of a delayed or wrong diagnosis can be very significant. On one occasion, a man awaiting referral to a specialist for further investigation of his memory problems lost £6000 of his family savings. His wife could see the mistakes he had made and acknowledged that he would never have made them when functioning in his usual capacity. Once a diagnosis of dementia had been reached she was able to establish an enduring power of attorney and negotiate through the bank that any cheques written by her husband over a set amount be forwarded to their solicitor for authorisation before being processed.

In a similar case, a man who, on several occasions, became lost and forgot where he had parked his car while out on business handed in his resignation one Friday afternoon. Having voluntarily made himself unemployed, and with no medical diagnosis at the time, this man did not qualify for any benefits, which resulted in his family experiencing severe financial hardship and anxiety as they tried to find the money from their savings to meet their day-to-day bills and outgoings.

In 1993 the Trades Union Congress (TUC) produced a briefing note which it had written in association with the Alzheimer's Disease Society. It pointed out that a number of people of working age do develop dementia, and stated the principle of the TUC to support workers who face dementia and their families. Not only is the working life of the person with dementia likely to be affected, but people who care for someone with dementia may also have to give up work to care full-time. The note highlighted that young-onset dementia can result in an occupational pension that is inadequate because it has to be claimed early. In seeking to enhance the entitlements of people with dementia, the following arguments were suggested:

1. Dementia is a chronic and fatal condition, so members with dementia will not draw their pensions for as long as other people who retire early
2. Early dementia is relatively rare. Therefore even if a precedent is set, it will not often have to be followed.

The briefing note also called for dementia to be recognised as grounds for early retirement because of illness, and that employers who learn that a former employee developed dementia while at work should reinstate the employee's rights and benefits.

Benefits

People with young-onset dementia and their carers qualify for statutory benefits in the UK. At the time of writing, these benefits include statutory sick pay and incapacity benefit, disability living allowance, invalid care allowance and a 'status discount' on their council tax bill. The accessibility of these benefits depends, however, on the following:

- Awareness of the existence of these benefits
- Understanding eligibility
- Competence in being able to complete the application forms.

Quinn (1996) describes how the process of applying for financial benefits can be very troubling: 'you feel as if you are begging … we've never asked for anything in our life'. Indeed, many carers believe that it is their duty to care for their relative, and the thought of being eligible for these benefits is alien to them. It can be difficult to convince some people of their entitlements. Filling out the necessary self-assessment forms can be time-consuming and difficult. Many of the questions seem designed for people with obvious physical difficulties rather than the implied care and mobility difficulties that a diagnosis of dementia may entail. Carers need to consider what would happen if they were not around to supervise or help. In one example, a man was physically able to wash and dress himself, but only because his wife prompted him to go into the bathroom, laid out everything necessary for him to wash himself, and supervised his choice of appropriate clothing. Without her assistance he did not initiate any personal hygiene activities and could not be relied upon to dress appropriately for the time of year.

Citizens Advice Bureaux, social workers, general practitioners and the Benefits Agency are among those who can assist in the claiming of these benefits. Helpline services such as Counselling and Diagnosis in Dementia (CANDID) are also assuming a greater role.

Social concerns

A diagnosis of dementia does not end within the confines of the family. It rapidly leads to friends and neighbours needing to be told, as well as the person's employer being informed. The bank, the Driver and Vehicle Licensing Agency (DVLA), building societies and solicitors also need to be informed.

Telling friends and neighbours of the diagnosis is difficult in its own right, partly because of ignorance about the disease and its causes. 'Surely he [or she] is too young to have Alzheimer's disease?' is a reasonable enough initial response to news of the diagnosis. Unsure how to respond or help, it is sometimes easier to stop asking how things are, to brush over any embarrassing signs of the disease, or to gradually stop visiting. Quinn (1996) illustrates one carer's view, who says, 'It's so difficult … people just don't know how to behave'.

Legal aspects

It is important that younger people with dementia and their relatives understand the need for long-term legal and financial planning. There are several strategies which can be employed to secure the overseeing of legal and financial issues for people unable to manage their own affairs. (Box 12.2).

Living wills

A 'living will' or advance directive is a statement about medical treatment, listing in advance people's wishes should they ever become unable to communicate those wishes or take part in decisions about their treatment. The British Medical Association (1992) issued a statement on advance directives in which living wills were seen as advantageous in stimulating dialogue between doctors and their patients, and as a means of providing relief to relatives while maintaining patients' autonomy. As a means of maintaining such autonomy, living wills may be particularly useful for people with dementia.

Police contact

Members of the public do not expect younger people to suffer from dementia. Unusual or inappropriate behaviour in younger people with dementia is more commonly interpreted as rudeness or drunkenness. Anecdotal examples of police contact with young people with dementia include a man repeatedly found wandering by the police, a man arrested for refusing to get off a bus and a woman in her 50s cautioned for

Box 12.2 Methods of obtaining legal protection for people with dementia

1. The Court of Protection. The court will consider applications made by anyone with a concern for an individual's financial wellbeing.
2. Appointeeship enables a designated person to claim social security benefits and allowances on behalf of someone who is incapable of doing so by reason of mental incapacity.
3. The Power of Attorney Act 1971 allows one person, the donor, to give authority to another, the attorney, to deal with the donor's financial affairs. Powers of attorney cannot be created by people suffering from mental incapacity and are cancelled once the donors become mentally incapable of managing their own affairs.
4. An Enduring Power of Attorney specifically authorises the attorney to continue even after the donor is no longer mentally capable of dealing with financial affairs. It has to be made while the donor is able to understand the process being agreed to. However, Jacoby (1993) explains how a person may be capable in law of understanding this process while at the same time being incapable of managing financial affairs. Hence mental illness per se does not preclude establishing an Enduring Power of Attorney.

The major advantage of an Enduring Power of Attorney for people in the early stages of dementia is that it allows them to exercise some degree of choice over who will eventually manage their affairs. Also, there is no delay in the management of their affairs as the legal matters have already been dealt with. This is particularly important for younger people with dementia as they often have dependants relying on continued access to moneys held in their name. Enduring Powers of Attorney are extremely useful in assisting people with dementia and should be made as early as possible (Holland, 1995).

The Public Trust Office has produced an explanatory booklet which describes the procedure under the Enduring Power of Attorney Act 1985, and this is available free upon request.

shoplifting. The police responding to younger people with dementia need to be informed in order to ensure that situations are handled with care and that people with dementia are not criminalised. Behaviour typical of people with dementia that may result in contact with the police can be summarised as follows:

- *Wandering*: defined as a 'tendency to keep on the move, either in an aimless or confused fashion, or in pursuit of an indefinable or unattainable goal' (Stokes, 1986), wandering poses serious safety concerns, especially if the person wanders off in bad weather, into remote areas or into busy traffic.
- *Driving offences and accidents*: research has shown an association between dementia and traffic accidents (Lucas-Blaustein, 1988; Gilley,

1991; O'Neill 1993). Younger drivers with dementia may represent an even greater individual risk, particularly if driving heavy goods or public service vehicles (O'Neill, 1993).

- *Shoplifting*: absentmindedness and forgetfulness associated with dementia may, on occasions, cause people to leave shops without paying for items.
- *Inappropriate sexual behaviour or indecent exposure*: dementia can be associated with sexual offences, although the prevalence is unknown (Lynch, 1988). In some people with dementia, social norms associated with dress and impulse control are often erased or forgotten. Repetitive behaviour such as fidgeting with zippers or buttons may be misinterpreted as deviant behaviour. Because judgment is often impaired, undressing in public or leaving one's household without proper clothing are common occurrences (Alzheimer's Association, 1994). Other inappropriate sexual behaviour may include the person with dementia making advances to a stranger. Alternatively, inappropriate advances or affection shown towards children may cause concern.
- *Aggression and violence*: dementia can cause aggressive and violent tendencies. In Pick's disease, for example, there is often a forensic history owing to violence, aggression or shoplifting (Brown, 1992). Emotional changes, irritability and explosive temper can also result in aggression.

Driving

In the UK a driving licence is valid until the driver is 70 years old, with the responsibility for reporting disability or illness being given to the driver. However, it is the duty of physicians caring for people with dementia to inform them of their responsibility to notify the DVLA that they have been diagnosed as suffering from dementia or a dementia-like illness (O'Neill, 1993). People with dementia will not automatically be forced to stop driving, but will require confirmation from a medical officer that they are safe to continue to drive. It is inevitable that the time will come when driving is no longer safe for practically all sufferers from dementia.

For younger and older people with dementia alike, being stripped of the right to drive can represent a significant loss. Although it is sometimes the case that sufferers willingly relinquish their car keys, complex situations in which sufferers refuse to accept that they pose any danger by continuing to drive are more common. The example of a man who turned up at a petrol station but was unable to remember how to fill the car up with petrol, unable to work the controls on the dashboard, and yet insisted to his wife that he was perfectly able to drive, demonstrates the difficulties that can arise.

If the family carer or other household members cannot drive, difficulties may arise regarding day-to-day mobility. When the person with dementia has a young family still at home, the need for a 'taxi' service to and from school, youth clubs and friends' houses is unremitting. The situation may be particularly acute in rural areas. In addition, the family carer may be stranded as a result of the sufferer's inability to drive. Lifts to friends' houses, evening classes, shops and local towns all cease, and using taxis is not only expensive but less convenient.

SUPPORT AND SERVICE GROUPS

Younger people with dementia and their carers often have difficulty in finding support that is appropriate. They fall outside the remit of many existing services in their area and there are very few services designed specifically for this group. Emphasis must be placed on the *age* of the person with dementia, rather than the name of the disease. It is not necessarily appropriate to put people of all ages with the same diagnosis of dementia into one care setting.

Services should be specialised in terms of offering care in an appropriate setting specifically for younger people with dementia. Moriarty and Levin (1995) highlight the increasingly important role that community services will play as the majority of people who develop dementia spend most of their remaining lives in the community. In terms of institutional provision, a study by Alzheimer's Support West Wiltshire (Fossey and Baker, 1995) concluded that specialised services should be provided in a domestic environment as similar as possible to that of a normal house. The study also found that the carers of younger people with dementia wanted respite, day and residential care to be integrated into the same setting, to reduce disorientation and confusion.

Services must be offered by people who have a thorough understanding of the care implications for younger people with dementia. Referring to the care of people with dementia in general, and not specifically to younger people, Kitwood and Bredin (1992) make the point that as yet there exists no coherent theory of the process of care for people with a dementing illness. Such an absence, they claim, is remarkable, suggesting that care practice is relatively ineffective without a coherent theory. In the place of any coherent body of theory there exists a considerable body of 'folklore and an abundance of tacit knowledge' (Kitwood, 1993). Kitwood (1993) argues that caring *needs* a theory – a 'grasp in consciousness'. Nursing, he claims, has hardly addressed the issue of caring for a person with dementia.

In addressing the issue of caring for people with dementia, the need for carer training must not be ignored. The understanding that health-care professionals and family carers *can* work together to achieve common goals in caring for people with dementia must be recognised and promoted. In recognition of the need for partnership between family carers and health-care professionals, the CANDID counselling service offers regular study days aimed at helping those involved in caring for a younger person with dementia to understand their situation more fully. An increasing number of study days are being arranged by independent and voluntary organisations with the intention of bringing health-care professionals and family carers together, to learn from each other and to share experiences of caring.

Family carers themselves are often young and still in work, and therefore benefit enormously from day care that is available early enough in the morning and late enough in the evening to enable them to continue to work. Whilst many carers find that they need to abandon full-time employment in order to care for their relative with dementia, others find that the 'escape' to work, where life goes on outside dementia, is a much-needed part of their life which they cannot afford, financially or emotionally, to relinquish. These issues are not specific to dementia care but are pertinent to younger carers in general. However, the need for specialist day care, available 7 days a week, was one of the findings of a report by Alzheimer's Scotland (1990) into the needs of younger people with dementia.

Almeida and Fottrell (1991) highlight the need for practical advice and guidance on the likely course of the illness as fundamentally important for the carers of people with dementia. Providing clear, factual information about the disease is one of the most important means of support it is possible to offer. The potential of support groups and services is maximised when they are based upon a clear understanding of the illness and where it is leading. Offering factual information about the illness allows the disease process to be understood. This in turn puts into context the reasons why people with dementia behave as they do. Fact sheets and advice sheets on a wide range of issues are available from agencies such as the Alzheimer's Disease Society and CANDID. It is vital that all decisions are based on the clearest possible picture of the disease and the future it is likely to bring. It was out of the perceived need of health-care professionals and family carers for practical advice and information that the CANDID service was developed.

A word of warning! Knowledge is constantly changing, as is our understanding of the diseases that cause dementia. In being willing to transfer their knowledge and understanding to others involved in the care of people with dementia, health-care professionals must also guard against diminishing the scope for new initiatives in dementia care.

Support groups

Support groups form another component of the wide range of services necessary in providing effective care for people with dementia and their families. The Alzheimer's Disease Society is the largest national support organisation in the UK for people involved in caring for someone with dementia. It lobbies for improved rights for carers, provides information and advice, funds research, provides some day-care facilities and is generally involved in raising the profile of people with dementia. On a more local level, the Alzheimer's Disease Society facilitates support group meetings in which people can share experiences, and can offer and receive help from each other. The Alzheimer's Disease Society support groups are not age-specific, though the Society does have a working party and specialist staff dedicated to the issue of young-onset dementia.

In an unpublished survey, I found that family carers rated the development of carer support groups as a top priority when forced to prioritise services. Through their work at the National Hospital for Neurology and Neurosurgery, the nurse counsellors became aware of the need for a support group for the carers of people with dementias other than Alzheimer's disease. As a result, the Pick's Disease Support Group was founded in the UK in 1995, to provide information and advice as well as regular meetings for health-care professionals and relatives involved in the care of people with Pick's disease, frontal lobe degeneration, Lewy body disease, corticobasal degeneration or Korsakoff's syndrome. In fact, the support group is open to anyone involved in caring for a person with an 'unusual' or rare dementia. The Pick's Disease Support Group currently has over 300 members, the majority of whom are under 65 years old.

Counselling and Diagnosis in Dementia

Established in 1995, CANDID is a unique service providing advice, information and support to health-care professionals and family carers on the wide range of dementing illnesses that may affect people below the age of 65 years. It aims to tailor advice to the specific needs of individual enquirers. The service is principally accessed by telephone, letter and electronic mail, but users can visit the CANDID office in person if they prefer. All advice is given by trained nurses, and where necessary appropriate issues are discussed with a consultant neurologist and psychiatrist.

The CANDID service is based at the National Hospital for Neurology and Neurosurgery, Queen Square, London. Enquiries relating to people registered as patients of the hospital are recorded in the patient's notes, and the general practitioner is informed of the enquiry and the advice given; in these cases advice can be specific and direct, as the patients and their social situations may be well known to the CANDID staff. Where the enquiry does not relate to a patient of the hospital, the advice given is more general, and many health-care professionals are themselves provided with information.

Many enquiries relate to the difficulties involved in obtaining a diagnosis, finding out about services or obtaining information about a particular disease. Questions regarding the hereditary nature of some diseases are also asked. It would seem that contact from carers is more frequent at certain 'critical' times: time of diagnosis, stopping driving, starting day care, and other periods of particular and identifiable change. The service aims to provide rapid feedback to all enquirers.

Teaching

Teaching is a vital component of the CANDID service. Study days highlighting the problems of younger people with dementia are organised on a regular basis, and there is considerable involvement in postgraduate medical and nursing courses. A regular forum has been established whereby professionals from different disciplines involved in the care of younger people with dementia meet to discuss common issues and share experiences. By running educational courses, CANDID is active in increasing the awareness of specific problems of younger people with dementia.

Research

Many enquiries concern recent research findings. The CANDID service operates within the Dementia Research Group at the National Hospital and so is ideally placed to keep abreast of current research.

National and international communication

A national data base of specialist facilities and services for younger people with dementia is being established and CANDID has used the Internet to establish global communication links, electronic mailing and World-Wide Web pages.

CONCLUSION

Although the prevalence of dementia rises with increasing age, it does also affect younger people. With growing awareness of young-onset dementia (defined here as dementia affecting people before the age of 65 years) and improved diagnostic procedures, the true prevalence of young-onset dementia will be revealed. Whilst many of the issues involved in the care of a person with dementia are the same regardless of age, some factors are of particular relevance when the person affected is relatively young. Family concerns and the implications for family members, and legal, employment and financial issues are recognised as causing particular difficulties.

The specialist Multidisciplinary Young Onset Dementia Clinic has been presented as an example of good practice. Its patient population has been used as the basis of the epidemiological breakdown of main causes of dementia. Whilst many of their needs are common to all service users, for example their need to be treated with compassion, dignity and understanding, younger people with dementia are described as a group who are in need of specific and appropriate service provision. The CANDID service has been cited as an example of specific service provision, which aims to develop care partnerships between professional carers and between patients, their families and those professionals.

The theme of this book, partnerships in caring, is reflected in the working of this clinic; it is an example of internal partnership, with a multidisciplinary team of staff and their particular clients working together. The CANDID service is seen to have a more external partnership role, with its aims to educate 'society' and to help people with dementia to live in and with that society.

Quinn (1996), discussing dementia care in the borough of Kensington and Chelsea, suggests that the way forward would be the appointment of a development worker who could work with both health and social services, and with local organisations on an interagency basis. It is suggested that this strategy might allow partnerships of care to be further developed into comprehensive services for younger people with dementia.

This chapter concludes with excerpts from a letter written by Shirley Nurock, the carer of a younger person with dementia (Nurock, 1994). It reinforces many of the issues raised here.

> *How does the younger person suffering from Alzheimer's disease, fully aware of the prognosis, ever come to terms with the implications of this devastating disease? Loss of job, loss of status and income, of self-esteem, of independence, loss of a future ... family ... that you may not knowingly see your children grow to adulthood, become a burden to them and your wife. No matter how determined to fight the illness, it is not like others, for there is no cure, no remission.*
>
> *For a doctor, the diagnosis of Alzheimer's is especially hard to bear. How to come to terms with the apparent indifference of other doctors, reluctant even to see you? With the lack of suitable facilities in the way of assessment, day or respite care? With depression? With the absence of outside emotional support in the early stages, coupled with the frustration of knowing that your mental faculties are failing, that people don't understand you and talk about you as if you were not there? How to accept that you, a physically fit and active man, are expected to spend your days sitting in a circle round a television set (which you can't understand*

anyway), surrounded by strangers 20 years your senior, because there is nowhere else to go?

How does the wife in her forties ever come to terms with the loss of a loved partner? Gone the shared memories, shared happiness, the future you had planned together. What remains? Coping with the practical aspects of bringing up a family, working and caring for a husband, with planning for a future which you don't want to happen, with its social, financial and legal burdens.

To bear the hurt of friends and family who vanish into thin air, the humiliation of always being dependent on others, the isolation of caring, this nightmare that nothing could have ever really prepared you for. To find the strength to battle for advice on caring, support, the benefits and services available – those services which never catch up with your needs. Alzheimer's is not a static illness. It requires continuous reassessment.

How to come to terms with the emotional side of the long bereavement? Anger – or grief masked as anger, guilt, depression, despair, frustration, numbness, disbelief, agony and ultimately horror as the disease progresses at a furious pace and you are forced into the role of bystander, overcome by the realisation of how ill you feel from stress and how deeply affected by pity and heart-rending sorrow at what is happening to this man...

How do children view the gradual loss of a father, he who they barely had time to know as he once was, for they have grown up with his increasing vagueness and forgetfulness? He cannot help with their homework or share in their successes – instead they must feed him. But this illness must not be allowed to stand in the way of their paths to independence...

The health authorities and social services should be made aware of the total lack of suitable services for this age group. Being told by the consultant that there were so few younger people with dementia in the borough that it wasn't worth organising anything for them, is an affront. Given funding and carefully trained, well-rewarded staff, it cannot be hard to provide a structured and coordinated specialist service within the framework that already exists for the elderly: a comprehensive package of resources which will follow from diagnosis to death; one that provides compassionate and flexible care to help the person with dementia, carer, and family come to terms with their fate.

Few in number, we do not deserve to be forgotten or ignored.

(From Nurock 1994, with permission)

REFERENCES

Almeida, J. & Fottrell, E. (1991) management of the dementias. *Reviews in Clinical Gerontology* **1**, 267–281.

Alzheimer's Association (1994) *The Alzheimer's Association National Public Policy Program.* Chicago: Alzheimer's Association.

[ADS] Alzheimer's Disease Society (1995) *Services for Younger People with Dementia.* London: ADS.

Alzheimer's Scotland (1990) *Mini Survey into Pre Senile Dementia.* Scotland: ADS.

Bell, J. & McGregor, I. (1991) Living for the moment. *Nursing Times* **87**, 18.

British Medical Association (1992) *Statement on Advance Directives.* London: BMA.

Brown, J. (1992) Pick's disease. In: *Unusual Dementias. Baillière's Clinical Neurology* **1** (3), 535–557.

Cayton, H. (1995) Directions. *Alzheimer's Disease Society Newsletter* March, 2.

Fossey, J. & Baker, M. (1995) Different needs demand different services. *Journal of Dementia Care* **3** (6), 22–23.

Gilley, D.W. (1991) Cessation of driving and unsafe motor vehicle operation by dementia patients. *Archives of Internal Medicine* **51**, 941–946.

Gray, A. & Fenn, P. (1993) The cost of Alzheimer's disease in England. *Alzheimer's Review* **4** (2), 81–84.

Harvey, R.J., Roques, P., Fox, N.C. & Rossor, M.N. (1996) Services for younger sufferers of Alzheimer's disease. *British Journal of Psychiatry* **168**, 384–385.

Holland, J. (1995) Enduring Powers of Attorney. *Alzheimer's Disease Society Newsletter* February, 6.

Husband, H. (1996) Sharing the diagnosis – how do carers feel? *Journal of Dementia Care* **4** (1), 18–20.

Jacoby, R. (1993) 'Medico legal issues in old age psychiatry'. In: Jacoby, R. & Oppenheimer, C. (eds) *Psychiatry in the Elderly.* Oxford: Oxford University Press.

Jorm, A.F., Korten, A.E. & Henderson, A.S. (1987) The prevalence of dementia: a quantitative integration of the literature. *Acta Psychiatrica Scandinavica* **42**, 740–743.

Kitwood, T. (1993) Towards a theory of dementia care: the interpersonal process. *Ageing and Society* **13**, 51–67.

Kitwood, T. & Bredin, K. (1992) Towards a theory of dementia care: personhood and well-being. *Ageing and Society* **12**, 269–287.

Lloyd, M. (1993) *Early Onset Dementia in the Maidstone Area of Kent Social Services.* Maidstone Hospital.

Lucas-Blaustein, M. (1988) Driving in patients with dementia. *Journal of the American Geriatrics Society* **36**, 1087–1091.

Lynch, S.P.J. (1988) Criminality in the elderly and psychiatric disorder: A review of the literature. *Medical Science and Law* **28** (1), 69.

Moriarty, J. & Levin, E. (1995) How to give carers a break. *Journal of Dementia Care* **3** (3), 20–21.

Newens, A.J., Forster, D.P., Kay, D.W., Kirkup, W., Bates, D. & Edwardson, J. (1993) Clinically diagnosed pre senile dementia of the Alzheimer type in the northern region: ascertainment, prevalence, incidence and survival. *Psychological Medicine* **23** (3), 631–644.

Nurock, S. (1994) The forgotten few. *Alzheimer's Disease Society Newsletter* October, 3.

O'Neill, D. (1993) Driving and dementia. *Alzheimer's Review* **3** (3), 65–68.

Quinn, C. (1996) *The Care Must be There.* London: Dementia Relief Trust.

Rice, K. & Warner, N. (1995) How much do psychiatrists tell their patients? *Alzheimer's Disease Society Newsletter* July, 4.

Rossor, M.N. (1992) Introduction. In: *Unusual Dementias. Baillières Clinical Neurology* **1** (3), 477–483.

Ryan, D.H. (1994) Misdiagnosis in dementia: comparisons of diagnostic error rate and range of hospital investigation according to medical speciality. *International Journal of Geriatric Psychiatry* **9**, 141–147.

Sainty, M. (1995) In sickness and in health. *Journal of Dementia Care* **3** (3), 65–68.

Stokes, G. (1986) *Wandering.* Bicester: Winslow Press.

Tobiansky, R. (1994) Diffuse Lewy body disease. *Journal of Dementia Care* **2** (2), 26–27.

TUC, (1993) *Alzheimer's Disease and Other Dementias: Workplace Issues.* London: TUC.

USEFUL ADDRESSES

Alzheimer's Disease Society, Gordon House, 10 Greencoat Place, London SW1P 1PH, UK

Alzheimer's Association, 919 North Michigan Ave, Suite 1000, Chicago, Illinois 60611–1676, USA

CANDID, The National Hospital for Neurology and Neurosurgery, Queen Square, London WC1N 3BG, UK

Pick's Disease Support Group, The National Hospital for Neurology and Neurosurgery, Queen Square, London WC1N 3BG, UK

Public Trust Office, Protection Division, Stewart House, 24 Kingsway, London WC2B 6JX, UK

Professional practice with people with dementia and their family carers: help or hindrance?

Charlotte L. Clarke

KEY ISSUES

- The study described here identified a theory of normalisation which explains one way in which family members responded to having a family member with dementia

- Family carers emphasised the continuance of their relationship with the person with dementia

- Professional carers, at times, emphasised the pathological aspects of the person with dementia and the caregiving relationship

- The study suggests that dementia care management could usefully focus on the interpersonal dimensions of families and care

INTRODUCTION

This chapter draws on data collected from family and professional carers about the care of people with dementia. The study found that family carers normalised their relationship with people with dementia, a process rarely validated by professional carers who sought to encourage compliance with a model which emphasised the pathological aspects of the person with dementia and the family's relationships. However, it is unnecessary and perhaps unhelpful to dwell on the inadequacies of professional care. I would prefer to use this opportunity more constructively and to examine the processes of exchange between professional carers and people with dementia and their families, in which a subtle level of 'unofficial' activity in exchanging knowledge is identified.

THE EFFECTS OF DEMENTIA ON FAMILY RELATIONSHIPS

When a family member suffers from a disease causing cognitive loss and behavioural alterations, such as dementia, the effect upon family members extends far beyond the need to provide physical care and far beyond the primary carer. Family members have also been characterised as victims of dementia; Zarit et al (1985) state that there is probably no other disease that involves families so much or has such devastating effects. The problems faced by family members in terms of their relationship with the person with dementia can be identified in two areas: the experiences of loss (Barnes et al, 1981; Gabow, 1989) and the adoption of altered roles within the relationship (Barnes et al, 1981; Cantor, 1983; Steinmetz and Amsden, 1983; Bonder, 1987).

It has been suggested, however, that these alterations in relationships and roles of family members are perceived more positively by some caregivers than others. Fitting et al (1986) interviewed 54 caregivers who had a spouse with dementia. An unexpected finding of the study was that 25% of the husbands reported having an improved relationship with their spouse with dementia since caregiving began. A possible explanation is the influence of reciprocity, repayment for the wife's earlier home-making and nurturing activities.

Gilleard (1984) reviewed a number of studies relating to carer stress and found that what appeared to cause most problems were factors that distorted or disturbed the relationship between the carer and the dependant. The complex web of kinship obligation (Qureshi and Simons, 1987; Ungerson, 1987), responsibility (Finch and Mason, 1993), reciprocity (Pratt et al, 1987), affection (Cicirelli, 1983) and mutuality (Hirschefeld, 1981; Motenko, 1989) is the emotional bond of family caregiving. It provides each situation with a unique mix of strength and fragility. For example, Hasselkus (1988) writes of the 'powerful invisible forces' that influence caring relationships, whilst Wuest et al, (1994) identified the process of 'becoming strangers' as family carers become estranged from the person with dementia.

Very often professional carers become involved with the person with dementia and the person's family, although it is important to note the assertion by Pitkeathley (1989) that 'the first thing to say about this relationship [between family and professional carers] is that for the great majority there is *no relationship at all*' (p. 81). It is in this area of the interrelationships between family carers, people with dementia and professional carers that the study described here can be located.

THE STUDY – A THEORY OF NORMALISATION

The study found that family carers responded to the challenge of a family member with dementia by engaging in a process of continually defining and redefining their lives together as normal for them. A number of components formed part of this process. In brief, the strategies of 'pacing', 'confiding' and 'rationalising' enabled carers to manage their relationship with the person with dementia (Clarke, 1995); family carers utilised this perception of their relationship when negotiating the involvement of professional carers (Clarke and Heyman, 1998); and, as described in this chapter, this definition of their normalised life influenced their relationship with professional carers.

Data were collected from 14 family carers by diary and interview, from 60 multi-disciplinary professional carers by questionnaire, and through 9 case studies, involving 9 family carers (by interview and diary) and their professional carer contacts (a total of 25 by interview). The data were analysed using the grounded theory techniques of constant comparison and movement between the empirical data and theoretical constructs (Strauss, 1987). It is important to note the distinction between the analysis of the data, to create a number of categories which describe the data content, and analysis at a theoretical level which seeks to 'make sense' of the raw data analysis through exploration of the relationship between the data and social policy, professional practice and other theoretical areas.

Emerging from analysis of the data was the way in which family carers worked to keep their lives in an established pattern and moreover sought to keep hold of the relationship that existed between themselves and the person with dementia. They tried to keep their lives as normal as possible. This is blindingly obvious once stated, but for me at least, had been totally obscured by the weight of literature and professional advice which emphasised the negativity of family caregiving. In seeking to understand how anything normal could emerge out of such an apparently dire situation I was then drawn to the theory of normalisation as a pre-existing theory (well known in the fields of learning disability and mental health) to assess the explanatory power it had for dementia care and family caregiving.

Normalisation

Originating in Scandinavia in the late 1960s in the field of learning disabilities, the theory of normalisation was popularised in America by the work of Wolfensberger (1972). It was the mid 1970s before normalisation influenced services in Britain in response to the need for an ideological framework which was based on human values and took account of the social context in which people lived. Normalisation was intimately linked to deviancy theories and the social implications of a devalued status. Blanket assumptions were made about what was normal and valued in society (Twigg and Atkin, 1994). Consequently, many of the service changes can be criticised for adhering to static normative values (those acceptable to and considered appropriate by the professionals who defined the normative values), rather than, as demonstrated in the present study, interpreting norms as flexible and individually defined.

Gilbert (1993) is critical of the assumption that locates the social reaction to deviance with the individual (and their stigmatising characteristics) rather than with the rest of society (who implement strategies for excluding deviants). This unequal distribution of power and control in the deviant-societal relationship limits implementation of normalisation, and fosters a paternalistic professional role (Tyne, 1992). Such criticisms are echoed in my study, in which people with dementia find their 'personhood' marginalised whilst their dementia becomes the preoccupation of professional carers. Gilbert (1993) advocates that emphasis be placed on materialism: the extent to which resources influence social and professional relationships and the social experiences of living with a disability. This is an important feature of much disability literature (e.g. Locker, 1983) and provides explanation for the work of Anderton et al, (1989), consisting of interviews with 30 Chinese-Canadians and Anglo-Canadians, in which they identify the 'ideology' of normalisation as specific to Western health-care systems.

Paralleling later development in the field of learning disability, normalisation has begun to emerge as a relevant concept in chronic illness and, in particular, for parents of children with chronic illness (e.g. Robinson, 1993). No mention is made in this context, however, of individual rights, of integrating people in a community, or of ideologies. What is in common in both fields is the influence of deviance and stigma, and the role of individually defined norms.

So what is this 'normal' life that people strive to achieve? What is beginning to emerge is a collection of research which informs an answer to this question. The few studies that have linked chronicity and normalisation have used grounded theory or phenomenological approaches. Thus, for the first time, normalisation is being articulated by the people whom it affects. It is now that individually rather than externally defined norms begin to emerge.

These ideas are very different from those of the early days of normalisation when the emphasis was on protecting rights. Perhaps, however, these two views are not incompatible with the position of the individual whom the concept seeks to represent. In learning disabilities, and to some extent mental illness (with their history of institutional, custodial care), individuals had no norms perceived to be of value. What needed protecting was not their existing lives but their right to a life not available to them at that time. Chronic illness more frequently involves individuals who are perceived to have had, and are trying to continue to have, a valued life, a life that is individually lived but determined by a variety of social characteristics.

The role of supporting the principle of normalisation in each instance is necessarily different. In chronic illness consideration must be given to how individuals achieve normalisation and how the provision of health and social care may support them. Answers to these questions must be sought from the interactionist perspective of normalisation to which the study described here contributes. The links with deviancy and labelling theories remain explicit in interactionist interpretations, but there is a shift to considering strategies for negotiating normalisation on an interpersonal level. This is an ongoing process of negotiation since disabilities are rarely static and obtrusiveness is situation-dependent (Strauss et al, 1984; Robinson, 1993).

There is a shift, then, from professionals attempting to implement norms on behalf of others to individuals seeking to attain their own norms for themselves. However, in both situations the norm to be achieved remains one perceived to be acceptable to others in society.

Knafl and Deatrick (1986) provide an analysis of the concept of normalisation as it is applied in chronic illness which moves beyond the deviancy-dominated work of Strauss et al (1984). They emphasise the cognitive process involved in normalising. Acknowledgment of the abnormality is made, but its social significance (its deviancy from social norms) is denied.

Robinson (1993) draws on grounded theory studies of the experience of repeated hospitalisations for parents of children with chronic conditions, and the evolution of relationships between people managing chronic conditions and health-care professionals. She describes the process of normalisation as a story developed by people with chronic illness (or the parents of a chronically ill child) in which events that support being normal are focused on, whilst events that do not support being normal are rendered irrelevant to this evolving story of themselves. A similar process is evident in my own study in which normalising is achieved, in part, through rationalising during which events and knowledge are selectively acknowledged and (moving beyond Robinson's work) selectively disseminated to others. In my study, rationalising also involves the selective attribution of events and information to the person or the illness, and selective comparisons to other people and situations. These also enable family carers to focus on the 'normality' of the person with dementia and their relationship.

THE PROCESS OF INTERACTING

The process of interacting is one of three social processes identified by my study. The process of interacting is concerned with the way in which professional carers work with people with dementia and their family carer. This process is influenced by, and in turn influences, the process of interfacing, in which family carers negotiate the involvement of professional carers – see Clarke and Heyman (1998) for more detail – and normalising, in which family carers work to define their lives with the person with dementia as normal for themselves – see Clarke (1995) for more detail. The process of interacting has a number of key components which are described below.

Transitory nature of professional carer involvement

Getting into care

Unlike caregiving by family carers, which occurs in the context of a continuing relationship, professional caregiving takes place as a response to a perceived need of the person with dementia and the family carer. Professional caregiving only commences when a potential health or social care need arises, and on most occasions professional carers have no preceding interaction with the person with dementia or family carer.

The reasons for professional carer involvement centre around either a therapeutic-diagnostic function or an instrumental function. From the therapeutic-diagnostic aspect, depending upon the nature of the service involved, professional carers perceive their involvement to be an important part of the management of the illness. 'Treatment' of the individual dominates the service interaction with the caregiving situation.

> So many illnesses can look as though they are dementia when they're not, and if some person is not assessed early on then someone can be left with a treatable illness which is not treated, so that's very much why we want to be in early.
>
> *Community Psychiatric Nurse (interview)*

In the alternative mode of initial contact, the instrumental function, professional carers perceive the commencement of their caregiving as occurring in response to a failure in family caregiving.

> Generally what's happened is there's been a breakdown of some kind. The informal carer may have been doing the job for a long, long time and then suddenly something's going wrong, if they're ill or hurt, then we tend to get the message to go in and pick up the pieces.
>
> *District Charge Nurse G (interview)*

However, professional carers perceive there to be benefits in prolonged contact with a family, acknowledging that effective services may not be best delivered by a 'hit and run' mode of delivery. Consequently, professional carers seek to base their care upon a developing relationship with the couple:

As the illness progresses, as the problems increase, then you can build up on [the early contact] and you've got a relationship formed.

Community Psychiatric Nurse (interview)

Getting to know people

One central feature of the family carer's work with the person with dementia is the carer's knowledge of, and therefore ability to relate to, the individual as a person rather than as someone who has dementia. This is crucial to the family carer's ability to normalise their relationship with the person with dementia.

This knowledge of the pre-dementing person is almost always denied to professional carers. Professional carers are therefore dependent on their own assessment of the person and the caregiving situation. Professional carers place great emphasis on becoming familiar with clients and caregiving situations. The process of assessing, or getting to know people, is a complex task. It is rarely completed in a single meeting and requires the ability to work on an individual level with people, establishing their knowledge base, perceptions and expectations:

Therefore it's very much an exploratory, sort of where they're at and what they're doing.

Social Worker T (interview)

You're sitting there thinking, is this the right time? Shall I [discuss the diagnosis]? Where are they in this illness? What's their feelings? What's their thoughts? What's their background?

Community Psychiatric Nurse (interview)

The time scale of getting to know people is emphasised by professional carers, again reflecting the need for a well-established relationship. In addition, the need for family carers and people with dementia to know the professional carer before some aspects of professional caregiving can function is acknowledged.

It takes several visits to decide what type of personality they have, exactly what they can remember, what they can, can't do. It takes a number of conversations with them before I can decide in what way I could perhaps be able to help them. It certainly takes, and I'm talking about all the clients, they've really got to know you very well before they will confide in you.

Domiciliary Care Worker (interview)

Family carers also work at knowing the family member they care for. This involves adjusting to intrapersonal and interpersonal changes, and presents difficulties in keeping hold of aspects of the person which make them that individual.

> It's a hard process to adjust your ideas about one of your parents from an intelligent woman who had a surprisingly wide idea of life and then to see her gradually deteriorate, and slip away, it doesn't seem right somehow.
>
> *Mr K, caring for his mother (interview)*

Assessment at home also extends beyond knowing the people with dementia to getting to know their family carers and making an assessment of their wishes and competence in caregiving and the support which they would benefit from. Assessment by professional carers goes beyond establishing the needs of the individual, to making decisions about the relationship of these needs to the resources available:

> We obviously make a judgment on the carer's capabilities and how much we would be expected to provide and balance that against what we can provide.
>
> *District Nurse I (interview)*

However, some literature indicates the failure of professional carers and services to fully assess and address family carer needs (Nolan and Grant, 1989; Pitkeathley, 1989), although this may have been ameliorated to some extent recently in Britain by the Carers (Recognition and Services) Act 1995.

In my own study, however, professional carers were ready to acknowledge that the process of assessment was sometimes traumatic for the people with dementia and their carers, often involving waiting for a diagnosis to be made, anticipating unpleasant tests and, as the following professional carer describes, being scrutinised and judged by others. Such an introduction to health and social care services would seem to militate against the joint venture into care necessary to support a partnership.

> I think people sometimes feel threatened, especially by assessment – what is it, am I going to be assessed? You know, 'Are they making judgments about me and my family?', so I suppose it could be pretty threatening to people in that respect.
>
> *Psychiatric Day Assessment Unit Sister (interview)*

Getting out of care

Once involved in providing care to a person with dementia and a family carer, two options are available to professional carers in the development of that situation: either continuation or discontinuation. If professional carer involvement continues it may, according to the nature of the service, change from a supervisory role to gradually increased instrumental input, until home caregiving is finally discontinued:

> Basically, you can't withdraw the service once you're started it.
>
> *Community Practice Teacher I, (interview).*

This pattern of care delivery over time was also found by Davison and Reed (1995) in relation to an older person's entry to sheltered accommodation.

Alternatively, the professional carer may seek to discontinue care, easing out of service provision or passing the provision on to another professional carer. Again, this differentiates the nature of professional and family carer relationships. Family caregiving is persistent, extending into residential care environments if necessary, albeit in a changed form. Professional caregiving is more specific in its purpose and therefore may withdraw at any time when it is perceived to be inappropriate by the family carer, person with dementia, professional carer or their organisation.

> The way we usually get out of it is when they're past the worst stages we ease them onto the home care service, or perhaps involve some member of the family that hasn't been involved before, who hasn't been too bothered, and get them involved because you have to ease out of it somehow, because there is such a demand and you only have so much time.
>
> *Domiciliary Care Worker (interview)*

For family carers the act of ceasing care was complex, wrapped as caregiving is in a mesh of family obligations. The sample of caregivers in this study were all co-resident carers and had therefore arguably 'chosen' to care. Some felt that the death of their dependant was the 'best option', whilst others could not contemplate ceasing home care.

> I can't see any situation where I would relinquish responsibility, no. I wouldn't take on that burden of handing her over to strangers, especially when you hear stories about these homes. I mean you've read these stories and no matter if she was a vegetable I still couldn't face that responsibility.
>
> *Mr K, caring for his mother (interview)*

Supporting home caregiving

A number of issues are addressed by professional carers when considering the support of home caregiving for people with dementia. These include the perceived benefits of homecare for the person with dementia: 44% of professional carers who completed the questionnaire in the study were uncertain whether helping the person with dementia to remain at home was best for the person with dementia, and a further 11% felt that it was not best for them.

> A dementing person may not appreciate his/her home environment therefore it is not necessarily the best.

> *District Nursing Sister A (questionnaire)*

Of the professional carers who completed the questionnaire, 88% felt that helping the person with dementia to remain at home was not necessarily detrimental to the carer's welfare. This is contrary to the functionalist literature which dominated the 1970s and 1980s and which suggested an inevitability about declining wellbeing when caregiving (e.g. Poulshock and Deimling, 1984; Haley et al, 1987). More recently, however, this body of research has been criticised for being 'probably ... more responsible for the creation of caregiving stress than are either caregivers or the recipients of their care' (Kahana and Kinney, 1991, p. 138). The professional carers completing the questionnaire adopted a more interactionist approach, emphasising the relationship context of caregiving as well as individual characteristics of the family carer:

> You try and support them so that they can continue to be informal carers, and continue to get a reward from it, whatever that might be.

> *District Nurse G (interview)*

Working with people with dementia

Getting on with it

The work carried out by professional carers was, not surprisingly, intended to meet the health and social needs of the person with dementia. The actual focus of care delivery depended on the identified needs of the person with dementia and the nature of the service involved, for example the district nursing service tended to be involved in aspects of physical care.

> We get her up in the morning, put her pad on, take her into the living room. Go in at lunchtime or just after. Change the pad and give her a wash. Then the evening service goes in, puts her to bed and changes the pad.

> *District Charge Nurse G (interview)*

It is in the area of meeting physical care needs, more than any other, that the work of professional and family carers intersect. Whilst assessment of the individual occurs in differing contexts and there may be variation in the needs identified, professional and family carers are often working with a similar purpose in meeting the physical needs of the person with dementia.

It's important he's clean and not smelly.

Mrs D, caring for her husband (interview)

Psychological and social care of people with dementia in the present study was addressed by both professional and family carers, again dependent upon the nature of the service and the perceived needs of the individual:

I think a lot of [the job] is to do with reassurance, that people aren't actually going mad.

Social Worker B (interview)

Professional carers identified a general need for people to be in a social environment:

It's just a generally accepted thing that geriatric nurses are told you've got to get people to interact.

Enrolled Nurse, Psychiatric Assessment Day Unit (interview)

However, family carers were able to make this care specific to the person's family and employment situation because of their personal knowledge of the person with dementia:

On a Sunday I like to make him nice for his niece coming. He'll say, 'Do I look nice?' I'll say, 'You look beautiful.'

Mrs P, caring for her husband (interview)

Promoting social and psychological care was seen by both professional and family carers to be a way of promoting the health and wellbeing of the person with dementia:

He loves to go to [the shopping centre], he loves watching people. He seems happy.

Mrs H, caring for her husband (interview)

If they haven't anyone there to talk to they would just go inwards. They like to talk of the same old memories they've always had. [Otherwise] they would just get worse quicker probably.

Domiciliary Care Worker (interview)

The meeting of care needs also involves the complex issue of risk management. Again, this is an area of care emphasised by both professional and family carers, although from differing perspectives. The recognition and management of risks is closely linked to normalisation and is based on the past knowledge of the person with dementia held by the family carer or the knowledge of dementia held by professional carers – see Clarke and Heyman (1998) for a more detailed analysis. One woman described how she likes to let her father go out for walks on his own occasionally, even though in the past he has disappeared for hours overnight and repeatedly been returned by the police:

> You see, I think [going out alone] is good for him. Just to be able to go out on his own sometimes because he's been so used to it.
>
> *Ms Y, caring for her father (interview)*

However, managing risks posed dilemmas for carers:

> I mean you're not supposed to keep people against their will, but you have a duty to keep people safe while they're here.
>
> *Enrolled Nurse, Psychiatric Assessment Day Unit (interview)*

Risk-taking for people with dementia extends beyond that of physical safety into psychological and social care. Professional and family carers place an emphasis in care on encouraging independence and discouraging the de-skilling of people with dementia. However, they also acknowledge the ease with which this fails to be achieved. Kitwood and Bredin (1992) and Sabat and Harré (1992) argue that people with dementia are, perhaps through näivety, depersonalised and deskilled by others.

> I can't believe that the person who lived in the community for 75 years and then comes into residential care loses all the skills even to the extent of putting a spoonful of sugar into the tea. This in a lot of cases is taken away from them, not maliciously, but 'I'll do it because it's quicker for me to do it than them'. But what the hell, they're not going anywhere.
>
> *Social Services Day Centre Officer (interview)*

Professional carers frequently said that they use the strategy of personalising a situation as a proxy for knowing the individual's wishes. Personalising was perceived to be one way of maintaining the rights of the person with dementia.

> If I'm with [person with dementia] I like to try and talk to him. I don't

like to think that if I couldn't talk that people are talking above me. I tend to talk through him.

Domiciliary Care Worker (interview)

Professional carers also discussed acting as advocates for people with dementia and their carers, protecting their rights within the systems of health and social care.

> I suppose I see a lot of what I do in terms of advocacy and representing people's rights. I do think people in hospital are very vulnerable, and I do think they can be manipulated very easily, and if you do have difficulty with memory, confusion or whatever, then it's easy for them not to get what they want because they don't know how to articulate it. I would say that part of my role is to do with advocacy and protection and ensuring the system plays fair and doesn't take advantage.

Social Worker B (interview)

Working with family carers

Maintaining or moving

Service interventions, and the intentions of professional carers when working with family carers, are either to 'maintain' the caregiving situation or to 'move' it. When intending to maintain caregiving, professional carers talk of the need to 'preserve' family carers, making them last as long as possible:

> You must keep them going whichever way you need to support them.

Domiciliary Care Worker (interview)

In the case of movement, a developmental model of care is used in which family carers are encouraged to progress through stages of the caregiving experience. Movement is used by professional carers in describing the response of a family carer or person with dementia to their caregiving situation:

> When [the family carer] in particular began to feel less stressed, I think at that point I did feel, well, this situation has moved, and one was beginning to see that it wasn't such an insoluble problem.

Social Worker T (interview)

There may be movement towards an acceptance of service input, or movement towards an acknowledgment of the probable future impact of the illness. Situations of non-movement were seen by the professional carers as a problem:

> I don't think [the family carer] accepts the prognosis that he's going to get a lot worse, don't think she accepts that at all.'
>
> *Community Psychiatric Nurse (interview)*

However, in seeking to normalise their lives, the family carers focused on what was normal (or redefined the abnormal as being within the limits of normality). Inevitably, conflicts of perception and priority arose between professional and family carers when the former focused on the problems and the latter focused on the normal. These issues affect the process of interfacing and also affect the continuance of professional carer contact (Clarke and Heyman, 1998).

Whether maintaining or moving, professional carers seek to support family carers by promoting the normalising strategies of pacing, confiding and rationalising (Clarke, 1995). For example, they acknowledge the need for family carers to 'let off steam', and offer education to empower family carers trying to rationalise their situation. Each of these strategies can be interpreted in terms of either maintaining activities (for example, respite care) or moving activities (for example, coming to terms with the disease).

Professional carers emphasise the need for family carers to preserve some aspect of their own life, of their own individuality, in order to maintain a life beyond caregiving. However, this may also oppose the process of normalising because it emphasises the abnormality of caregiving and the person with dementia.

> I think it's about keeping a door open for them and offering them something, and actually somewhere in the future trying to get them to reinvest back in life, which can be a very emotional thought for anybody.
>
> *Community Psychiatric Nurse (interview)*

Professional carers sought to help the family carers rationalise by providing them with education in managing the person with dementia. In these ways professional carers sought to promote movement in family carers' understanding and control of their lives. However, professional carers seek to move family carers towards rationalising in relation to the perceived 'facts' of dementia. Family carers use rationalising in relation to what is perceived to be normal for their relationship and the person with dementia. Kitwood and Bredin (1992), however, argue that there is a lack of correlation between the 'facts' of dementia, or its pathology, and the lived experiences of the disease. The medicalisation of dementia and caregiving relationships is perpetuated by the professional carer's orientation to the disease at the expense of the relationship between the person with dementia and the family carer.

> Demented is just a word. They [family carers] don't know what it involves, the problems, etc. They think they're starting to forget things, they don't realise part of the brain dies and they're going to get worse. Lack of understanding, really.
>
> *Social Services Day Centre Officer (interview)*

However, medicalisation of the person with dementia is also perceived to have benefits for the family carer since the imposed structure enables carers to regain some control and understanding of the situation. This is also a feature of the process of normalising (Clarke, 1995) when family carers selectively acknowledge information and selectively attribute behaviours either to the person who has dementia or to the disease.

As when caring for people with dementia, professional carers emphasise the need for a well-established relationship in working with family carers.

> They're very difficult areas to broach [e.g. sexuality] so the relationship has to be quite long-standing. Sometimes I dip my toes in, I think, right, back off for a few weeks, you're not ready for that yet.
>
> *Community Psychiatric Nurse (interview)*

> I can say things to him [the family carer], if he looks a bit grubby, I'll say, 'That's rotten, you'll show me up if any of your friends see you going out like that!' He just takes it as a joke, 'Righto, I'll get it off'. We have a very good relationship.
>
> *Home Carer (interview)*

DISCUSSION

The care of people with dementia is guided by the assessment, identification and management of need. However, the needs that are identified and prioritised are determined by the knowledge base of the carer. Clarke and Heyman (1998) compare the knowledge base of family carers, based on the particular caring situation and the individual who has dementia, and the knowledge base of professional carers, which is based on the pathology of dementia and the experiences of caring for others who have dementia.

Professional carers work within a framework of care which is inevitably restricted to the application to individuals and specific care situations of a generalised knowledge base of dementia. Such a collective and pathologically driven system of care can be characterised by:

- An emphasis on the individual, locating the problems of dementia with the affected person rather than with non-dementing people – this has been strongly argued against by Kitwood and Bredin (1992) and denies the social construction of health-care problems
- Assessment that seeks to expose the individual's deficits, a stance argued against by Perkins and Tice (1995)
- A 'hit and run' mode of service delivery with problem-led interventions which are cognisant of an assumed trajectory of continual decline
- Ignoring the family dynamics (or even encouraging divisiveness) in the care situation (Pitkeathley 1989; Clarke, 1997).

This is the framework for professionally dominant care, as discussed in Chapter 1. The potential for a negotiated partnership in care is minimal. However, as the research presented here demonstrates, family carers use a different framework: the emphasis is shifted from the individual with dementia to the relationship between them, from the disease of dementia to the dynamic of the family, from an orientation to the future to that of the past and present, from being problem-centred to being individual and relationship-centred (Clarke, 1995).

Health-care professionals constitute an important interactionist influence on the family carer's normalisation of the person with dementia and their relationship together. However, my study found that health-care professionals were oriented towards problems and possible future events, and towards the dementia rather than the person. This orientation is evident in the process of interacting by which professional carers provide care for the person with dementia on a problem-led basis, and for the family carer in a way that promotes 'movement' along a medicalised pathway of inevitable decline and increasing service usage. For example, whilst involvement in educational or therapeutic activity and information receipt may facilitate normalisation, it may also merely emphasise the abnormal (Knafl and Deatrick, 1986). Such concerns feature strongly in the process of interfacing in which the 'costs' of service intervention are weighed up. For example, Mr O (who cares for his mother) felt that attending a carers' support group would deny him the opportunity to do something he wanted to do and merely emphasise his role as a caregiver. That health-care professionals can have a major and frequently negative impact on normalisation is found both in this study and by Robinson (1993):

> As one woman put it, health care professionals are oriented towards 'servicing your illness' rather than 'getting on with life'. (p. 20)

Assessment and care that are problem-led undermine the work of people with dementia and their family carers. This approach exposes what they have sought to hide (Keady and Nolan, 1994a; Robinson et al, 1997) and may fail to acknowledge the strategies implemented by people with dementia and their families to manage their situation. My research identified three strategies used by family carers to help them maintain a normalised relationship with the person with dementia. Firstly, and most visibly used by family and professional carers, was the strategy of 'pacing' Pacing allows the family carer and the person with dementia to limit their involvement with each other, either physically or emotionally. However, some forms of pacing, such as respite care, remove people with dementia from their 'normal' environment and so interrupt the process of normalising.

> The hospitals are good, they take him for a month and they give me him back for a month.
>
> *Mrs P, caring for her husband (interview)*

A second strategy employed is that of confiding, enabling family carers to convey – and therefore 'offload' – some of the anxiety they may experience about caregiving, and to help them identify and manage some of their problems:

> Sometimes I get tired like and a bit down, I don't show it. I only talk to one person, and that's the Lord.
>
> *Mr C, caring for his wife (interview)*

Thirdly, family carers use rationalising to cognitively manage the person with dementia and to normalise their relationship by a process of selective acknowledgment (of information and behaviour of the person with dementia), selective attribution (to individual or illness), and selective comparisons (to other people or an ideal state):

> She's not that far gone. She's quite witty and quite sharp some of the time.
>
> *Mr O, caring for his mother (interview)*

Through normalisation, family carers are seeking to manage the impact of dementia in a way that protects their relationship and protects the personhood of the individual with dementia. The danger of undermining this activity is that it may fracture the family and establish an antagonistic relationship between the family and professional.

The dichotomy, however, between the perspectives of family and professional carers is theoretical only, and the characteristics presented above become caricatures in practice. Family carers are indeed concerned with problems and future events, albeit in terms of their impact on family exchange and dynamics. Family carers do not find it easy to focus on the person rather than the dementia, and normalising requires continual work to 'hang on' to the individual and their relationship.

> Somewhere in that body is the [husband] I married, but he's slowly going, and you know that you know, and you think to yourself, 'Never mind, somewhere in there he's there,' but it's like looking after a baby.
>
> *Mrs U, caring for her husband, (interview)*

Professional carers demonstrate in practice a greater sensitivity to the individual and the family than is suggested by the framework of pathologically led care. However, this is a level of care that is poorly acknowledged not only in theory but also in policy. Professional carers had to work against 'the system' to deliver the care that they felt was appropriate. For example, one social worker kept people 'on the books' for longer than normal to facilitate any later contact; one community practice teacher 'hid' the need for support and comfort for the family carer under the more instrumental reason for contact of bathing the person with dementia.

In shifting to a family-centred approach to care, professional carers are, however, hampered by a number of factors. Firstly, they may meet only the person with dementia or the family carer. For example, day and residential respite care and assessment unit staff may have minimal contact with the family carer, although respite care is arguably delivered for the benefit of the carer (Twigg, 1989). One social worker described her approach to this problem for Mrs D, who cares for her husband:

> She's never been to the residential home, she won't have anything to do with it. And so gradually one's trying to introduce both of them to stop this sort of separateness. I'm hoping that she might come with me to bring Mr D out and then she can actually look at it and he might not feel he's being pushed out and she might know a bit more about where he is and start to meet staff and have a point of contact between them.
>
> *Social Worker (interview)*

Secondly, professional care intervention may be focused on a recognition of obligations in risk management, on behalf of both themselves and the person with dementia. One social services day centre officer was concerned about Mr N's inclination to 'escape' from the day centre:

> We're very much at risk because he's our responsibility when he's here.
>
> *Social Services Day Centre Officer (interview)*

It's very unsafe for [the person with dementia] being upstairs. I personally refuse and I don't allow the auxiliary to bring her downstairs because it's too unsafe to bring her downstairs and I won't put us at risk.

District Nurse (interview)

Family carers interpret risk with a baseline of the individual as an independently functioning person, able to take risks, able to judge the wisdom of those risks, and with the right to self-determination in deciding to take that risk, like Ms Y's father (mentioned above) who was allowed to wander from the house at any time of the day. Professional carers judge risk-taking in relation to their knowledge of the illness; consequently, people with dementia are perceived to be unable to make judgments and unable to maintain their own safety. They need to be protected, from themselves as much as anything else (Like Mr N, for example, who was physically contained within the day centre).

Many of these issues of an individual's rights defy a single answer because of the multiple perspectives involved. Furthermore, the rights of the person with dementia are tangled inextricably with the rights of the family carer. Mrs P, for example, cares for her husband and protects his sense of personal worth, but perhaps at the expense of his sense of self-determination because of the medication used to sedate him. Mr O cares for his mother but wishes she was in residential care, so perhaps her sense of self-determination is maintained only at the expense of that of her son. Mrs M cares for her husband but refuses his access to health and social care professionals, so perhaps she is maintaining her own sense of self-determination and personal worth at the expense of professional carer contact from which her husband might benefit.

Thirdly, professional carers are denied a knowledge of the individual and family because they have no shared history with them. Instead, they seek to apply their professional knowledge base of dementia to individuals. McKee (1991) argues that it is the movement between aggregate and individual knowledge that is the hallmark of humanistic health-care practice. Assessment may focus on the exposure of problems, but this is modified by attempts to know the family and by applying their own humanity as a proxy in the situation. Professional carers seek to learn about the family through sustained contact with them. By personalising the situation, professional carers seek to respond to their own wishes interpreted as a substitute for those of the person with dementia and the family carer:

Well, I would want to know [about illness].

Enrolled Community Psychiatric Nurse (interview)

Family carers reject care and advice that is insensitive to the individual situation and may consequently reject overtures from professional carers for closer contact:

> I've only met [the family carer] once. She refused to come to the reviews we had. When the occupational therapist went to visit she just clammed up and wouldn't answer any questions, wouldn't cooperate. She didn't come to any support groups, I spoke to her a couple of times on the phone but she seemed to get into a rage.
>
> *Enrolled Nurse, Psychiatric Assessment Day Unit (interview)*

Policy guiding the practice of health and social care professionals needs to recognise and support the activities of professional carers working with family carers and people with dementia in a way that shifts the emphasis away from the individual, the disease and the problems, to the family and their strategies for managing any deficits. Further, there is a need to shift from a functionalist view of normalisation, supporting what is societally valued, to an interactional perspective, supporting what is individually and family centred.

Continuity in professional carer is an essential aspect of achieving this approach. The family carers in the study greatly valued professional carers with whom there was sustained contact, as well as professional carers who worked *with* them rather than *for* them. Continuity of carer allows the professional carer access to the knowledge base of the family and the person with dementia, and thus allows care to move away from the pessimism of continual decline in dementia to the optimism of sustained family relationships which promote the wellbeing of the person with dementia.

Similarly, assessment in dementia care needs to recognise the full range of activity currently undertaken by some professional carers. A shift from the functional and cognitive ability of the individual, with its pathological focus, to assessment of and by the family (Keady and Nolan, 1994b) and the dynamics of the relationship between family carers and the person with dementia, will create opportunities to learn about individual care situations and will facilitate a collaboration in care management between the professional carers and whole family.

Dementia care and normalisation

Here is a challenge: to refocus dementia care management on its interpersonal dimensions. To achieve this may mean letting go of some aspects of current professional thought and practice. There is a need to question the use of health-care interventions that reinforce the abnormality of caregiving and the pathology of dementia.

The interpersonal aspects of dementia care cannot be discussed without reference to the work of Kitwood. From the interactionist standpoint that 'persons exist in relationship', he argues that as cognitive ability disintegrates, so interrelationships must take over if 'personhood' is to be maintained (Kitwood and Bredin, 1992), a view also supported by Sabat and Harré (1992). Kitwood also argues (Kitwood and Bredin, 1992; Kitwood, 1993) for relative wellbeing in dementia and identifies four 'global sentient states' which must be protected if wellbeing is to be maintained: a sense of personal worth, a sense of agency (control of personal life or self-determination), social confidence and hope. This pushes professional practice with people suffering from dementia into new arenas. It relates to the early definitions of normalisation from the field of learning disability, which emphasise human rights.

Any intervention will best support normalisation if it acknowledges the family carer's knowledge base as at least equal to (although very different from) a professional knowledge base. A powerful care intervention will arise from judicious use of both these knowledge bases, with the aim of retaining the person with dementia as primarily a person, and fulfilling the needs of the family carer. Hasselkus (1988) argues that professional and family carers need to recognise the context of meaning in which their expertise is embedded, and challenges carers to make these meanings accessible to each other. My own study, however, has demonstrated that at times family and professional carers have fundamentally different orientations in the purposes of their care.

Services that emphasise the interactional, relationship basis of family caregiving are developments strongly supported by my study. One example is the therapeutic use of family systems theory in which no single person is regarded as different or pathological, but the whole social system is regarded as one unit. This perspective is addressed by Forchuk and Dorsay (1995) in relation to nursing theory, but in relation to dementia care it remains relatively unexplored. Notable exceptions include the work of Bonder (1987) and Benbow et al (1993) and a valuable review is presented by Richardson et al (1994). Family systems theory offers considerable potential when working within an interactionist framework with dementia sufferers and their families, but is, as yet, largely untapped.

CONCLUSION

Three clear trends emerge from the development of the theory of normalisation: the transitions from functionalism to interactionalism, from fixed societal norms to ever-changing individually defined norms, and from health-care professionals as instigators to potential underminers.

Normalisation has been used in several substantive areas of health care. Originally developed in the field of learning disability, it has proved to be a major ideology shaping service developments since the 1960s. Normalisation has also been perceived as a relevant concept in the field of mental health and, more recently, in chronic illness and for parents caring for a chronically or terminally ill child. The study described in this chapter contributes to its application in a further substantive field, that of family caregiving to someone with dementia.

The role of health-care professionals is identified in this study as potentially undermining the process of normalising, an issue addressed by family carers in the process of interfacing and operationalised in the process of interacting. This seems to be an unnecessary complication in the complex role of caring for someone with dementia, and as such is a contradiction for the 'caring' professions.

REFERENCES

Anderton, J.M., Elfert, H. & Lai, M. (1989) Ideology in the clinical context: chronic illness, ethnicity and the discourse on normalisation. *Sociology of Health and Illness* **11**, 253–275.

Barnes, R.F., Raskind, M.A., Scott, M. & Murphy, C. (1981) Problems of families caring for Alzheimer patients: use of a support group. *Journal of the American Geriatrics Society* **554**, 80–85.

Benbow, S.M., Marriott, A., Morley, M. & Walsh S. (1993) Family therapy and dementia: review and clinical experience. *International Journal of Geriatric Psychiatry* **8**, 717–725.

Bonder, B.R. (1987) Family systems and Alzheimer's disease: an approach to treatment. *Physical and Occupational Health in Geriatrics* **5**, 13–24.

Cantor, M.H. (1983) Strain among caregivers: a study of experience in the United States. *Gerontologist* **23**, 597–604.

Carers (Recognition and Services) Act (1995) London: HMSO.

Cicirelli, V.G. (1983) Adult children and their elderly parents. In: Brubaker, T. (ed.) *Family Relationships in Later Life*. London: Sage.

Clarke, C.L. (1995) Care of elderly people suffering from dementia and their co-resident informal carers. In: Heyman, B. (ed.) *Researching User Perspectives on Community Health Care*. London: Chapman & Hall.

Clarke, C.L. (1997) In sickness and in health: remembering the relationship in family caregiving for people with dementia. In: Marshall, M. (ed.) *The State of the Art in Dementia Care*. London: Centre for Policy on Ageing.

Clarke, C.L. & Heyman B. (1998) How families and professional carers appraise risks for people with dementia. In: Heyman, B. (ed.) *Risk, Health and Healthcare: A Critical Approach*. London: Chapman & Hall.

Davison, N. & Reed, J. (1995) One foot on the escalator: elderly people in sheltered accommodation. In: Heyman, B. (ed.) *Researching User Perspectives on Community Health Care*. London: Chapman & Hall.

Finch, J. & Mason, J. (1993) *Negotiating Family Responsibilities*. London: Tavistock/Routledge.

Fitting, M., Rabins, P., Lucas, M.J. & Eastham, J. (1986) Caregivers for dementia patients: a comparison of husbands and wives. *Gerontologist* **26**, 248–252.

Forchuk, C. & Dorsay, J.P. (1995) Hildegard Peplau meets family systems nursing: innovation in theory-based practice. *Journal of Advanced Nursing* **21**, 110–115.

Gabow, C. (1989) The impact of Alzheimer's disease on family caregivers. *Home Healthcare Nurse* **7**, 19–21.

Gilbert, T. (1993) Learning disability nursing: from normalisation to materialism – towards a new paradigm. *Journal of Advanced Nursing* **18**, 1604–1609.

Gilleard, C.J. (1984) *Living With Dementia – Community Care of the Elderly Mentally Infirm*. London: Croom Helm.

Haley, W.E., Brown, E.G., Brown, S.L., Berry, J.W. & Hughes, G.H. (1987) Psychological, social and health consequences of caring for a relative with senile dementia. *Journal of the American Geriatrics Society* **35**, 405–411.

Hasselkus, B.R. (1988) Meaning in family caregiving: perspectives on caregiver/professional relationships. *Gerontologist* **28**, 686–691.

Hirschefeld, M.J. (1981) Families living and coping with the cognitively impaired. In: Copp, L.A. (ed.) *Recent Advances In Nursing: Care of the Aging.* New York: Churchill Livingstone.

Kahana, E. & Kinney, J. (1991) Understanding caregiving interventions in the context of the stress model. In: Young, R.F. & Olsen, E.A. (eds.) *Health, Illness and Disability in Later Life – Practice, Issues and Interventions.* Newbury Park: Sage.

Keady, J. & Nolan, M. (1994a) Younger onset dementia: developing a longitudinal model as the basis for a research agenda and as a guide to interventions with sufferers and carers. *Journal of Advanced Nursing* **19**, 659–669.

Keady, J. & Nolan, M. (1994b) The Carer-Led Assessment Process (CLASP): a framework for the assessment of need in dementia caregivers. *Journal of Clinical Nursing* **3**, 103–108.

Kitwood, T. & Bredin, K. (1992) Towards a theory of dementia care: personhood and well-being. *Ageing and Society* **12**, 269–287.

Kitwood, T. (1993) Towards a theory of dementia care: the interpersonal process. *Ageing and Society* **13**, 51–67.

Knafl, K.A. & Deatrick, J.A. (1986) How families manage chronic conditions: an analysis of the concept of normalisation. *Research in Nursing and Health* **9**, 215–222.

Locker, D. (1983) *Disability and Disadvantage: The Consequences of Chronic Illness* London: Tavistock.

McKee C. (1991) Breaking the mould: a humanistic approach to nursing practice. In: McMahon, R. & Pearson, A. (eds) *Nursing as Therapy.* London: Chapman & Hall.

Motenko, A.K. (1989) The frustrations, gratifications, and well-being of dementia caregivers. *Gerontologist* **29**, 166–172.

Nolan, M. & Grant, G. (1989) Addressing the needs of informal carers: a neglected area of nursing practice. *Journal of Advanced Nursing* **14**, 950–962.

Perkins, K. & Tice C. (1995) A strengths perspective in practice: older people and mental health challenges. *Journal of Gerontological Social Work* **23**, 83–97.

Pitkeathley, J. (1989) *It's My Duty, Isn't It? The Plight of Carers in Our Society.* London: Souvenir.

Poulshock, S.W. & Deimling, G.T. (1984) Families caring for elders in residence: issues in the measurement of burden. *Journal of Gerontology* **39**, 230–239.

Pratt, C., Schmall, V. & Wright, S. (1987) Ethical concerns of family caregivers to dementia patients. *Gerontologist* **27**, 632–638.

Qureshi, H. & Simons, K. (1987) Resources within families: caring for elderly people. In: Brannen, J. & Wilson, G. (eds) *Give and Take in Families: Studies in Resource Distribution.* London: Allen & Unwin.

Richardson, C.A., Gilleard, C.J., Lieberman, S. & Peeler, R. (1994) Working with older adults and their families – a review. *Journal of Family Therapy* **16**, 225–240.

Robinson, C.A. (1993) Managing life with a chronic condition: the story of normalisation. *Qualitative Health Research* **3**, 6–28.

Robinson, P., Ekman, S.-L., Meleis, A.I., Winbald, B. & Wahlund, L-O. (1997) Suffering in silence: the experience of early memory loss. *Health Care in Later Life* **2**, 107–120.

Sabat, S.R. & Harré, R. (1992) The construction and deconstruction of self in Alzheimer's disease. *Ageing and Society* **12**, 443–461.

Steinmetz, S.K. & Amsden, D.J. (1983) Dependent elders, family stress, and abuse. In: Brubaker, T. (ed.) *Family Relationships in Later Life.* London: Sage.

Strauss, A.L. (1987) *Qualitative Analysis for Social Scientists.* Cambridge University Press.

Strauss, A.L., Corbin, J., Fagerhaugh, S. et al (1984) *Chronic Illness and the Quality of Life*, 2nd edn. St Louis: Mosby.

Twigg, J. (1989) Not taking the strain. *Community Care* **77**, 16–19.

Twigg, J. & Atkin, K. (1994) *Carers Perceived: Policy and Practice in Informal Care.* Buckingham: Open University Press.

Tyne, A. (1992) Normalisation: from theory to practice. In: Brown, H. & Smith, H. (eds) *Normalisation – A Reader for the Nineties.* London: Routledge.

Ungerson, C. (1987) *Policy Is Personal – Sex, Gender and Informal Care.* London: Tavistock.

Wolfensberger, W. (1972) *The Principle of Normalisation in Human Services.* Toronto: National Institute on Mental Retardation.

Wuest, J., Ericson, P.K. & Stern, P.N. (1994) Becoming strangers: the changing family caregiving relationship in Alzheimer's disease. *Journal of Advanced Nursing* **20**, 437–443.

Zarit, S.H., Orr, N.K. & Zarit, J.M. (1985) *The Hidden Victims of Alzheimer's Disease: Families Under Stress.* New York: University Press.

Developing partnership in the work of community psychiatric nurses with older people with dementia

Trevor Adams

KEY ISSUES

- Community psychiatric nurses make an important contribution to the care of people with dementia and their families

- Community psychiatric nurses work according to a process consisting of assessment, planning, intervention and closing

- The work of community psychiatric nurses specialising in dementia consists of monitoring, networking, counselling and information-giving

- There is a lack of partnership between the community psychiatric nurse, the family and the person with dementia

- Community psychiatric nurses need to develop partnership through research and practice

THE DEVELOPMENT OF PSYCHIATRIC NURSING WITH PEOPLE WHO HAVE DEMENTIA

In Britain, community psychiatric nursing with older people with dementia developed as a speciality in the late 1960s through the work of community psychogeriatric teams, for example at Severalls, Oxford and South Manchester (Whitehead, 1970; Leopoldt et al, 1975; Ainsworth and Jolley, 1978). Barker and Black (1971) described their work on one of these early teams in the Buckinghamshire integrated domiciliary psychogeriatric service as consisting of 'mainly counselling and advising relatives on problems of care and management and, very important, giving sufficient time to their problems, however trivial'. In addition, their work included the coordination of relief beds and the provision of a night sitting service. Whilst their work was ambitious and, no doubt, filled a gap in service provision, not all of the Buckinghamshire service roles have been taken on by community psychiatric nurses (CPNs) in other areas. Lancaster (1984) describes her work as a community psychiatric nurse as consisting of liaison, coordination and consultancy in addition to the more accepted roles of clinician, assessor, therapist and educator. While these descriptions of practice are interesting and worthwhile, it must be noted that they are anecdotal and not based on empirical findings.

Empirical studies of the work of CPNs with older people with dementia are few in number. Tough et al (1980) identified the tasks undertaken by CPNs with older people based in five health centres. However, the study did not distinguish between confused and non-confused clients, so there is no indication of the composition of the sample with regards to the clients' mental state. This makes it difficult to extrapolate the study results to the work of CPNs with older people with dementia.

Three developments in the UK have had an important bearing on the work of community psychiatric nursing with older people with dementia. Firstly, changes in health and social policy have located the provision of care to older people with chronic health and social problems (such as dementia) with the social services (DoH, 1989). This may have given rise to a decrease in the number of CPNs specialising in older people, the first decline since the development of specialist services for older people in the 1960s. This raises two issues: firstly, people with dementia often have a variety of physical problems, and therefore it seems appropriate that the responsibility to provide care should be located with agencies who are experienced at providing health-related care; secondly, Brooker and White (1997) found that there had been a substantial increase in the number of CPNs working with people with 'severe and enduring' mental health problems. This term did not include people with dementia. This raises the further issue: is not dementia severe and enduring enough to be considered under this term?

A second important development in the late 1980s was the setting up of the Admiral Nurse Service (Jarvis et al, 1992). The original service was based in north-east Westminster but it has now been extended to a number of other areas, primarily in the London area. The service was established to offer practical and emotional support for families and other people who care for people with dementia (Greenwood and Walsh, 1995). The philosophy of the Admiral Nursing Service is that traditional CPN services have not addressed the needs of families, as they care for their relatives with dementia. As we have seen, this is not a new approach to working with older people with dementia, and indeed specialist CPN services for older people have – from the time of Barker and Black (1971) – been based on the principle of 'care for the carer'; nonetheless, the Admiral Nursing Service has created considerable interest within dementia care.

The third approach was a study undertaken by the Centre for Study in Dementia Care at the University of Portsmouth relating to the development of an advanced nurse practitioner in dementia. This also had important implications for the development of community psychiatric nursing as a speciality within mental health nursing (Rolfe and Phillips, 1997). The study established a new role of advanced nurse practitioner (ANP) in dementia, which consisted of service development, liaison and collaboration with other services, education, outreach, health education and early intervention. This new role was evaluated through the use of an action research methodology through interviews with patients and family carers. It was found that many of the staff who took part in the study recognised the existence of an unidentified and potentially large group of sufferers from the early stage of dementia who are not known to services; that the ANP was as much valued by other health-care professionals as she was by nurses, and that the ANP provided an alternative to the general practitioner for both assessments and clinical interventions. These findings have important implications for the development of CPN work with people with dementia, as they suggest that through the development of ANP there is a likelihood of benefits to clients as well as possible cost benefits.

THE STUDY

Method

Thirteen cases were taken from the caseload of four CPNs working with older people with dementia. Each case consisted of an older person with dementia. Data were collected by observation and interview. One visit per case was observed using a predesigned observation schedule based on the researcher's experience as a practising CPN; this listed phenomena which the researcher might note in the interaction between the CPN and the client and/or caregiver. Following the observed visit, further data were collected by means of an in-depth interview with the CPN. Again, a predesigned schedule was used to initiate question areas. However, the bulk of the interview consisted of the family carer responding to various probing questions that arose from earlier answers to predesigned questions within the interview schedule.

The data collected in the form of transcripts and field notes were analysed using a form of grounded theory as described by Dey (1993). The validity of the data was checked using three methods:

1. comparing the results obtained in the study with the earlier views of the researcher – the change in views suggesting the researcher did not merely read his own views into the findings

2. asking the CPNs to say whether the codes and categories generated in the data analysis were consistent with what they had said
3. asking two CPNs working with people with dementia in other geographical areas to comment on the findings of the study.

These three measures generally found the findings of the study to be valid. However, it needs to be said that the CPNs working in other geographical areas said that their work had much in common with that of the CPNs in the study: nevertheless, they did report that they undertook other forms of work that were different, such as advocacy, and received clinical supervision.

Data presentation

Following analysis of the data the findings were gathered together under four headings: the CPNs' working environment; the CPNs' method of working; the orientation of the CPNs' work; and CPNs and carers.

Working environment

The CPNs for older people were based in two rooms within the day hospital for older people with mental health problems within a large mental hospital. There were four CPNs and each had responsibility for a specific geographical area. The CPNs took referrals from any source and had the following criteria for acceptance: clients should be 70 years of age or over, with a mental health problem, or under 70 years old and chronically confused.

Methods of working

The work of the CPNs is a process consisting of four parts: assessment, planning, intervention and closing (Fig. 14.1). These parts correspond to some of the stages represented in the nursing process as described by a number of writers including Yura and Walsh (1978) and Ward (1985). Their work did not include an evaluation stage, as it was not something that the CPNs identified as being a part of their working process. However, in reality, it may well be that evaluation was an ongoing activity that tended to merge with planning and had no separate identity of its own. The nature of evaluation in the work of CPNs would be a worthwhile area for further study, as evaluation is often neglected among nurses. The stages of the CPNs' work were not separate but rather merged together. For example, assessment occurred over the first few visits and continued even after the intervention had started.

Assessment   During the assessment stage, the CPN decides whether to accept the case. The CPNs operate an open referral system which receives

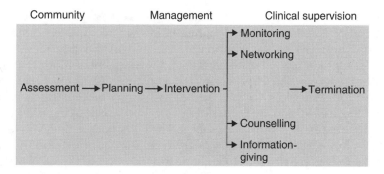

Figure 14.1 Community psychiatric nursing with older people with dementia and their families.

referrals from a wide variety of sources including general practitioners, social workers and doctors working in the psychiatric sector. It needs to be recognised that the cases are referred to the CPNs by agencies that are already aware of the existence of the service. The open system does nothing to find cases, but rather waits for cases to be referred; consequently, people who are chronically confused and their relatives may have to wait months or years before their general practitioner refers them to the CPN service. This raises the problem of putting people with dementia and their families into contact with specialist services when they need them, and highlights the need for services to be proactive in attracting new cases.

A variation of Roper's model of nursing as suggested by Thomas (1988) was used to elicit information on the client's and the carer's physical and mental states and social circumstances. The CPNs claimed that they used this model to underpin their practice; in reality, however, the CPNs based their work on a completely different set of ideas. These ideas were not understood explicitly by the CPNs, but were implicit. This understanding of an implicit rather than an explicit model may be linked with the work of Benner and Tanner (1987), who argue that 'expert' nurses (that is, experienced nurses) make use of intuitive knowledge in their nursing practice. The CPNs did seem to be using an intuitive basis to their work, which was shown in the methods of data collection used in the study. When asked the question, 'How does the model help you?' one of the CPNs commented, 'It helps us to identify nursing problems'.

Assessments were carried out on an informal basis, usually in the client's home. The assessment was not confined to the first visit but continued over the first few visits. These visits also provided time when the CPN could get to know the client and the family carer. During the period of assessment the CPNs asked numerous questions about the physical and mental state of the client and the carer, together with their social circumstances. These visits were friendly and conversational rather than bureaucratic. The assessment documentation was completed later in the office, on the basis of the information elicited in the interview. As the assessment took a few visits to complete, the assessment tended to merge with other stages of the CPN work such as planning and intervention.

The way in which the CPNs assessed cases may be illustrated by CPN A's visit to Mrs Jackson, a 57-year-old carer who was looking after her 67-year-old moderately confused husband. The CPN had visited Mrs Jackson about 10 days earlier when she was at home with her husband; however, Mrs Jackson was reluctant to talk about the situation to the CPN with her husband present. Consequently, CPN A made a second appointment to see Mrs Jackson when her husband was in day care and Mrs Jackson could take a day's leave from her employment. During the interview, CPN A asked Mrs Jackson various questions about the difficulties she had been encountering with her husband. These questions were open-ended and gave Mrs Jackson the opportunity to say exactly what she wanted. Moreover, CPN A's informal and relaxed style of questioning allowed Mrs Jackson to have some say over the agenda of the interview. Some of the questions that CPN A asked built upon information she had already gained during the first interview. Her questions allowed the interview to progress into new and unexplored areas. Some of CPN A's questions enabled Mrs Jackson to give vent to her anger and frustration with her situation.

Throughout the interview, CPN A tried to build up a picture of the situation that Mrs Jackson was facing. However, whilst it appeared that Mrs Jackson fitted in with the CPN's line of questioning, she really had an agenda of her own, which was related to finding out whether the CPN could help her get hospital-based day-care provision for her husband. This had become an important issue to Mrs Jackson as the private carer was finding it increasingly difficult to manage her husband's behavioural problems, notably his wandering.

Although this assessment interview was different from those in other cases, in that the carer was particularly assertive and proactive, it does illustrate various phenomena. Firstly, the CPN collected data relating to the history of the situation. Secondly, the CPN collected data relating to physical, psychological and social aspects of the situation. Thirdly, the CPN was concerned with the welfare of the carer and with her responsibilities in meeting the needs of the client. This third phenomenon is as interesting as it is disturbing, and is dealt with more fully later in the chapter. However, suffice it to say at this point that the assessment is a political event where various interested parties are given the opportunity to put forward their points of view and to put in a bid for what they want.

Planning The CPNs planned the way in which they believed they could best contribute to the case. In spite of being supplied with special forms on which they could write a care plan, the CPNs said they planned their casework as they assessed and visited their clients and carers. One CPN told me:

> I do it [planning] in my head an awful lot ... I do have a care plan for each client but often there is more in my head than is written down ... once you see a client you have an idea how often that person is going to need visiting and [I] keep that information in my head.

Indeed, the CPNs viewed writing care plans as a hindrance to their work in that it wasted time. One CPN said that it took an hour to complete the care plan properly. This presented the CPNs with a problem; as another CPN said:

> I can either go and visit someone and actually do something, or I can sit here for the afternoon and write.

Also, the written care plan only contains a fraction of the work that the CPNs do with clients and their carers; as one of the CPNs put it, 'We do much more than is written on the piece of paper [the care plan]'. The care plan was usually written out some time after the 'mental' plan had been made, and there was some temptation to produce a written care plan retrospectively, after the CPN had completed the intervention. Essentially, the CPNs could see no point in writing the care plans. As one CPN put it:

> Because we are all experienced, you know after spending an hour with clients and we know what is necessary and we don't need to ... sit down and write it really.

Intervention The CPNs undertook a wide variety of tasks in their work with clients and carers. These tasks can be categorised under various modes of intervention. One such mode of intervention referred to by the CPNs was 'monitoring'. Usually monitoring referred to visiting clients or carers to see whether their physical or mental condition had deteriorated. If deterioration had occurred, the CPN reassessed the case and reviewed the intervention being given. If necessary, a referral to another, more appropriate agency was made. Less frequently, monitoring referred to specific checks made on various aspects of the client's or the carer's life – for example, whether clients were eating well enough or were keeping themselves clean. These two ways of understanding monitoring were combined in the response of one of the CPNs, who said, 'I am basically monitoring the home situation to see how she is coping. To assess her and see if she is going downhill, how well she is coping.'

Another example of monitoring may be seen in the work of CPN C with Mrs Roberts, an 80-year-old woman who was being looked after by a neighbour living two doors away. The neighbour had known Mrs Roberts for many years and was very willing to help Mrs Roberts by doing small tasks such as making her breakfast in the morning and collecting her pension from the post office. The situation was rather precarious, because Mrs Roberts was liable to leave the gas on, had a history of hallucinations and was also inclined to neglect herself. A large part of the CPN's work with this case was monitoring, which consisted of checking whether there had been any deterioration in Mrs Roberts' condition with a view to referral to another agency, and making sure that Mrs Roberts was having her basic daily needs met.

Another mode of intervention was that of 'networking'. Sometimes networking was directed towards mobilising the family, so that giving care did not fall upon just one family member. The use of networking to mobilise dormant family resources may be illustrated in CPN Ds work with Mrs Bollinger, a 78-year-old, moderately confused woman who was living alone. The CPN commented that she had

> ...spoken to the niece to try and get the family involved in actually being a support to her [the carer]. It is a problem with the family because the only time when the family want to know anything about [the client] is when he is very ill. And the rest of the time, she [the carer] is left on her own with nobody. So I have spoken to the niece and said it's fine when [the client] is in [respite care] but she really needs support all the time.

At other times, networking was directed towards mobilising formal caring agencies such as the social services and the private sector. An illustration of this form of networking may be seen in CPN B's work with Mr Hindle, a 73-year-old man who was looking after his moderately confused wife at home. Mr Hindle had been finding some aspects of caring for his wife difficult, particularly her wandering and outbursts of aggression. As part of the intervention, CPN B arranged for Mrs Hindle to be assessed at the day hospital where she was offered day care for 3 days a week. After a few weeks, CPN B arranged for Mrs Hindle to have 2 weeks of respite care on a ward for older people with mental health problems within the hospital. However, Mr Hindle was still finding caring difficult, so finally CPN B contacted the social worker who had been involved in the case at an earlier stage, to see if she could arrange an assessment for Mrs Hindle regarding a permanent place in a residential home. Mrs Hindle was initially admitted to a local authority home for a period of assessment and then admitted on a permanent basis following a meeting between CPN B, the social worker and the officer in charge of the home.

Sometimes, networking is required more quickly; for example when there is an emergency requiring additional resources to which the CPN does not have direct access. This was the case when CPN A visited Mrs Phillips, a woman in her 70s looking after her blind and moderately confused husband. Mrs Phillips had had a fall earlier that day which had confined her to bed. Because she thought CPN A would visit, she waited before telling anyone that she was finding the situation difficult. The CPN described the situation as follows:

> When I arrived at one o'clock [Mr Phillips] was wandering around in his pyjamas, not being able to have anything to eat. She [Mrs Phillips] was in bed, unable to get up. So, it was a matter of assessing that situation, you know, taking the appropriate action really.

I asked the CPN what this action was; the reply was that it was 'to get him admitted to the respite care ward'. Occasionally, networking does not proceed because the other parties do not believe that they have anything to offer. An example in the study was when one of the CPNs cited difficulties in referring 'suitable' cases to the day hospital when differences of opinion may be encountered relating to the issue of what constitutes 'suitable'.

Another mode of intervention was counselling. This was a wide concept that included a number of ways of interacting between the clients and/or carers. The aim of counselling was to help the clients and carers by listening and talking to them. However, there were various dimensions to counselling as it was used by the CPNs. One of these dimensions related to the duration of the interaction, for example whether the counselling was on a short-term basis, e.g. in response to a crisis, or long-term. This may be illustrated by CPN A's visit to Mrs Scott, a carer looking after her mildly confused husband. Mrs Scott's situation was exacerbated by a cardiovascular accident she sustained 3 months earlier which left her with a right-sided paralysis and some speech impairment. The CPN visited the couple as the result of an urgent referral to the CPN service that someone had left on her desk. The anonymous note said that Mrs Scott was 'very depressed' and that she was finding things difficult at home. When CPN A reached the house, she found Mrs Scott with her husband in the living room. When CPN A asked Mrs Scott how she had been finding things lately, Mrs Scott burst into tears and was in that state for most of the 40-minute interview. Her husband looked on, apologetic about his wife's tears, but because of his obvious confusion, he did not know what they were caused by. The CPN's intervention was a response to a crisis and was designed to help Mrs Scott ventilate some of the despair she was feeling at a time when things were exceedingly difficult. As such, it was a crisis intervention which might possibly be required again, depending upon whether Mrs Scott's situation or her response to the situation changed.

Another dimension was the nature of the counselling. Various models of counselling were used as a basis for the interventions and included crisis intervention, grief counselling and supportive psychotherapy. Counselling was mostly directed towards the carer, as in the example of CPN A's counselling of Mrs Scott. However, occasionally counselling was directed the client. This happened in CPN D's intervention with Mrs a 75-year-old woman who had been living alone since her husband died 3 months earlier. Mrs Spencer had been moderately confused for over a year but had become depressed and lethargic since her husband died. Consequently, CPN D counselled Mrs Spencer using grief counselling as a framework for her intervention.

Another dimension to the CPNs' counselling was the extent of emotional expression by the client or the carer. This ranged from high levels of emotional expression, for example as displayed by Mrs Scott when she was visited by CPN A, to low levels of emotional expression, often described by the CPNs as 'supportive counselling'. The latter form of counselling, relating to low levels of emotional expression by the client or the carer during visits, seemed to overlap with the CPNs' idea of support. The CPNs tended to conflate the two ideas of counselling and support. This was apparent when the CPNs were asked what they thought was the aim of their intervention in a particular case, they replied that it was 'supporting the wife – counselling, really.' Moreover, there seems also to be a relationship between support and the idea of networking. Support was seen as something that could be gained by the client or the carer as the result of satisfactory communication about the client or carer between the various people, systems or agencies available to meet the needs of the client or carer at a particular time. For example, CPN C's work with Mrs Roberts, used earlier to illustrate networking, could also illustrate 'support' in the visits of the CPN. In addition, the idea of support was used by one of the CPNs to describe the help a carer was receiving – 'I think that the neighbours are quite supportive of her' – and as such, highlights the extent to which support received by clients and carers is related to intercommunication within and between people, systems and agencies.

The CPNs' work also included the giving of information. This took a number of forms. Sometimes it consisted of giving the carer (never the client!) information regarding the features and course of the dementia. For example, one of the CPNs explained the use of this form of information-giving as follows:

> I found that the first few visits was to try to explain to him [the carer] why … Mary [the client] is behaving as she is.

At other times, information-giving was concerned with telling carers about the range of services that were available in their locality. For example, one of the CPNs said to me that they 'told [a carer] about all the information about social services, available in the community and … what help he could get, and now he's having a District Nurse'. This example illustrates how information-giving can be a precursor to networking-oriented interventions by the CPNs or, indeed, the carers themselves. Information-giving could also be concerned with giving practical advice on the management of difficult behaviour. This information was usually given verbally but was sometimes supplemented by a booklet – most commonly *Who Cares?*, published by the Health Education Council. However, when I discussed this aspect of their work with the CPNs, I received the impression that they tended to undervalue the knowledge they had built up in dealing with practical management problems of confused old people, knowledge gained through many years of experience on care units for older people. My observation of the CPNs' practice gave me the impression that this expert knowledge was well received by carers. Another aspect of the CPNs' expert knowledge that should not be ignored is their influence upon the carer as a role model. This role was communicated to the carer by the CPN in various ways, primarily in the way the CPNs themselves talked about – and talked to – the client. A more specific form of information-giving consisted of providing carers with information about the implementation of community care in the locality. This was often needed because of reports in local newspapers about the imminent implementation of community care, which caused the carers anxiety about whether they might lose services such as respite and day care. As such, the CPNs were often called upon to give information on these matters and to reassure the carer as necessary.

Closing cases When the intervention was complete, the CPNs closed their involvement with the client and/or carer. The CPNs told me that they always prepared family carers for the time when CPN visits would no longer be considered necessary, by telling them at the beginning of their involvement that they would eventually close the case. The example of CPN B's final visit to Mr Hindle illustrates a visit in which the CPN ended a case. When CPN B explained to Mr Hindle that he was not planning to visit him again, Mr Hindle invited the CPN to call round any time he was in the area, to have something to eat. The CPN was somewhat taken aback by this remark and did not really know how to respond. The interaction seemed to imply that Mr Hindle had begun to see CPN B's visits partly as a social occasion. The CPN commented about the relationship with Mr Hindle, saying:

> It is difficult to draw a line between friendship and professional because of the type of client group that we are dealing with ... the ongoing problem being dementia, you get involved in visiting them a lot more and more over a period. So that you can't help building a lot of professional involvement on a friendship basis. I feel that you can get more out of the carers by being friendly than being too stiff-collared professional ... they don't feel relaxed enough to be open because you are so professional.

The CPNs told me that they usually left their telephone number with the client when they terminate cases:

What I tend to do is to is … We don't ever leave [the case] as final, we always say, 'obviously I won't be visiting on a regular basis as I have been doing, but if you need to contact, you can phone me at any time and I will come back again', and I think we all do that.

The orientation of the CPN's work

Throughout their involvement with the people with dementia and their family carers the orientation of the CPNs was towards the family. In cases where there was no informal (i.e. unpaid) carer, interventions were focused on meeting the needs of the client. However, when there was an identifiable informal carer looking after a client at home, the CPN focused upon the needs of the carers. In such cases the resolution of the carer's needs provided the overriding rationale for the CPN's intervention.

This may be illustrated by comparing two cases within the sample. One case is that of CPN D's work with Mrs Spencer, which we noted earlier. As Mrs Spencer's husband had recently died and she did not have any relatives living nearby, CPN D focused on helping the client come to terms with the grief she had encountered after the death of her husband as a means of minimising her confusion. In addition, CPN D monitored the situation, particularly whether Mrs Spencer had been looking after herself, and also to link her with the home care service. This was very different from the focus of the CPN's work with Mr Sackville, who was looking after his moderately confused wife at home. In that case, as with every other case in the sample where there was an informal carer, the intervention was focused on helping the carer cope with the client at home.

The relationship between CPNs and family carers

Although the CPNs visited clients in their homes in a professional capacity, much of the talk between the CPN and the carer was friendly rather than professional in nature. Items of interaction such as the friendly nature of the welcome of the CPNs by the clients and carers; the tone of voice adopted by the CPNs; the informal way in which the CPN sat down beside the client or carer and the way in which the CPN began to talk about matters unrelated to the care of the client seemed to indicate an element of friendship in this 'professional' relationship. For example, the performance of light tasks by CPN A for Mrs Phillips was interesting. During the visit A was very friendly with Mrs Phillips and they seemed to chat together more like friends than anything else. Some of the tasks that CPN A performed for Mrs Phillips were not, strictly speaking, part of her job as a CPN, but seemed more like acts of friendship. Indeed, it seemed at times that the relationship between CPN A and Mrs Phillips was more like the relationship between a daughter and mother. The CPN commented that she did not believe that there was any conflict between her style of relating to Mrs Phillips and her role as a CPN, but added, 'I think it's a grey area, where they merge to some extent'.

PARTNERSHIP
Developing practice

The data collected in the study gave various insights about the nature of the partnership between the CPN, the family and the person with dementia. Lack of partnership was displayed in four main areas.

Firstly, when a member of the family was involved in the case, the main attention of the CPN was directed towards that family member rather than towards the person with dementia. The CPNs treated primary family carers as the main resource that would enable community care to work (Twigg and Atkin, 1994). In this way, the user of the service was invariably understood to be the primary family carer rather than the person with dementia. This contrasts markedly with the way other areas of service provision to people with mental health problems understand the 'user' and the 'client'. In these areas, the 'user' is the person with the mental illness, not the family carer. This approach takes a considerable amount of power away from the person with dementia by depriving them of the right to participate in decisions about the provision of their own care. Moreover, it tends to encourage the development of a strong alliance between the CPN and the family carer; though this may be supportive to the family carer, it may not be in the interests of the person with dementia. It may simply be the case, however, that family carers are exploited themselves through their desire to see that the best is done for their dependent relatives and by virtue of strong emotional bonding. As a result, they end up taking on more of the care (and stress) than they are really capable. As Ungerson (1995) claims, 'these policies are driven largely by ideas of reducing expenditure – namely that it is cheaper and more cost-effective to care for people in the "community"' (p. 39). This, of course, serves the interests of the state, as continued family support delays the time when the state has to pay for the provision of residential or hospital care. It may be for that reason therefore that the CPNs focus on the primary family carer in their work with people with dementia who live at home.

Secondly, the CPNs had little understanding of the family systemic nature of dementia (Chapman, 1996). The theoretical model of dementia care commonly adopted by the CPNs related to stress and coping. However, in practice this model served to bring to light only those problems faced by the primary family carer, not by the whole family. The failure to develop an adequate understanding of what was happening within the family as a whole meant not only that the full implications of the situation were hardly ever recognised, but also that the problems encountered by the family and the resources available within the family were never adequately appreciated. There are a variety of theoretical models of dementia care relevant to CPN practice that would facilitate a family systemic approach, such as those offered by Zarit et al (1987) and Boss (1988). The work of Hanson (1989, 1997) has provided a theoretical basis for dementia care which applies a general systems perspective within a framework of social constructionism. Benbow et al (1993) provide an excellent review of the use of family therapy in the context of dementia care. Above all, without the use of a theoretical model of dementia care that takes full account of all the family, there can be no idea of partnership.

Thirdly, there was little attempt by the CPNs to deliver therapeutic interventions to the person with dementia. Because the attention of the CPNs was on the primary family carer, and also because of the widespread pessimism regarding the effectiveness of therapeutic interventions in dementia, the person with dementia was hardly ever seen as a legitimate target for such intervention. This narrow approach harks back to the therapeutic nihilism of former times; the only difference being that nowadays older people are given custodial care within the community rather than in a mental hospital. Woods (1996), Droës (1997) and Cheston (1997) review various therapeutic interventions that may benefit people with dementia; many of these interventions could be used by CPNs.

Fourthly, the CPNs gave little consideration of the differing perspectives of the family members. Various family members inevitably become involved in the care of people with dementia, and they all have their own perspective, their own agenda and their own voice (Globerman, 1996; Perry and Olshansky, 1996). Whilst this is a particularly important issue, it has been neglected in the professional and academic literature. The prevailing emphasis on the dyadic relationship between health-care professionals and the primary family carer has done much to privilege the primary family carer at the expense of other family members (and no doubt also the person with dementia). However, each member of the family will have a different way of seeing things; consequently, there is a need for CPNs to recognise the 'multivocal' nature of dementia care, which highlights the need for CPNs to hear the voice of everyone involved in the care of people with dementia – not just the voices of the primary carer, the doctor or their own! The primary way in which the voices of people with dementia and their families are heard is through listening to the accounts they give about what has happened and is happening to them.

Typically, CPN practice has only taken notice of the account offered by the primary family carer and has designated that as the 'right' one. However, each account given by a family member will be shaped by what that person wants from the situation. The theoretical basis for this position lies in ethnomethodology and conversation analysis (Garfinkel, 1967;

Sacks, 1992). From this position, various writers such as Potter (1996) and Edwards (1997) have argued that language is not a transparent medium – one cannot see reality through language – but rather that language is a performative medium and that through language people accomplish particular actions. Therefore, within the context of partnership, CPNs need to recognise that what is said by family members is merely their representation of the situation at that particular time and is shaped by the context in which it was said.

Developing research

Having examined the work of community psychiatric nursing with older people who have dementia, it is now possible to put forward some areas of research that may contribute to a better understanding of partnership in this type of practice. Various writers have made recommendations for the development of research in mental health nursing (White, 1994; Gournay, 1995). However, many of these recommendations are too general and give little attention either to the speciality or the issue of partnership.

Firstly, the study highlights the fact that the community psychiatric nurses interviewed paid only lip-service to nursing models such as Roper's model, and suggests their practice was based on a completely different set of ideas from those outlined by nursing models. This raises the questions of what are these ideas, how do they affect practice and how do they relate to the idea of partnership? It may be worth while to undertake further studies directed towards a better understanding of the ideas that underpin the work of CPNs with this particular client group, and how they guide and direct practice.

A particularly interesting area of study would be that of 'risk assessment' in the care of people with dementia in the community (Clarke, 1997). Community psychiatric nurses by virtue of working in environments that are less controllable than hospital wards often have to make decisions that are not 100% safe and involve some element of risk (though it should be pointed out that hospital wards themselves are not 100% safe). One family I worked with contained a somewhat manic old woman with dementia who was looked after by her two sons, one living nearby and the other living abroad. Every day their mother travelled long distances to markets in various towns. Quite clearly this posed various risks: for example, she could have got lost or come to some physical harm. Did she really require the increased supervision that would be obtained if she was moved (against her will, screaming and kicking) to sheltered accommodation? However, was it safe for an 80-year-old woman with dementia to go from town to town every day by bus? The decision made in consultation with her family and other members of the multidisciplinary community mental health team was that for ethical and pragmatic reasons the woman would be allowed to remain in her own home; however, this involved a risk which in the end might have meant her coming to some harm.

The idea of 'partnership' highlights the importance of including the person with dementia and all the family members in the assessment. This was noted in a document (DOH, 1990) guiding the implementation of the NHS and Community Care Act 1990, which asserted that:

> Both service users and carers should therefore be consulted – separately, if either of them wishes – since their views may not coincide. (p. 28)

A similar perspective is contained within the Department of Health document *Assessing Older People with Dementia Living in the Community.* (DOH/SSI, 1996), which advocated that:

> Involving both user and carer appropriately is essential and requires expertise. On the one hand, assessments of older people with dementia are sometimes made on the basis of the views of the older person. On the other hand, assessments sometimes ignore the views and needs of the carer of an older person with dementia. (p. 20)

Consequently, ways of enhancing decision-making by people with dementia, their families and CPNs, including risk assessment, should be developed through empirical research.

A second area of research suggested by the study relates to the stage at which CPNs should end their involvement with their cases. At present, there is no consensus regarding when and how community psychiatric nurses should discharge people from their caseloads. A better understanding of these processes could lead to improved methods of case management, for example through the development of measures and guidelines that would help prevent premature discharge of cases and reduce the cost of unnecessary community psychiatric nursing involvement. Indeed, these areas should also take in the concept of partnership, as it would be inappropriate for a CPN to end an involvement with a client without consultation with the family.

Thirdly, the study suggests that innovative approaches to practice embodying the idea of partnership should be developed. This would mean that rather than adopting a dominant position in their relationship with the family, CPNs could work 'alongside' families as they sort out the problems they have experienced regarding the onset of dementia in one of their members. One approach that may be used is that of advocacy. Killeen (1996) describes advocacy in the context of dementia care as 'making the case for someone, or a group of people, or helping them to represent their own views, usually to defend their rights or to promote their interests. Various writers describe different types of advocacy that are available for people with dementia (Burton, 1997; Dunning, 1997). The approach would enable CPNs to help families sort out their problems by guiding and representing families through the provision of services that are available for people with dementia.

Fourthly, the study found that the CPNs employed a number of interventions that helped family caregivers looking after older people with dementia. However, it is important that the cost-effectiveness of work with these caregivers is identified, particularly in terms of the total effect of the health outcome, bearing in mind that it is not just the primary carer who will incur problems associated with the care of the person with dementia, but the whole family. However, Collins et al, (1994), in a review of the effectiveness of various therapeutic interventions with families caring for older people with dementia, comment that 'there is a dearth of studies in an area of urgent interest to clinicians'. More recently, this dearth has been partly offset by three important papers. The first by Davis (1996), critically reviews studies relating to the effectiveness of psychosocial interventions directed towards relatives caring for people with dementia and sets these interventions within a typology. The second, by Zarit and Edwards (1996), provides an excellent review of the theoretical perspectives relating to providing family care, and discusses the various theoretical approaches that may be used with carers. The third, by Cuijpers and Nies (1997), provides a critical review of psychosocial interventions to carers of people with dementia, and argues that there is a need to enhance the methods that have been used previously in studies evaluating the effectiveness of interventions to these family carers. What these three studies do *not* show is whether the interventions are effective when they are delivered by community psychiatric nurses. Therefore, it would be worth while to undertake studies that would examine the effectiveness of interventions provided by CPNs to older people with dementia and their family carers. Such interventions could include psychosocial approaches, various counselling techniques (such as cognitive techniques and grief counselling) and the use of innovative techniques such as telephone services.

In addition, the study described in this chapter revealed that most of the work of CPNs relates to long-established cases of dementia. Consequently, it would be worth while to examine the effectiveness of early intervention by CPNs. The need to identify cases of dementia early in its development has recently been highlighted by the Alzheimer's Disease Society (1995). Illife (1994) points out the problem that many family caregivers spend a long time caring for a relative with dementia on their own before coming into contact with specialist services. Illife (1994) argues that the responsibility is placed upon general practitioners who 'too often ... are seen to be ignoring carer's concerns, attributing dementia behaviour to "old age"'. It would therefore be worth while for CPNs to develop approaches that would bring older people with dementia and their family carers into contact with specialist services (Gunstone, 1983). Various strategies designed to facilitate early intervention have been developed in experimental projects and include telephone help lines; the distribution of educational literature; case-finding; locating community psychiatric nursing teams in primary health-care centres; and helping general practitioners understand the benefits of early referral to specialist services for older people with dementia (Hugo et al, 1985; Goodman and Pynoos, 1990; O'Donovan, 1995).

CONCLUSION

This chapter has examined the role of community psychiatric nurses working with people with dementia and their family carers. Whilst there are no doubt limitations regarding their work, the chapter outlines ways in which community psychiatric nursing with people with dementia may develop. Above all, the chapter has asserted that the way forward for CPNs within the speciality is through the development of partnership, as outlined in *Working in Partnership* (DOH, 1994). However, what is at issue is not the necessity of partnership but rather the politics implicit in dementia care; the chapter focuses on the issue of where the power and control should lie: with the primary family carer, the rest of the family, the CPN or the person with dementia? This is an important issue for community psychiatric nursing which has not yet been addressed. It is hoped that this chapter will encourage discussion on these issues that will in turn facilitate enhanced community psychiatric nursing care.

REFERENCES

Ainsworth, D. & Jolley, D. (1978) The community psychiatric nurse in a developing psychogeriatric service. *Nursing Times* **74** (21), 873–874.
Aire, T. & Isaacs, D. (1978) The development of psychiatric services for the elderly in Britain. In: Isaacs, A.D. & Post, F. (eds) *Studies in Generic Psychiatry*. New York: Wiley.
Alzheimer's Disease Society (1995) *Right From the Start*. London: Alzheimer's Disease Society.
Argyle, N., Jestice, S. & Brook, C.P.B. (1985) Psychogeriatric patients: their supporters problems. *Age and Ageing* **14**, 355–360.
Audit Commission (1986) *Making a Reality of Community Care*. London: HMSO.
Barker, C. & Black, S. (1971) An experiment in integrated psycho-geriatric care. *Nursing Times* **67** (45), 1395–1399.
Benbow, S., Marritt, J.A., Morley, M. & Walsh, S. (1993) Family therapy and dementia: Review and clinical experience. *International Journal of Geriatric Psychiatry* **8**, 717–727.
Benner, P. & Tanner, C. (1987) Clinical judgement: how expert nurses use intuition. *American Journal of Nursing* **87** (1), 32–31.
Boss, P. (1988) *Family Stress Management*. London: Sage.
Brooke, C & White, E (1997) Report on community psychiatric nursing (unpublished report). University of Sheffield and Keele.
Burton, A. (1997) Dementia: a case for advocacy? In: Hunter, S. (ed.) *Dementia Challenges and New Directions*. London: Jessica Kingsley.

Chapman, A. (1996) Empowerment. In: Chapman, A. & Marshal, M (eds) *Dementia: New Skills for Social Workers* London: Jessica Kingsley.

Cheston R. (1997) *Psychotherapeutic work with people with dementia: a review of the literature.* (unpublished paper). University of Bath.

Clarke, C.L. (1997) Risk knowledge and reasoning in family and professional carers of people with dementia. British Society of Gerontology Conference, September 1996, Liverpool, UK.

Collins, C., Given, B. & Given, C. (1994) Interventions with family caregivers of persons with Alzheimer's disease. *Nursing Clinics of North America* **29** (1), 195–207.

Cuijpers, P. & Nies, H. (1997) Supporting informal care-givers of demented elderly people. In: Miesen, B.M.L. & Jones, G. (eds) *Care-giving in Dementia: Research and Applications.* London: Routledge.

Davis, L.L. (1996) Dementia caregiving studies: a typology for family interventions. *Journal of Family Nursing* **2** (1), 30–55.

[DoH] Department of Health (1989) *Caring for People: Community Care the Next Decade and Beyond.* London: HMSO.

[DoH] Department of Health (1990) *NHS and Community Care Act: A Brief Guide.* London: HMSO.

[DOH] Department of Health (1994) *Working in Partnership: A Collaborative Approach.* London: HMSO.

[DoH/SSI] Department of Health/Social Services Inspectorate (1996) *Assessing Older People with Dementia Living in the Community: Practical Issues for Social and Health Services.* London: HMSO.

Dey, I. (1993) *Qualitative Data Analysis.* London: Routledge.

Droës, R.M. (1997) Psychosocial treatment for demented patients: overview of methods and effects. In: Miesen, B.M.L. & Jones, G. (eds) *Care-giving in Dementia: Research and Applications.* London: Routledge.

Dunning, A. (1997) Advocacy and older people with dementia. In: Marshall, M. (ed.) *State of the Art in Dementia Care.* London: Centre for Policy on Ageing.

Edwards, D. (1997) *Discourse and Cognition.* London: Sage.

Garfinkel, H. (1967) *Studies in Ethnomethodology.* Englewood Cliffs: Prentice Hall.

Gilhooly, M. & Whittick, J. (1989) Expressed emotion in caregivers of the demented elderly. *British Journal of Medical Psychology* **62**, 265–272.

Gilleard, C. (1984) Emotional stress amongst the supporters of the elderly Mentally Infirm. *British Journal of Psychiatry* **145**, 172–177.

Gilleard, C. (1996) Family therapy with older adults. In: Woods, R. (ed.) *Handbook of Clinical Psychology of Ageing,* pp. 561–573. London: Wiley.

Globerman, J. (1996) Motivations to care: daughters- and sons-in-law caring for relatives with Alzheimer's disease. *Family Relations* **45**, 37–45.

Goodman, C.C. & Pynoos, J. (1990) A model telephone information and support program for the caregivers of Alzheimer's patients. *Gerontologist* **30**, 3.

Gournay, K. (1995) Reviewing the review. *Nursing Times* **91** (18), 55–57.

Greenwood, M. & Walsh, K. (1995) Supporting carers in their own right. *Journal of Dementia Care* **3** (2), 14–16.

Gunstone, S. (1983) Mental health nursing. The scope of prevention. *Nursing Times* **79** (37), 42–43.

Hanson, B. (1989) Definitional deficit: a model of senile dementia in context. *Family Process* **28**, 281–298.

Hanson, B. (1997) Who's seeing whom? General systems theory and constructivist implications for senile dementia intervention. *Journal of Aging Studies* **11** (1), 15–25.

Hirst, S.P. (1989) Gerontic nurse specialists: an examination of their roles with dementia sufferers and their caregivers. *Clinical Nurse Specialist* **3** (3), 105–108.

Hugo, M., Goldney, R., Skinner, E., Katsikitis, M. & Pilowsky, I. (1985) Using screening instruments in community psychiatric nursing for the elderly. *Australian Journal of Advanced Nursing* **2** (2), 13–147.

Illife, S. (1994) Why GPs have a bad reputation. *Journal of Dementia Care* **2** (6), 24–25.

Killeen, J. (1996) *Advocacy and Dementia.* Edinburgh: Alzheimer Scotland Action on Dementia.

Jarvis, J., Jason, J. & Butterworth, M. (1992) *The Admiral Nurse Project: a service for carers of people with a dementing illness; a critical appraisal of the clinical service from the carers' point of view.* London: Dementia Relief Trust.

Lancaster, C. (1984) Community psychiatry in Bloomsbury, 2. Adjusting to old age. *Nursing Times* **80** (43), 26–27.

Leff, J.P. & Vaughn, C.E. (1980) The interaction of life events and relatives' expressed emotion in schizophrenia and depressive neurosis. *British Journal of Psychiatry* **136**, 102–104.

Leopoldt, H., Robinson, J.R. & Corea, S. (1975) Hospital based community psychiatric nursing in psychogeriatric care. *Nursing Mirror* **141** (25), 54–56.

Mental Health Act (1959) London: HMSO.

Morris, R.G., Morris, L.W. & Britton, P.G. (1988) Factors affecting the emotional wellbeing of the caregivers of dementia sufferers. *British Journal of Psychiatry* **153**, 147–156.

The National Health Service and Community Care Act (1990) HMSO. London.

O'Donovan, S. (1995) Hold the line for carer support. *Journal of Dementia Care* **3** (4), 20–22.

Perry, J. & Olshansky, E.F. (1996) A family coming to terms with Alzheimer's disease. *Western Journal of Nursing Research* **18** (1), 12–28.

Potter, J. (1996) *Representing Reality.* London: Sage.

Pottle, S. (1985) Developing a network-orientated service for the elderly and their carers. In: Treacher, & Carpenter, J. (eds) *Using Family Therapy.* Oxford: Blackwell.

Rafferty, M. (1993) Mental health and the elderly. In: Wright, H. & Giddey, M. (eds) *Mental Health Nursing.* London: Chapman & Hall.

Richardson, C. (1997) Family therapy. *Current Opinion in Psychiatry* **10**, 333–336.

Rolfe, G. & Phillips, L.M. (1997) The development and evaluation of the role of an Advanced Nurse Practitioner in dementia – an action research project. *International Journal of Nursing Studies* **34** (2), 119–127.

Sacks, H. (1992) In: Jefferson, G. (ed.) *Lectures on Conversation* (2 vols) Oxford: Blackwell.

Thomas, M. (1988) Care plan for a confused person, based on Roper's activities of living model. In: Collister, B. (ed.) *Psychiatric Nursing: Person To Person.* London: Arnold.

Toner, H. (1985) *A Handbook for Carers of Dementia Sufferers: Does it Really Work?'* Paper presented to PSIGE Meeting, Glasgow, May.

Tough, H., Kingerlee, P. & Elliott, P. (1980) Surgery-attached psychogeriatric nurses: an evaluation of psychiatric nurses in the primary care team. *Journal of the Royal College of General Practitioners* **30**, 85–89.

Twigg, C. & Atkin, K. (1994) *Carers Perceived.* Buckingham: Open University Press.

Ungerson, C. (1995) Gender, cash and informal care. *Journal of Social Policy* **24** (1), 32–52.

Ward, M. (1985) *The Nursing Process in Psychiatry.* London: Churchill Livingstone.

White, E. (1994) Research priorities for community psychiatric nursing. *Mental Health Nursing* **14** (1), 14–16.

Whitehead, A. (1970) *In Service of Old Age.* Harmondsworth: Pelican,

Woods, R.T. (1996) Psychological therapies in dementia. In: Woods, R.T. (ed.), *Handbook of the Clinical Psychology of Ageing.* London: Wiley.

Yura, H. & Walsh, M.B. (1978) *The Nursing Process: Assessing, Planning, Implementing, Evaluating,* 3rd ed. Appleton-Century-Crofts.

Zarit, S.H. & Edwards, A.B. (1996) Family caregiving: research and clinical intervention. In: Woods, R.T. (ed.) *Handbook of the Psychology of Ageing.* Chichester: Wiley.

Zarit, S.H., Anthony, C. & Boutselis, M. (1987) Interventions with caregivers of dementia patients: comparison of two approaches. *Psychology and Aging* **2**, 225–232.

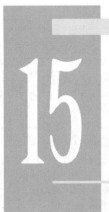

Attitudes towards dementia care: education and morale in health-care teams

Tracy Packer

KEY ISSUES

Qualitative interviews undertaken on a team of care workers on a unit caring for older people with dementia, revealed a number of significant issues. The five issues covered in this chapter offer an insight into how care workers perceive working in this area:

- Perceptions of aging and dementia

- The effect of community care policies on the function of the unit

- The person with dementia from a care worker's perspective

- The effect of challenging behaviours and the impact of aggression

- The consequences of stereotyping the unit and the question of public relations

INTRODUCTION

Since the 1960s there has been considerable research into how health-care professionals feel about working with older people. Many of these studies concentrate on the knowledge and attitudes of student nurses (Dellasega and Curriero, 1991; Stevens and Crouch, 1992), or put forward numerous variables that may affect the knowledge and attitudes of nurses generally. These variables include age, educational level, length of service, and the importance of a close relationship with an older person (Campbell, 1972; Taylor and Harned, 1978; Robb, 1979; Brower, 1981, 1985; Bowling and Formby, 1991). Owing to the difficulty of defining what constitutes 'attitude' and 'knowledge', there has been and will continue to be a great deal of inconsistency between individual studies. In the unlikely event that a generic group of statistically significant variables could be identified, managers will not be afforded the luxury of selective recruitment – at least, not in the UK while the health service is in the throes of yet another crisis in nurse recruitment and retention (Leifer, 1995). In any case, the moral and ethical arguments about selecting health-care workers on the basis of variables that are subject to flux over any given time have yet to be seriously considered.

Many knowledge and attitude studies have involved the use of standard measurement tools such as Kogan's Attitude to Old People scale (KOP) (Kogan, 1961), Palmore's Facts of Ageing Quiz (PFAQ) (Palmore, 1977, 1980, 1981) or the Oberleder Attitude Scale (Oberleder, 1962). These tools can be used as a one-off measurement of knowledge and attitudes, or applied before and after educational programmes to evaluate their effectiveness.

Meanwhile, the incidence of Alzheimer's disease and related dementias in the population over the age of 75 years is increasing (Jaques, 1992). As dementia is a problem predominantly – if controversially (Wilcock, 1983) – thought to be related to increased age, it is perhaps surprising that there is a dearth of knowledge or attitudinal studies undertaken within this area of care. In a study of American baccalaureate nursing students it was noted that 'knowledge about Alzheimer's disease was not found to be related to knowledge of ageing' (Edwards et al, 1992). This particular study used a very specific, multiple-choice knowledge score, the Alzheimer's Disease Knowledge test or ADK (Diekmann et al, 1988).

However, it is worth noting that as a response set bias has been linked with the KOP score (Silverman, 1966), it could be hypothesised that the PFAQ and ADK are also open to criticisms of a similar bias, since they are often used in the same way. It was suggested as long ago as 1961 that a response set bias may occur in these kinds of tests 'due to a need for approval (Crowne and Marlowe, 1961). One isolated study measured a knowledge and attitude score (KOP) against a score that measures a need for approval (McCabe, 1989). The test used was the Marlowe Crowne Social Desirability Score (MC-SDS) (Crowne and Marlowe, 1961). McCabe continued by suggesting that the respondents of this postal survey ($n =$ 255) may have felt a 'need to portray an image of the ideal nurse which reduces the likelihood of expressing negative attitudes towards older people.' In this study, the denial component of the MC-SDS had a significant positive relationship to the attitude score, allowing the inference that the attitudes of the respondents were not as positive as the KOP score indicated (McCabe, 1989). McCabe's study indicates that whilst such scales may be useful for discussion purposes when evaluating standardised education programmes, most knowledge and attitude studies using them may not have seriously considered the participants' need for approval. It would be difficult to know whether high scores are an indication of good memory or good practice. These scales alone may be ineffective in identifying the nature of attitudes or practical care delivery outside the classroom environment. Many of these studies have tended to be impersonal and large-scale, using questionnaires before and after the education programme to evaluate attitudes (Gunter, 1971; Robb, 1979; Snape, 1986) or else postal data collection (McCabe, 1989). The opportunity to discuss issues that might affect attitudes amongst individuals working in the field of elderly or dementia care could have been limited by the sheer size of the groups involved. In the much smaller study described in this chapter, qualitative information was offered by individuals working in an environment caring for older people with a dementing illness. Whilst generalisations beyond this group of participants should be treated with caution, the insights offered should contribute significantly to the future planning of attitudinal studies in this field. These insights can also contribute towards the future management of education, morale and health-care worker development within the field of dementia. Perhaps it is time to stop looking for generalised characteristics that can be attributed to the ideal care worker, and to start maximising the skills and potential that individuals already possess.

THE STUDY

Following the distribution of the two knowledge questionnaires to all members of the multidisciplinary team ($n = 28$), staff were invited during two staff meetings (or in writing if they could not attend) to take part in a tape-recorded interview with the researcher. Whilst these interviews were intended to be entirely voluntary and their contents were given anonymity, the researcher was aware of the pressure that participants could have felt they were under to attend. The participants were given no prior knowledge of the questions they would be asked, therefore they were not expected to sign a consent form until the interview had been completed. They then had the ultimate power of veto on the use of the tape and its contents. No-one who attended for interview exercised this right. In case of team members who might have objected to taking part, but were concerned about the opinions of other colleagues or superiors, the opportunity was provided to attend a given appointment but not to undergo the interview process. Full confidentiality was offered in the case of such a decision being taken.

A series of questions were complied, which considered a wide range of themes. Two of these questions asked the participants for their definitions of 'old age' and 'dementia'. The remaining questions were not entirely prescriptive. (Box 15.1), and the nature of the interviews allowed the respondents to determine the extent of the coverage and the relevance of

> **Box 15.1**   Core interview questions
>
> - What would be your definition of old age or ageing?
> - How would you define dementia?
> - What do your colleagues in other specialities think about your work?
> - What skills do you think are needed in dementia care?
> - What are the positive aspects of your work here?
> - What are the less positive aspects of your work here?

each theme to themselves. This also helped to determine the order of the questions which followed and the overall duration of the interview. All participants were discouraged from discussing the content of their own interview with colleagues who had not yet attended; this was intended to reduce the risk of peer pressure within the team influencing the development of any particular topic or point of view during the interviewing process. The interviews were required to gain detailed information that would help in the interpretation of the final analysis of the questionnaire data, in particular to identify the presence of reduced morale and less than positive attitudes towards those for whom the workers were caring. This was increasingly important in order to assist the newly recruited dementia development nurse to identify an appropriate educational support package, and a realistic development plan for the unit. The more frank the participants were during the interviews, the more they would be able to contribute towards this plan. In the event, data analysis was based on the responses of 23 members of the team or 82% of the sample ($n = 28$). The semistructured nature of these interviews may have been a contributing factor to the variability of the time taken to complete them. The shortest lasted 15 minutes, and the longest lasted 1 hour 30 minutes. The total interview time for the entire team was approximately 14 hours and 30 minutes.

Interview responses

Defining old age

It was important to establish some sense of how members of the team viewed older people, and defined old age, before delving more deeply into the nature of dementia and the people it affected. This first question, which had previously been taken for granted by the researcher as relatively straightforward, proved to be quite problematic. Many respondents spent considerable time deliberating over how to answer this, and several asked if they could come back to it later in the interview. A member of the multidisciplinary team said:

There is a positive side as well as a negative side ... with old age often comes wisdom and insight and sometimes patience, there can be a wealth of things, but on the other hand it's where you just ... well, everything just disintegrates really ... it's also a time when you become aware, when you can actually reflect. So there is a positive side to it, I know a lot of very elderly people that are extremely interesting and still have a zest for life, so it's not all one-sided. It's not all dementia, and it's not all where everything collapses ... there is a positive side.

Respondent D

I think it's generally a decline of the body isn't it? It could just be a natural process, basically you're falling to pieces, I suppose, and wearing out gradually.

Respondent P

These following responses from a trained and an untrained member of staff respectively were notable:

Well, the definition I hope it would be [is] to go into old age with all your faculties and your health to a certain extent, and just share it with your partner, but it's not that easy. I think that's what everybody hopes for but it's not like that sometimes, it just doesn't always happen that way ... it's very rare if it does actually.

Respondent O

I think old age is really depressing and you're getting old ... Yes, we're going around strong now and that's all right, but when you reach about seventy-five, eighty; you start saying 'My God, what next!' I find it really depressing.

Respondent J

There were, however occasional glimmers of hope for the image attributed to those who are older; the following contributor came across as the most forceful of these:

My mother is eighty-six, she is absolutely wonderful. She is looking after herself and she still lives on her own, she does the garden and she goes out ... My children tell me I'm old and think, 'Act your age not your shoe size, Mum!' Some people don't get old, do they? Some people are old at thirty ... from the time they're this high [hand gesture indicates a small distance off the floor], what was it my husband said to me? 'You're not going to grow old gracefully, are you?' I said, 'Certainly not!' ... He thinks [being old] means sitting back in your corner with your shawl and your knitting ... and I think that's really crazy ... I said, 'No way, my mother's not growing old gracefully, why should I?' I think you should go kicking and screaming, personally ... into old age.

Respondent I

What was striking was that over and over again, old age and being older seemed to be associated strongly in the respondents' minds with chronic disease, physical frailty and disability. There were also a number of occasions when an individual's general outlook on life was considered to be a crucial factor affecting how old that person felt, and how old the person appeared to be to others. Surprisingly, associations with cognitive impairment and psychiatric illnesses were less apparent than it had been anticipated. It is not clear why the team overwhelmingly associated cognitive disability with *abnormal* ageing processes, but their clinical area was a specialist admissions ward for older people with a diagnosis of some kind of dementing illness, and it is possible that the team felt that this, by definition, exempted people admitted to the unit from the umbrella of the normal ageing process.

Life experiences, intelligent conversations, memories of an age gone by and general wisdom were aspects of getting older that were often referred to positively during the course of these interviews. On the other hand, the possibility of physical wellbeing was often dismissed or not even considered. On the few occasions that it was noted, the individual referred to was described as lucky, unusual or surprising, and very much the exception to the rule. Nobody mentioned the possibility that a majority of older people were very physically active, and capable of getting on with their lives with minimal medical or institutionalised intervention – that this was in fact part and parcel of what normal ageing was all about (Jacques, 1992).

These findings were a little surprising coming from professional care workers specialising in dementing illness. On a day-to-day basis they were surrounded by people with moderate to severe cognitive disabilities, and often significant physical disabilities. These disabilities ranged from mild difficulties to a need for total assistance in all matters regarding activities of daily living. Spending a large part of their daily lives with older people who have moderate to severe dementia had supported (and possibly reinforced) their belief systems regarding physical ability, but had not undermined their general views regarding cognitive disability, that such cognitive disabilities are not part of the normal ageing process. It would have been interesting to consider the responses to the same question of professional care workers on a general elderly admissions unit. How normal or unusual would they perceive even the slightest level of cognitive disability in an older person?

Last, but not least, if professional care workers view physical disability and frailty as a normal part of being older, what chance for rehabilitation has a person who has a dementing illness and a physical disability? It could be argued that low expectations of a person's true ability may lead to reduced success in rehabilitation, misunderstanding of a person's needs, and ultimately placement in an area that cannot meet the needs of the person concerned. This only contributes further to a speedy decline in general wellbeing for the individual concerned.

Defining dementia

Having established the general view of the team regarding their perception of what it is like to be older, the interview participants were then asked to provide their definition of dementia. On the whole, it had been noted that cognitive impairments had not been attributed to those who aged 'normally'. It was not surprising, therefore, that in response to this question, memory loss and its effects seemed foremost in people's minds. This was, after all, a unit where everyone admitted to it had some kind of dementing illness.

Just how did the team members perceive the person with dementia, and what sort of generalisations were evident in their responses? Their answers would provide a useful and appropriate guide to the more general educational needs of the team.

Many people interviewed had much to say on what constituted 'dementia', and found it difficult to pin down a specific concept regarding the nature of dementia. Often people with dementia were referred to as 'they', 'dements', 'dementia people' or 'the old and confused'. This apparent distancing of the person with dementia from the rest of humanity may go some way towards explaining why many respondents reiterated that such people did not know what was happening to them, and could not be responsible for their own actions. Attributing someone's 'antisocial' behavioural responses to a dementing process is much simpler and easier than accepting that behaviour as a valid attempt at communicating a need. To be able to go further and identify the need, then challenge deep-rooted care practices in order to accommodate it, takes perseverance and courage in the face of one's own deficits. The whole process involves great risk at both a personal and an organisational level.

Occasionally the physical needs of people with dementia were likened to those of children, thus removing any of the responsibilities afforded a sentient adult, and subsequently justifying their behaviour in terms of their lack of reason:

> ...They're old and they're confused, and they say all sorts of dotty things that really don't matter anyway. I know that you're not supposed to treat them like children ... but in lots of ways they are

like children ... they don't know, they don't understand ... they don't know why they are the way they are and why they are not at home or where ever they think they ought to go ... they don't understand ... so they basically need lots of TLC [tender loving care], don't they ... they can't hold anything in their brains ... in a way it's almost a going back ... a going back to before your brain worked properly or before it was fully developed ... all the incontinence and all those things is like going back to children, aren't they.

Respondent I

Anybody that has some degree of memory loss which can be very mild or very chronic of which it then affects their ability to do anything ... and care for themselves in any way, shape or form.

Respondent E

It's a decline in the person's ability to remember ... to reason ... and to learn to cope, I think.

Respondent O

In fairness, there were a number of responses indicating concern for the feelings of the person with dementia. In the first of the extracts below, the speaker suggests that people with dementia may have some insight into their deterioration, and not only hints at an awareness of difficulties for the relatives, but the person with dementia as well.

...Alzheimer's dementia is basically when the brain cells ... [are] gradually fading out, I can't think of the word ... decreasing, and it's all very disturbing for the patients and it's a really terrible thing for the relatives.

Respondent P

From my point of view my job is just making the patients feel comfortable ... general wellbeing for them. I know there's an awful lot of research into dementia and I know they're hoping to find a cure, so I hope that things are going to be improved. It's a very sad illness, a progressive illness that must be very hard on the patient and on the relative ... it's like a deterioration of the brain ... and memory loss.

Respondent F

Finally, this speaker provided food for thought:

Some people look upon it as being a handicap to a person, I don't look upon it as being a handicap to a person ... I think [for] some people it's a process of life ... it's unfortunate but it's just part of life for some people and as you would deal with crisis in your life ... it's just another crisis that you have to deal with. Sometimes it's the actual person suffering ... it's just a condition that my mum and dad might suffer with ... you just try and support them as best you can and explain things as things happen really. Even with Alzheimer's you can't say this is definitely going to happen really, because nothing is ever definite ... you can't give a timetable, say ... how long somebody's going to dement.

Respondent T

At first glance this response may appear to be rather missing the point, and devoid of understanding about the magnitude of a diagnosis of dementia, but there is something in what the respondent is saying: there should be more to caring for this client group than mere 'crisis management'.

The concepts of offering support, education and effective communication are realistic, as is a philosophy of care that is flexible and adaptable, rather than concrete and unchanging. The remaining interview questions sought to establish just what was the likelihood of such achievements in this particular team, and what other factors might hinder these developments.

The impact of community care

The development of the community care policy in the UK did not explicitly feature in any of the questions that the respondents were asked in the interview. However, almost half of the respondents had something to say on what they considered the effects of community care to be. No cues or prompts were used to elicit these responses, and it became clear that the policy changes regarding community care were a significant issue for the whole team. In view of the importance of these changes to the provision of dementia care, it is worth examining the views the respondents expressed regarding this matter. These views form an integral part of the framework of care within which health-care staff work.

Some respondents expressed dismay over the way in which people in their care had been treated. They explained how members of the older generation may have risked their lives for their country in two world wars, worked hard all their life and contributed willingly to a national pension scheme. However, these contributions to society appeared to be worthless in terms of the quality of care they received in their later years.

I think it's wrong ... they closed all these wards here ... where did they put all these old people? It's wrong, I just don't think it's right. They've worked all the days of their life to help build this country up and then they get swept under the carpet and that's it … forgotten about. If you've got money then you're OK, but if you haven't it's not nice … it's a Catch 22, isn't it?

Respondent B

I would just say that … a lot of the people that stay at home should have more help … they don't get enough help. You have the ninety-two-year-old looking after the ninety-year-old, it's not on. You work all your life, surely you should be able to live comfortably to the end of your days? That's how I see it … It can't continue like this, it'll have to change.

Respondent W

The average length of stay for a person on the unit was far longer than had been anticipated as appropriate for an acute area providing medical treatment and an assessment service. This may have been due in part to the lack of suitable community resources that would enable people to return to their own homes. This issue was identified by a number of the respondents:

It seems [that] the last couple of … five, six months the patients don't go nowhere. They stay here and they don't go nowhere … going on and…

Respondent U

As soon as [the patients] leave, we get reports that 'Ooh, 'they're fine' … 'cos they're in a different environment. That's the only thing at the moment is the amount of time a patient stays on the ward … the long-stay ones [patients] are interfering with the new ones coming on … we seem to concentrate on them, then the new ones are getting neglected … that's the only thing at the moment because they are staying too long.

Respondent Q

It seemed that most of the frustration of the care workers was on account of their own feelings of lack of usefulness. While the patients continued to 'block' beds, there was little the team could be seen to be doing once the medical treatment and assessment had been completed. The staff did not appear to be equipped with the skills and insight to deal with the ongoing care of a person who could not be discharged 'out of sight and out of mind', and would not suddenly 'get better' as a result of their actions. As the development of community care had effectively forced this state of affairs upon them, the resulting increased length of stay was not considered to be a great help, either to themselves or for that matter to the people to whom they provided care.

During the interviews the unit was likened to a nursing home on more than one occasion, and through the tone of voice and the body language it was clear that this was an undesirable progression. It was obvious that nursing-home care was regarded with great distaste, which explained their reservations concerning the slide away from acute care. It was clear that the team was worried about its image.

The respondents repeatedly referred to issues of staffing and money. In some cases these issues seemed to bear the brunt of the blame for the perceived deterioration of care services for older people. The extracts that follow offer a small glimpse of the thought processes within the team as a whole:

> A lot of things are not quite as good as they could be; [they could be] solved by money, couldn't they, but that's true of the entire Health Service, let's be fair. I mean ... all right, more staff ... and then it's all money, isn't it? More staff is probably one of the things that would help ... it's just a question of being able to spend more money on this place.
>
> *Respondent I*

> We've not had proper staffing on that side [social work] to encourage the move on ... it's the staffing I think mainly, because we've had too many social workers in the last couple of years, I think we've had five or six ... something like that. I mean they seem to be coming and going.
>
> *Respondent Q*

Although socioeconomic factors may well have contributed in some part to the problem, it is worth considering the possibility that certain areas of current caregiving practices could shoulder some responsibility. The remainder of the interview responses were able to shed some light on this issue.

The person with dementia

In the midst of the political and economic dilemmas facing service providers, there are, of course, the people with dementia – that is, the people for whom a needs-led service is provided. The interview participants were asked what skills they believed were necessary to enable professionals to care for a person with dementia. In response, the unanimous conclusion was that patience was the most desirable quality. Several people spoke at length about the value and need for this, and disclosed thoughts about their own internal conflicts while developing such a skill:

> I think you have to have a special patience, and you do have to have a different outlook. You've got to because [otherwise] you wouldn't be able to stay there … it is very different. It probably will sound sugary, but I honestly do think that you do have to have special qualities to work with dementia patients. Through that you get to know people's strengths and weaknesses and that is a very important thing. For me personally, it makes you look at things in a different light. You begin to get people's attitudes and I think I'm more tolerant and less demanding, I can accept weaknesses more than I used to.
>
> *Respondent D*

References to children and childcare cropped up on numerous occasions. It was thought possible that those who had children would be more able to develop strategies to work with people who had dementia, although no-one was able to develop this theory beyond pure conjecture. This belief may be grounded in the opinion that like children, people with dementia are not autonomous, and cannot always be responsible for what they do. This helps reinforce both deliberate and unintentional objectification, which can sometimes take place in this care setting. It also discourages care workers from investigating the reasons for a person's behaviour. If people with dementia are viewed as incapable of autonomous or responsible actions, then in view of this belief system, their actions are seen to be meaningless.

Alternatively, the perception of the world from a 'child's eye view' may well be very different from what we imagine. It is possible that the skills that parents develop to interpret the world and events in it in a meaningful manner to their children, could well be appropriate to use with people who have dementia. The allusion to childcare should not be dismissed out of hand, as there may be much that can be gained from examining this concept much more closely.

> I think you need loads of patience. It wouldn't be any good if you got irritated, forget it, don't even bother, because you can't get irritated with them [patients] because they can't help it … they are not doing it on purpose, are they? It's like children, you just can't get irritated – all right you do, but you mustn't. You have got to bite your tongue. I think patience has got to be one of the prime qualities you need. They need to be treated like human beings, to be treated nicely, and spoken to nicely and not anybody to get ratty with them.
>
> *Respondent I*

I don't like likening children to people with dementia, although I suppose that I do tend to think that someone who has had children is able to deal with that sort of behaviour easier … but that's a personal feeling of mine. I don't know whether it would bear out, but I do feel that people who have had children … are more aware of that patient's needs.

Respondent S

Several participants in the study spoke openly about the sense of frustration they felt at times. Despite specifying that patience was an absolute necessity when dealing with this client group, they acknowledged that losing your temper was not difficult at all, and was in fact quite understandable at times! The difficulty was in trying not to portray that feeling to the person with dementia, either verbally or non-verbally.

Some participants clearly recognised that people with dementia could very quickly establish what sort of mood care workers were in and how much time they had to spare within seconds of turning up. Other care workers maintained that people with dementia did not know or understand what was going on around them, and were not responsible for their responses. This contrast of views is illustrated in the next two extracts:

If you are relaxed [or] if you are anxious … you're tense, the patients do pick it up … If you relax and you smile they smile as well, but if you are tense, if you are angry and you are sort of engrossed with yourself, I think they pick things up … you'll be surprised at what you get if you smile at that minute.

Respondent L

It's more pressure working with the dementia, more than the person who isn't demented … because you have so much to put up with, so much to be thinking about, so much abuse from some of the patients, then you just ignore everything really. I think it's the pressure working with them, but you know they can't help it … they have just gone confused.

Respondent J

Throughout the interviews, participants offered vignettes to illustrate care practice on the ward. There were a few occasions when an apparently inappropriate outburst was met with a prompt and skilful response. However, there were many times when the sheer frustration of unsuccessfully trying to find out what was wrong on repeated occasions had almost become too much for the care worker concerned. A widespread, formalised support system for care workers in similar circumstances has yet to be addressed. However, the increasing use of clinical supervision suggests that it might be an ideal tool with which staff can work through their frustrations and anxieties in this speciality (Wright et al, 1997). Respondent M in the next group of extracts offers a vivid glimpse of the trials and tribulations experienced by both care workers and people with dementia.

> [There's] a particular patient, his mind is on the go but you can't actually get him to do anything. You can't put a puzzle in front of him because he can't channel … it's all over the place, it's haywire. He wants to do something, he's frustrated and angry. He wants something but there's nothing. What can you give him to occupy him – *what*? You can't even sit down and talk to him to occupy him. You can *not* entertain the man, there's nothing you can do.
>
> *Respondent M*

> I think if you're going to go in there and say, 'Oh, come on, Mr X … come on … get up … get your clothes on …' 'it's going to be a different kettle of fish if you go in and say, 'Oh, good morning, George' (or Fred, or whoever), 'how are you this morning?' and take time just to sit on the edge of the bed and have a little chat with them first, and then say, 'Would you like to get up?'
>
> *Respondent R*

There are numerous hindrances to successful care giving, some less obvious than others. The trained member of staff quoted below who was particularly insightful, had undertaken a series of courses, and developed useful communication skills in the day-to-day work on the unit. It was unfortunate that those skills could not be utilised as effectively while filling in paperwork. This often removed a positive role model from the care arena, leaving enthusiastic but less skilled care workers to learn by trial and error. This situation was not ideal for any of the parties concerned, particularly the people with dementia.

> I do think that the nursing process, you know, the legalities of all those things, does hamper the work on the ward, because I think that the people who are skilled at doing those types of things [ward work] aren't necessarily the people that are able to do them because they've got other jobs to be doing.
>
> *Respondent E*

Lastly, but no less significantly, a number of the respondents talked of the difficulty in knowing whether what they were doing was making any difference, or even whether it was the right response in the first place. At the very least this suggests a need for increased training in non-verbal as well as verbal communication skills. All too often care workers expect verbal feedback, and often miss the very blatant messages that are being given without the use of language. If they are unaware of the messages they themselves are often sending out, they cannot be expected to understand the messages of others.

> You do get interrupted, you can't just continue and do your job. You can't get on with anything because you're constantly being stopped by the patients. Also you don't get any feedback from them ... you can ask them if they want something and they don't really give you a proper reply, so it is quite difficult.
>
> *Respondent D*

The issue of receiving feedback is a critical one. Care workers need to reflect upon what they have achieved and how they have achieved it, in order to learn by the experience and carry those skills onwards. This is particularly relevant when reflecting on events that have caused concern. Dementia care mapping is a useful tool that assists staff in interpreting the information people with dementia can give us (Kitwood and Bredin, 1993). It also encourages those who are using the method to critically examine and evaluate their own skills and practice. This helps place the person with dementia firmly in the centre of the care milieu.

The care environment

When the interview respondents were asked about the positive aspects of their work on the unit, very few of the respondents could think of an appropriate response. Some of the respondents turned the question into a joke, others asked if they could move on to the next question and the remainder thought long and hard before making a response. The most positive aspect care workers could think of was the relationship they were able to build up with the families of their patients. The carers' support group was also cited as an example of something positive and after that suggestions dried up. In the interview none of the respondents offered any positive statements that related directly to the person with dementia. On the other hand, the request for the respondent's views on other aspects of working on the unit were quick and specific. Every respondent reported that the behavioural problems and aggression of the patients were by far the most difficult aspect of their work. One respondent said:

> Occasionally you get violence, I won't say there's so much violence here you can't actually work in it, but the problem is [that] it's not actually recognised that dementia patients can be quite aggressive. A

lot of people don't realise that and are amazed really ... these people should realise that to be chased by an eighty-four-year-old man is not funny ... if [the chaser] was someone who was twenty-two or twenty-three, then psychologically it would be terrible.

Respondent G

This respondent highlighted an area which is very contentious, and no less so in this team, where the issue of aggression is not only in need of recognition from outside the unit, but by staff within the work area as well. Much of the difficulty with this appears to lie in the conceptual understanding of the term 'aggression'. Can aggressive behaviour be attributed to people with dementia, purely because of their given diagnosis? In other words, is dementia being equated with aggression? Alternatively, is *all* aggressive behaviour related directly to the dementing person's frustration, owing to their continuing loss of communication skills and general disempowerment? One respondent commented with regard to the ability of a dementing person to comprehend what is going on around them:

You often hear people say, 'Ooh, they're quite happily demented', but my experience of patients on this ward is that they're not happily demented. They've got a lot of insight, even patients who find it very difficult to communicate ... they've got an awful lot of insight into what is going on with them ... the things they come out with really shake me at times, and a patient that really hasn't made a lot of sense in their speech will suddenly come out and say, 'I think I'm going mad, there's something wrong with me ...' you know, that sort of thing, and I really do get upset.

Respondent R

On initial reading, the following extract appears to show that dealing with challenging behaviour and aggression really is a major consideration. However, on further examination, it becomes clear that rather different but related issues are emerging. These extracts vividly illustrate one of the underlying problems:

Well, about five o'clock there's an hour ... and we nicknamed it the 'sundown syndrome', but there's about an hour they'd [the patients] be really terrible on a late shift. I've not done a night shift but I've heard that some of them do get quite nasty ... Recognition that it does happen for a start, not a denial. If you get someone who's had a black eye, then the next morning someone's saying, 'that person's not aggressive' that is so silly. We've all been hit yet we get somebody turn around and say, 'They've just got a behaviour problem'. They are not, they are aggressive. It would be nice for it to be recognised, that yes, we have aggressive patients and perhaps … if it's not improved in six weeks then something has got to be done, because we are at risk and we are always going to pick up the tab if anything happens to us.

Respondent Q

I think it's a lack of understanding and insight on how to handle … quite honestly, I think some of them take it very personally, half of your staff that can handle and another half that can't handle … then it's lack of information being fed through.

Respondent N

In the preceding extract, the respondent talks of the need for colleagues to control their own feelings and emotions when working with a person with dementia who is angry. Health-care workers who take outbursts against themselves to heart are seen as not being able to 'handle' themselves or the situation very well. Those dealing with an outburst in an impersonal manner, however, are 'handling' both themselves and the circumstances well. Ironically, this situation reinforces the perception of people with dementia that needs to be challenged. In dealing with challenging outbursts, there is a fine line between professional distance and empathetic understanding.

The boundary between expression and aggression in dementia care has been blurred so much that it is often difficult for staff to understand what is meant by the term 'aggressive' (Stokes, 1987). If there has been a breakdown in communication between a care worker and a person with dementia, it is possible that aggressive behaviour may result. Some care workers would not describe this person as aggressive, but would note the aggressive response and describe it as frustration which results following misunderstandings. Other care workers would have no hesitation in describing the person as aggressive, as after all, the response was an aggressive action. This dichotomy only serves to confuse care teams and the individuals within them. If they have not made their personal definitions of 'aggression' clear, the resulting communication breakdown within the care team may lead to suspicion, mistrust and animosity.

Another factor to be seriously considered when dealing with the issue of aggression is the level and type of support (both formal and informal) that individuals can expect to receive once they have been involved in an incident that has resulted in an aggressive outburst. The following respondent was particularly honest when disclosing her thoughts on the matter:

I don't think we're so forgiving of one another because there's some people that feel happy to deal with those types of patients. Some people are not so happy and I think … if you were to turn around and say, 'I don't want to do that', then some people see you as being a failure. I think there's too much of that … some people are very willing to say, 'Oh, look, I got it wrong, I did that really badly' or 'I need some help'. The vibes I get … is that it is just *not* the thing to do, that you have to battle on regardless.

Respondent E

This highlights the importance of a support system that moves into action in the very environment where the aggressive incident happens. All care workers should be aware of the need for understanding and peer support, long before external departments become involved in the matter. It is critical that any such incident is evaluated in a thorough manner, so that all possibilities for learning more about a person are considered. This helps the person with dementia as much as the care worker concerned in the incident. Of course, training and any number of frank discussions around such an issue, are also an essential adjunct to this emotive area of care.

A great degree of honesty and frankness should be encouraged when sharing strategies for the management of aggression. Many care workers are frightened and lacking in confidence. Other health-care workers have reservations about their own responses when threatened by a person with dementia. Some feel that their own standing as a skilled professional is compromised if such an outburst occurs against them. Either way, none of these feelings should be driven 'underground' where they cannot be addressed, and may in the long run contribute to a very real dilemma. Some care workers commented:

Behaviour … violence … having not ever come across that sort of thing before, it was very, sort of, alien and I wasn't quite sure what to expect. I wasn't quite sure what my reaction was going to be … I think that was more frightening than anything. I think your automatic reaction is sort of … if somebody goes for you, to go back … to either protect yourself or … I didn't know what my reactions were going to be.

Respondent O

I won't say that if a patient goes for me I won't feel aggression in return, because sometimes you do feel aggressive towards them. If somebody whacks you one, you are bound to feel a bit aggrieved, aren't you? It's natural.

Respondent T

I would rather that they [the care workers] walked away from a patient and turned around and said to them, 'I'll be back' and then come away and vented it some, rather than vent it on the patient. I realise that that's easy for me to say because I'm not there when they are being thumped, and when they are being spat at or shouted at.

Respondent D

[The] other different members of staff on the ward, they've all got a different way of thinking about how to handle a different approach ... a lot of people in the ward have been with Alzheimer's and dementia for years and years and years, and I've been here a year, so my experience is, 'Ooh, who do I follow?' Who's got the best [approach]?' – 'Who's right?' – 'Who's wrong?' ... I'm very confused on that one.

Respondent M

Undergoing more formalised training programmes can be important and useful, but only if the people who do so find it relevant to their own experience. Much of the training offered regarding aggressive behaviour is aimed at an audience who will be familiar with control and restraint measures. This is less appropriate when working with frail people who have dementia. Training should focus on communication skills. One respondent expresses a succinct view on this matter:

I don't know what they can teach you, I think a lot of it is common sense. I mean obviously if you are going to stand there with attitude on your face, and looking rather aggressive, you're going to get into more trouble than you are if you can relax with someone and talk quietly to them. I'd be quite happy to go to training if it would be of benefit.

Respondent R

Finally, ignoring the issue will not make it go away. Reducing the amount of aggressive incidents on a unit takes time, commitment and honesty from all members of the team. If it is ignored, patient care will deteriorate, staff sickness will escalate, and recruitment and retention of staff will become even more difficult than they may already be.

One last pause for thought on this matter is provided below. If members of staff are regularly leaving their workplace expressing feelings like those heard in this extract, then no time can be wasted on dealing with the matter:

When there are patients being aggressive ... hitting ... sometimes I can't cope, but I do ... it's too stressful, I just can't wait to get out of the place.

Respondent B

Peer perceptions of dementia care

The staff on the unit provided a variety of views regarding the general perception of their work. It was overwhelmingly considered to be negative, although there were different opinions as to why this might be the case. There was an acceptance that the care of older people in itself was not taken seriously as a good career option. The general assessment, rehabilitation and psychiatric wards for old people are housed in a separate building 3 km from the main hospital. This 'natural' division from the mainstream of care delivery was seen to support that opinion in a covert way. Staff who had undertaken bank or agency work prior to working on the unit, and staff who continued to do so, emphasised that this view was rife in many areas within the National Health Service (NHS) Trust.

> I did bank work around the hospital and there was bad vibes about the ward from different nursing staff … they were saying, 'Ooh, you don't want to work on that ward, it's not very nice. The patients are not very nice.' I've had some friends that have done some agency and come on, and they've seen it and they've wondered … why am I working with patients like that?
>
> *Respondent A*

> Care of [the] Elderly sometimes has got a slight stigma in nursing, especially some people say, 'Ooh, you're not working there, are you?' but some people don't fully understand what we do, it's just a figure of speech really … I suppose they regard it as a hard job, which Care of the Elderly is, the kind of patients they are, it's hard work. Perhaps it's because they [colleagues] feel sorry for you, that you have to work so hard or something like that. I've never really come to grips with how it's seen.
>
> *Respondent P*

> Oh, they [colleagues] say they couldn't work here, it's too much like hard work … too much lifting.
>
> *Respondent W*

In some cases it was thought that 'care of older people' and certainly 'dementia care' was simply too much like hard work – not just because of the sheer physical effort that was often involved, but also because of the amount of emotional labour too. On a number of occasions during the interviews, staff talked of being seen as 'martyrs'. Although this term is not meant to be derogatory, it does help to reinforce the view that there is nothing to be gained from the endeavours made in this field but pain and disillusionment, both for the person with dementia, and for any care worker in that field daring to challenge the status quo. The following statements reflect the general view.

> The comments I usually get is, 'How can you work there?' 'How can you stand it?' 'Haven't you got marvellous patience.' That sort of thing which makes you feel a little bit of a martyr, but I'm not.
>
> *Respondent S*

> I think most of them think, 'Ooh, how could you cope with that?' ... One of my friends is doing sort of children's nursing, ICU, that type of thing ... and it's all hip ... I suppose some of it is looking after old people but it's more than that. Mental illness in any sense gets bad press, I think, because people don't understand it, and they see demented patients as being aggressive all the time. It's not seen as nursing because you're not there with the drips, the temps you know ... and that's what people perceive as being nursing.
>
> *Respondent E*

There was, however, an alternative view observed by some people: this was the accusation that their job was actually easier than the work taking place in other areas of care. Anybody could become good at undertaking physical labour and maintaining personal care, if they elected to do so. The perceived absence of complex equipment, or obvious patient recovery, reinforced this. Here the very nature of nursing was under fire. This can be reflected back on the numerous allusions to nursing-home care, made (throughout these interviews) by the team members themselves. What was striking was that during this line of thought, not one person was able to offer a seriously considered argument countering this point of view. Some people almost appeared to believe this view themselves, and those who did not, could not identify what skills they themselves had to offer in this area of care. It became clear that until the team members could believe this themselves, these types of widespread opinions would continue to undermine any fragments of positive contribution that the team felt it had to offer.

> Sometimes they don't believe that it's actually as hard work as we make it out to be. It's not appreciated as being hard work on here. They've got it easy, so ... I find it sad [that] people have said to me, 'Ooh, it's easy on [named ward], what are you complaining about?' Well, it's not the fact that I'm complaining about the ward because, at the end of the day you've got to do the work, and you do the work

to the best of your ability, but what I'm saying is that we should have more acclaim for what we do.

Respondent T

Apart from the widespread opinions regarding the relative ease of caring for this client group, there were also some feelings that reflected the effect of more deep-rooted beliefs. Management strategies and recruitment policies prevalent throughout the country had helped reinforce the low status of care in this speciality. Outside the unit, it was thought that staff only worked there because they were desperate for a job, or because it was easier to get a higher grade in that area of care. This commonly held belief needs to be proved or disproved, and if it is found to be true, then the reasons for it must be considered. It is likely that there is more to this than meets the eye, and if the reasons for it are not related to the acceptance of lower standards because of recruitment difficulties, then this must be widely publicised. This is a view that is damagingly perpetuated, and if it is a myth it must be finally dispelled once and for all. If it is not a myth, then such practices must be challenged and eliminated. Staff in the field have enough to contend with, without being held to ransom by such views.

[There's] a friend of mine … in his opinion, and from a lot of people's opinions that I've heard, they feel that this is not an area that people choose to work in. People end up working in it, not by choice [but] because there's a job going, or a grade coming up that you want. I think part of it stems back to a couple of years ago when all students qualified, they always got jobs in their own Trust. It was felt that the ones who were the best able to, got put over on the main [hospital] campus, and then the ones that didn't get the jobs would come over here because they were virtually guaranteed … because there was such a high turnover of staff, and people always got jobs here. That's carried on, people haven't got rid of that opinion.

Respondent G

The respondents seemed to be fairly evenly split over the way they dealt with the onslaught of inaccurate views about their ability. Some of the respondents made efforts to further their endeavours by talking publicly about how good they believed the ward to be. However, other members of staff were clearly not happy about being on the unit, and publicised this fact both on and off the unit. This in itself appeared to damage morale even further. This contrast is seen in the extracts below.

You probably get irritated with people outside because of their lack of understanding. You can get quite frustrated with people who make comments, and you're trying to keep a good standard up for those patients because they cannot do it for themselves and so it's important.

Respondent D

Angry ... angry, actually, because there is a lot that I get out of it so I anticipate that everyone else should ... it doesn't always work like that. I tend to blow the trumpet on the ward, about dementia and what's being done...

Respondent Q

...the people that are there [on the ward] that ... makes it feel worse because they keep saying, 'Oh, I don't want to be here', and I just think, 'Well, why don't you leave if you don't really enjoy the job that much ... why don't you leave?' ... because it doesn't help my morale.

Respondent H

It became clear that the way the team perceived itself was not solely dependent upon factors within the working environment. The views of professional colleagues around the hospital had a very influential effect on the image of the ward within the NHS Trust. Generally, the care workers on the unit were not equipped with the insight and knowledge to enable them to identify the skills that made them good at what they did. They were consequently unable to stand their ground and defend their motives for working in dementia care. This was possibly a result of the prevailing stereotypes existing within health care. Whilst a considerable amount of work has been undertaken by writers such as Tom Kitwood to break this stereotypical image of dementia and dementia care, nevertheless it is important that more work is developed and adequately funded to replace negativity frameworks with new and positive images relating to the care of older people with dementia.

CONCLUSION

Care workers working with people with a dementing illness need to have enough skills to identify the medical, functional and environmental limitations that may impinge upon the abilities or actions of the person with dementia. The existence of all of these skills in people working with dementia is currently taken for granted.

There are key issues that need to be addressed in any area where people with dementia are receiving care. People responsible for staff recruitment, service provision, change management and skills development in dementia care should systematically review these issues regardless of whether they believe there is an existing 'problem' or not.

Although the study described in this chapter was relatively small, sufficient work has been undertaken to suggest that the views expressed by the respondents are similar to those of other health-care workers with older people.

In order to improve the quality of life for people with dementia in an institutional setting, I would suggest that the principles of 'personhood' (Kitwood and Bredin, 1991) should be applied throughout that care setting. This would help care workers recognise wellbeing and the early indicators of ill-being in those for whom they care. It is important, therefore, that care workers fully understand that in being able to do this, they will build significantly upon their own care skills and knowledge. Perhaps more importantly, both they and people with dementia will be able to develop deeper and more mutually supportive relationships with each other.

The hierarchy of the care team, however formal or informal, should encourage an environment where frank and honest exchanges of values and feelings are encouraged. Only when sensitive and controversial issues are explicitly discussed can they have an impact upon the delivery of care. Dementia care is just as challenging as other speciality areas, with professional carers in the field often confronting their own personal fears and insecurities on a daily basis. It is important they are supported and assisted to identify, recognise and promote their own skills. It is also important that they are not allowed to believe that working with people with dementia is devaluing and demoralising as the result of either their own ignorance and misunderstanding, or perhaps more importantly, the ignorance and misunderstanding of other health-care workers.

REFERENCES

Bowling, A. & Formby, J. (1991) Nurses' attitudes to elderly people: a survey of nursing homes and elderly care wards in an inner-London health district. *Nursing Practice* **5** (1), 16–24.

Brower, H.T. (1981) Social organisation and nurses attitudes towards older persons. *Journal of Gerontological Nursing* **7**, 293–298.

Brower, H.T. (1985) Do nurses stereotype the aged? *Journal of Gerontological Nursing* **11**, 17–28.

Burnard, P. (1991) A method of analysing interview transcripts in qualitative research. *Nurse Education Today* **2**, 461–466.

Campbell, M.E. (1972) Study of the attitudes of nursing personnel towards the geriatric patient. *Nursing Research* **20**, 147–151.

Crowne, D.P. & Marlowe, D. (1961) A new scale of social desirability independent of psychopathology. *Journal of Consulting Psychology* **24**, 349–354.

Dellasega, C. & Curriero, F.C. (1991) The effects of institutional and community experiences on nursing students intentions toward work with the elderly. *Journal of Nursing Education* **30** (9), 405–410.

Diekmann, L., Zarit, S.H., Zarit, J.M. & Gatz, M. (1988) The Alzheimer's Disease Knowledge Test. *Gerontologist* **28**, 402–407.

Edwards, R.M., Plant, M.A., Novak, D.S., Beall, C. & Baumhover, L.A. (1992) Knowledge about aging and Alzheimer's disease among baccalaureate nursing students. *Journal of Nursing Education* **31** (3), 127–135.

Finnerty-Fried, P. (1982) Instruments for the assessment of attitudes toward older persons. *Measurement and Evaluation in Guidance* **15** (3), 201–209.

Gunter, L.M. (1971) Students' attitude towards geriatric nursing. *Nursing Outlook* **19**, 466–469.

Jacques, A. (1992) *Understanding Dementia*, 2nd edn. Edinburgh: Churchill Livingstone.

Kitwood, T. & Bredin, K. (1991) *Person to Person: A Guide to the Care of Those with Failing Mental Powers*. Essex. Gale Centre Publications.

Kitwood, T. & Bredin, K. (1993) *Evaluating Dementia Care: The DCM Method* Bradford: Bradford Dementia Research Group.

Kogan, N. (1961) Attitudes towards old people: the development of a scale and an examination of correlates. *Journal of Abnormal and Social Psychology* **62**, 44–54.

Leifer, D. (1995) Recruitment crisis. *Nursing Standard* **10** (15), 18–19.

McCabe, B. (1989) Ego defensiveness and its relationship to attitudes of registered nurses toward older people. *Research in Nursing and Health* **12**, 85–91.

Oberleder, M. (1962) An attitude scale to determine adjustment in institutions for the aged. *Journal of Chronic Disease* **15**, 915–923.

Palmore, E. (1977) Facts of aging. *Gerontologist* **17**, 315–320.

Palmore, E. (1980) The facts of aging quiz: a review of the findings. *Gerontologist* **20**, 669–679.

Palmore, E. (1981) The facts of aging quiz: part two. *Gerontologist* **21**, 431–437.

Robb, S. (1979) Attitudes and intentions of baccalaureate nursing students towards the elderly. *Nursing Research* **28** (1), 43–50.

Silverman, I. (1966) Response set bias and predictive validity associated with Kogan's attitudes towards old people scale. *Journal of Gerontology* **21**, 86–88.

Snape, J. (1986) Nurses' attitudes to care of the elderly. *Journal of Advanced Nursing* **11**, 569–572.

Stevens, J.A. & Crouch, M. (1992) Working with the elderly: do student nurses care for it? *Australian Journal of Advanced Nursing* **9** (3), 12–17.

Stokes, G. (1987) *Common Problems with the Elderly Confused: Aggression*. Bicester: Winslow Press.

Taylor, K.H. & Harned, T.L. (1978) Attitudes toward old people: a study of nurses who care for the elderly. *Journal of Gerontological Nursing* **4**, 43–47.

Wilcock, G.K. (1983) Age and Alzheimer's disease. *Lancet* **346**.

Wright, S., Elliott, M. & Scholefield, H. (1997) A networking approach to clinical supervision. *Nursing Standard* **11** (18), 39–41.

16

Partnership in dementia care: taking it forward

Charlotte L. Clarke

INTRODUCTION

This chapter has just one purpose, but it is a purpose to which the whole of this book has contributed. That is to set out one way (and there are no doubt others) of working towards a model of professional care for people with dementia and their families which allows a partnership in care. To do so is necessary so that we can know not only how to develop practice in this area, but also are able to recognise when we have achieved it.

The importance of two factors obstructing the development of such a partnership has become apparent in the preceding chapters: these factors are discrimination and reductionism in the approach to contemporary dementia care. In developing practice there is therefore a need to shed such negative and unhelpful aspects of our professional practice. There is a need to develop instead practices that are:

- Non-discriminatory
- Non-reductionalist.

Just two words – easily written and said, but perhaps not so easily done. Indeed, it is notable that these two areas are defined in negative terms, for I do not believe that the current state of dementia care practice allows us to be more optimistic. Let us start at least by striving to eliminate what we should *not* be doing.

NON-DISCRIMINATORY DEMENTIA CARE

Contemporary dementia care practices, and the care of family carers, are underpinned by discrimination. How can such a bold statement be made? Let us look at the evidence from this book alone, much of which is derived from empirical research. Chapters 1–3 are concerned with the construction of dementia, and in particular the dominance afforded to the 'medical' view of dementia, and consequently dementia care, at the expense of other ways of knowing about dementia. Chapters 4–6 are concerned with the value placed on people with dementia – so little, it seems, that books need to be written to encourage us to remember that they are indeed people in their own right (e.g. Kitwood and Benson, 1995). Chapter 7 is concerned with the role played by research in keeping the person with dementia silenced. Chapters 8–12 are concerned with various groups who find themselves disadvantaged by the social and political structures in which we all live, namely confused older people in residential and nursing care homes; family carers who are wives of someone with dementia; male family carers; people experiencing the early stages of dementia; and younger people with dementia. Chapters 13 and 14 are concerned with the way in which the needs of family carers are privileged, at times, over the needs of the person with dementia. Chapter 15 is concerned with the ways in which care staff themselves feel devalued as a result of working with older people with dementia.

Mental health status

Barnett (1997), in a study evaluating a service for people with dementia which privileged the perceptions of these users themselves, describes the marginalisation of people with dementia in the management of their own care and how they are 'sidelined from the collaborative process' which (potentially) exists between service agencies and family carers. She describes this marginalisation as emanating from the perceived lack of insight of people with dementia, although insight is so defined by professional staff as to inevitably exclude people with dementia. However, Barnett (1997) found that, erroneously, staff linked insight with the ability to communicate, to the detriment of their care:

> The 'one-way street' of care, which proceeds from not recognising the awareness of clients with dementia, penalises them as their communication skills decrease, and excludes the crucial individual information which could support truly person-centred care. And by not listening to what clients themselves have to say we shut ourselves off from their wisdom. (p. 4)

To develop practice in this area we need to find ways of hearing and learning from people with dementia. They must not be marginalised because of 'their' communication difficulties, a point affirmed by Frank (1995). This is a complicated area, however, and in Chapter 8 Jan Reed describes the marginalisation of confused older people in residential and nursing homes by other residents who are concerned to protect their own identity as being 'not confused'. This situation is compounded by the approach of the care staff who seek to ensure equity between those who are confused and those who are not. In Chapter 6, Anne Whitworth, Lisa Perkins and Ruth Lesser have provided an example of how communication strategies can be developed to facilitate collaboration. Further, we need to suspend 'our' understandings of normative values (such as the emphasis placed on orientation to time, place and person in interventions such as reality orientation) and exist with people with dementia irrespective of the parameters of comprehension. In Chapter 5 Jane Crisp provides useful and practical steps which can be taken to achieve this.

Increasingly, information is available about *how* to communicate with people with dementia, and we may at last be moving beyond the point of needing to ask whether we *can* communicate. For example, Killick (1997) describes his work as a writer with the Dementia Services Development Centre at the University of Stirling in which he works with people with dementia to put their ideas and thoughts into words. Kitwood (1997) has identified six 'access routes' by which people may 'gain insight into the subjective world of dementia' (p. 15). These are listed in Box 16.1.

In seeking to prevent the marginalisation of people because of their status as someone with dementia, it is worth bearing in mind the guidelines (now dated but still awaiting full implementation) of the King's Fund publication *Living Well into Old Age* (King's Fund Centre, 1986):

- People with dementia have the same human value as anyone else irrespective of their degree of disability or dependence
- People with dementia have the same varied human needs as anyone else
- People with dementia have the same rights as other citizens
- Every person with dementia is an individual
- People with dementia have the right to forms of support that do not exploit family and friends.

Many of these points are debated by Malcolm Goldsmith in Chapter 4. He considers, among other ethical issues, the rights of people with dementia

---

Box 16.1 Kitwood's 'access routes' for understanding people with dementia

- Through accounts that have been written by people who have dementia.
- By careful listening to what people say, in some kind of interview or group context.
- Attending carefully to what people say and do in the course of their ordinary life.
- Consulting people who have undergone an illness with dementia-like features.
- Through the use of our own poetic imagination.
- Through the use of role play, actually taking on the part of someone who has dementia and enacting it in a simulated care environment.

to make their own choices. Central to these considerations, he argues, is whether someone with dementia is perceived to have any 'personhood' (Kitwood and Bredin, 1992) or whether the dementia has resulted in a death of 'self' – an issue succinctly debated by Sabat and Harré (1992). Similarly, Sweeting and Gilhooly (1997) identify the 'social death' of someone with dementia who is no longer regarded as a whole and valued person. This tension is also explored in Chapter 3 by Michael Hill and indeed forms a core thread through most of the chapters. If we recognise the personhood of people with dementia then we implicitly value them and respect them despite their mental health status.

Dependency

Western society places a high value on independence, and dependency is seen to be undesirable. In Chapter 3 Michael Hill argues that this binary division is too simplistic and that all individuals regardless of their needs are dependent on others. It is far more appropriate to consider dependency as a range of interdependency states, which change over time. In this way the ideas of reciprocity, discussed in Chapter 1, are inevitably crucial mediators in the experience of dementia and family caring. The meanings of dependency held by older people have been rarely explored, notable exceptions being Reed and Payton (1996) and Langan et al (1996), although these studies did not include people with dementia.

I am often struck by a quote of unknown origin about the expectation on people to 'slide gracefully from a state of independence to a state of gratitude'. This, for me, typifies the state of passivity and powerlessness into which dependent people are placed by others. The 'disengagement theory' postulated by Cummings and Henry (1961) has fuelled this contentious perspective in relation to older people and has received much criticism for confusing the intrinsic changes associated with becoming older with the effect of society upon older people – the 'structured dependency' described by Townsend (1981). However, irrespective of age, this powerlessness is rejected by people with disabilities themselves (Dalley, 1993). Just as institutional care has become an untenable form of caring for people because of the restrictions it places on people's choices and control over their lives, so care within a family is now beginning to be seen as similarly debilitating for people (Parker, 1993). Dalley (1993) states:

> The straitjacket of dependency on the altruism of close kin or the isolation of living alone with minimal community care support may be as oppressive as the old forms of institutional care. (p. 19)

Further, Dalley (1993) argues that community care 'simply confirms the model of dependent people as dependent, and carers as carers. It represents an ideology of compulsory altruism, passivity and individualism' (p. 19). This, to some, may appear to be an extreme view but it should be considered in the light of the argument expressed by Kevin McKee in Chapter 7: that our interpretation of 'quality of life' has become synonymous with 'quality of care'. Whilst the adequacy of care for people with dementia is rightly evaluated and challenged, be it by family or professional carers, we must not assume that this means that we are judging the quality of life of people. Indeed, their quality of life may at time be compromised by their care, and in Chapter 13 I question the appropriateness of some health and social care interventions for people with dementia and their family carers.

Thus the disadvantages experienced by people by virtue of their status as a dependent person cut across society at multiple levels: from social and economic policies that perpetuate passivity and poverty, to interpersonal interactions that are coloured by our lack of knowledge about the meaning of dependence to people with dementia. These issues must be tackled at the level of social policy as well as professional practice before there can be a move towards developing partnerships of equality.

Age

Discrimination against older people is a well-recognised social phenomenon, but in dementia care this results, paradoxically, in discrimination against younger people with dementia as well. Because dementia has been seen as a disease of 'old age', and even worse as an inevitable part of growing old (as discussed by Phair and Good, 1995), it has been subject to societal judgments about the appropriateness of investing substantial sums of money in research, teaching and practice. Indeed, in Chapter 4 Malcolm Goldsmith describes the disparity in research funding in Britain: £10 per person with dementia being spent on research, £109 per person with heart disease, £474 per person with cancer and £15 000 per person with AIDS.

Compounding the age-related discrimination, dementia care interventions have been narrow in their range because of the therapeutic pessimism surrounding the management of dementia. This has resulted in care management strategies which emphasise containment, behaviour management and, critically, a shift away from caring for people with dementia to caring for their family carers – a focus perhaps seen as far more amenable to successful intervention in reducing stress and improving coping strategies.

However, such a pessimistic approach to dementia care has had a consequential impact on the care of younger people with dementia. Dementia care has matured in a market of older people and the needs of younger people with dementia have not had a place in this until very recently. As Chapter 12 by Jill Walton describes, the needs of these younger people with dementia are, at times, quite different, but the resources available are underdeveloped. Indeed, they are located in just a few specialised centres, such as the CANDID service in Britain which she describes.

Age has not always been seen as a criterion for demarcating sections of a population. Macintyre (1977) identifies the end of the twentieth century as the time when older people in Britain became a 'special case', as the industrialisation of society imposed an age-related structure on work practices and therefore on economic and social participation. The view of dementia as being a disease of old age is no longer tenable, as evidenced for example through the work of Jill Walton – it is a disease of people, not of older people. There is a need to ensure therefore that research, education and practice reflects this; for example, the teaching of dementia care should not be restricted to courses about older people.

Other important age-related issues concern the position of family carers and professional carers. The stereotypical family carer as someone who is middle-aged (and I may add, female) has obscured the presence of the many older people who care and the unknown number of very young carers. In Chapter 15 Tracy Packer identifies the impact that caring for older people with dementia has on the morale of health-care workers, of their attitudes of caring for people and their own educational needs. Their perception of their work as low-status results in their being unable to identify and therefore articulate the skills that they need to work with people with dementia, to the disadvantage of the development of care services. An acknowledgment of the unrecognised skills of those working with people with dementia is a good starting point in developing those skills and care practices.

Gender

Issues of gender in the experience of dementia have not been addressed to any depth by research, and so we can only speculate on the impact it may have. However, in dementia care and in particular in the care of family members, discrimination on the grounds of gender is clearly evident. In Chapter 9 Christine Carter links care *in* the community to care *by* the community, to care by women in the home. She is not alone in doing so. Dalley (1993), for example, states that 'community care, then, is based on an ideology of familism which in turn rests on a gendered division of labour within the domestic sphere' (p. 18). This gendered division of labour is double-edged: women experience societal assumptions about their caring nature and in practice are expected to assume unquestioningly the mantle of primary family carer – and they are not expected to need much assistance to do this; men who are carers find services more attentive to meeting their needs and providing practical assistance, but may lack the social networks and societal 'permission' to undertake the role (Clarke and

Watson, 1991). The assumption that it is women who care has been to the detriment of recognising, and developing services for, the substantial number of men who do care (Arber and Ginn, 1990).

Dalley (1993) argues that caring is the 'currency of social transactions', particularly in marriage and domestic life. Consequently the distinction she makes between women as carers for and about others, and men as carers about but not for others, compromises the value of caring as currency within such gender-defined caring roles. Ungerson (1987) distinguishes between the life courses of men and women carers, highlighting the importance of full-time paid work for men which 'blots out' other calls on their time, whilst women experience a 'conglomeration of continuous demands, emanating from different sources' (p. 204). To assess carer need and implement professional interventions which rest assumptively on gender-defined roles of family carers will result in our being insensitive to the actual needs of individual carers and therefore offering inappropriate interventions.

There is a need for us to challenge our gendered expectations of family carers. Christine Carter in Chapter 9, for example, found that women who cared for their husbands were expected to be involved unquestioningly in their caring roles, and little attention was paid by health-care professionals to the impact of caring for their husband upon their marital relationship. Liz Matthew, in Chapter 10, found that there was a tension for male carers between involving and remaining close to their wives, and distancing themselves from them emotionally with the resultant losses associated with losing a partner in life.

Culture

Little has been written about dementia and dementia care in the context of culture, and we need to ask whether it varies across different populations, for example across different ethnic and socioeconomic groups. It appears likely that the meanings that we commonly attribute to dementia are specific to industrialised cultures. It is in complex, economically structured societies that concepts of age, gender and mental health status affect an individual's experiences. For example, only in societies in which people 'retire' from paid employment or are unable through illness to participate in employment do the precursors to designating someone as 'different' exist. In Chapter 13, I discuss the ideological position of normalisation of dementia care as being possibly culture-specific, Anderton et al (1989) finding that Chinese-Canadians, unlike the more affluent Anglo-Canadians, were unable to accommodate (and normalise) someone who was not economically self-sufficient.

Phair and Good (1995) describe the assumption that carers from ethnic minority groups 'all live in extended families and look after their own' as unfounded. Their lack of usage of statutory services, they argue, is probably due to the inappropriate nature of the services rather than a lack of need for support. Indeed, Norman (1985), studying older people in a second homeland, found them to be particularly disadvantaged in service provision. Askham et al, (1997), investigating the health and social services provision for older people from black and minority ethnic populations in England and Wales, identify the ambiguities that exist in current social policies between treating people as 'individuals' and being respectful of group identities such as ethnic background.

Whilst dementia is indiscriminate in affecting people whatever their background, in relation to care needs Arber and Ginn (1997) write of the 'leverage' that possession of financial, material and cultural resources may have in mediating the need for family care (irrespective of the degree of disability). These resources are 'intimately bound up with class' (Arber and Ginn, 1997):

> We suggest that the working class are doubly disadvantaged both by being more likely to be called on to provide care to elderly parents at an earlier age, when it conflicts with the demands of employment, and by having less material resources with which to ease their caring burden. (p. 151)

NON-REDUCTIONALIST DEMENTIA CARE

In responding to the discriminatory nature of understanding dementia and dementia care, as described above, we need to widen the focus and look at the context in which these events take place. Much of the contemporary drive in health care adopts a reductionist approach, seeking an understanding of more and more minute aspects of our lives, with the resulting risk of failing to notice the purpose and implications of what is being done. Rather as different species of animals have varying degrees of peripheral vision, so we must let our sight absorb the images that surround our central concerns.

People with dementia do not live in a void, divorced from the rest of society and their family, and dementia care is only one part of their whole lives. If we are to work in a partnership with them then there is a need to respect these other dimensions of their life, so that care may be sensitive to their needs and their voices may find an avenue for expression. Key issues are those of the biography of the individual and their family, the focus for care interventions, and interpretations of 'health' such that we move towards notions of wellbeing in a number of dimensions.

Biography

One of the first areas that demands wider scrutiny is that of the biography of the person with dementia. The processes of developing a biography, the impact of dementia upon it, and the subsequent strategies for the readjustment of one's own biography need to be explored. Two current studies touch upon this, namely Robinson et al (1997) in Sweden and, in Britain, John Keady and Jane Gilliard in Chapter 11, and also Keady (1997). Note how crucial is the intimate knowledge of a person's life in the work of Jane Crisp in Chapter 5, and in Crisp (1995), when she writes of being better able to understand her mother because of their shared lives together. It is, I argue elsewhere (Clarke and Heyman, 1998), this intimate knowledge of the lives of people with dementia that makes the knowledge of their family carers so crucially important to their care. It complements the knowledge of health and social care professionals and we cannot afford to let it go unrecognised.

There is a need to utilise care assessment and management strategies which will allow us to access the life of the person with dementia. Life review and reminiscence therapy serve the double purpose of allowing the person with dementia to recall their past, and seek self-affirmation from so doing, and of allowing us a route into their lives. Innovative methods can be used to capture the individual's sense of personal history, for example making life history videos (Hargrave, 1994) and multisensory approaches which use a variety of media (Murphy and Moyes, 1997). Moreover, the need of professional carers to come to know the person with dementia through a close and sustained working relationship is necessary to develop care that is sensitive to the individual's needs (as I discuss in Chapter 13).

The family carers' perspective of the person with dementia must be sought, reflecting as it does their own particular version of the life, wishes and strengths of the person with dementia. Two important studies are those of Keady and Nolan (1994), who developed an assessment framework with the family carer as the primary informant (although this does concentrate on assessing carer need), and of Anne Whitworth, Lisa Perkins and Ruth Lesser, reported in Chapter 6, in which the communication strategies of people with dementia and their family carers are assessed.

It is important, though, not to equate biography with the past. The past is merely one component of an individual's biography and we need to recognise the impact that society, including receipt of health and social care, can have in shaping the individual's present and therefore future. Discriminatory practice, as described previously, is inclined to deny people with dementia a future as a valued person and risks curtailing their self-esteem, sense of self and negotiation of biography. Such practice only affords people a future couched in the negative terms of inevitable medical decline. It is important to note the emphasis in Chapter 11, by John Keady and Jane Gilliard, that people with dementia do *not* want much information about their future from health-care professionals – the very thing that many professional carers feel is important to impart to individuals and their family carers (Clarke and Heyman, 1998).

Research activity must also reconsider the part it plays in isolating the person with dementia in the present, with little recognition of the person's past or future aspirations. In Chapter 7 Kevin McKee argues that some (more quantitative) research 'reduces' the person with dementia to nothing more than a number, with no biography or sense of the person at all. Stevenson (1996) provides a useful critique of methodologies for psychiatric nursing practice and in particular highlights the need for them to be sensitive to the lay perspectives of people with dementia and their family carers. Qualitative methods need to be recognised as a fruitful way of achieving this and therefore valued in terms of the information they can provide, a point also made by Murphy and Longino (1992) in relation to older people.

Focus of care

The ambivalence about whether the person with dementia or the family carer is the target of care interventions is discussed in Chapter 1. There is undoubtedly a tension for services between the perceived therapeutic pessimism surrounding the care of people with dementia, and the more optimistic outcomes of 'relieving' family carers of their burden – in itself a narrow interpretation of the family carers' role, which dismisses the relationship between them and the person they care for (Kitson, 1987; Orona, 1990; Clarke, 1997).

The approach to dementia care that emphasises the burden of a single family carer recognises other family members not as carers but as supporters or antagonists to the primary carer. However, restricting our understanding of family caregiving to that of one primary carer fails to recognise the intrafamily dynamics of families caring for someone with dementia. Perry and Olshansky (1996) found that there were differences in how each family member defined and found meaning in the situation. Particularly important for addressing a partnership in dementia care is the process by which family members were found to construct the continuing biography of the person with dementia by comparing that person's present and previous characteristics, redefining the individual's identity and rewriting their own relationship with the person with dementia (Perry and Olshansky, 1996).

The perception of family caregiving as being undesirable and even harmful to the carer's own health (the approach adopted by community psychiatric nurses in the study described by Trevor Adams in Chapter 14), together with social critical interpretations of dependency (discussed earlier in this chapter), portray the situation of people being cared for at home as one of despair and despondency. However, some services move beyond this interpretation. Dalley (1993), for example, emphasises the collective responsibility for caring in a community and writes of the need to reverse policies that promote individualism and the consequent dependency of one individual on another. Also, people with dementia can be self-sufficient in some environments, for example Malmberg (1997) describes the emergence of 'group homes' for people with dementia in Sweden; homes which comprised a small number of tenanted flats with shared kitchen and living room facilities.

An alternative perspective on the focus of care, one that allows partnerships to be promoted, recognises the person with dementia and the whole family as being bound together by indivisible ties of kinship which have contributed to the creation of the biography of each. Health and social care professionals can respect and work with these ties of interdependency. Indeed, failing to do so reduces the ability of professional carers to work in partnership. Elsewhere I argue that professional carers need to protect the relationship between the person with dementia and the family carer (Clarke, 1997), and other work articulates the difficulties that arise when the relationship is not respected. For example, Christine Carter in Chapter 9 found that the experiences of women caring for their husbands with dementia centred around the rights, responsibilities and expectations of the marital relationship.

A number of approaches to practice emphasise the unity of family structures. Friedemann (1993) describes three levels of family nursing: the individual level, in which the family is viewed as the context of the individual; the interpersonal level, in which the family is regarded as a number of dyadic and triadic units; and the systems level, in which the family has its own structural and functional components which interact with outside environmental factors. Similarly, family therapy (which, like family nursing, is particularly popular in the USA) (Richardson et al, 1994) and family systemic practice (Perry and Olshansky, 1996) conceive of the family as a unit rather than as a series of individuals.

Health status

Earlier in this chapter we considered the discrimination against people by virtue of their mental health status. In following on from that point we need to consider what alternative ways there are of attributing states of health and illness. This book is not the place for lengthy debate about the nature of health and illness, and there are many other books that do justice to this enormous subject – Rogers (1991) is one useful example. There is a need, though, to look beyond the label of the psychiatric illness and broaden our interpretation of the individual's health status. In Chapter 3 Michael Hill provides an account of the shifts from biomedicine to consideration of the social and psychological health of an individual, termed 'biopsychosocial medicine' by Engel (1977). Indeed, the philosophy of 'holistic' care is now subscribed to by most health-care professionals, even though its influence may not always be evident in practice. However, other aspects of the health of people with dementia have received relatively little attention, for example sexual health (Archibald, 1995, 1997) and spiritual health (Barnett, 1995; Froggatt and Moffitt, 1997).

In research, and often in practice, the voice of the person with dementia is heard only through the proxy of the family carer. To assume that the perspectives of the family carer and the person with dementia are congruent is misguided. The lay interpretations of dementia held by family carers, and their experiences of dementia care, have been the subject of considerable exploration since the 1980s (e.g. Wilson, 1989; Wuest et al, 1994), but the perspective of the person with dementia has received little attention. One exception is the work of John Keady and Jane Gilliard, discussed in Chapter 11, who detail the experiences of people in the early stages of dementia. In professional practice, there is a need to develop therapeutic exchanges with people with dementia and their carers which truly afford them a voice to describe to us, the health and social care professionals, their own individual experiences, the meaning that dementia has for them and the tolerance that they have in their lives for professional intervention (Clarke and Heyman, 1998).

Kitwood and Bredin (1992) argue that it is more appropriate to consider the experience of health, rather than seek to rectify all traces of medically defined illness. They call for a sense of wellbeing to be the goal in dementia care. Wellbeing, they propose, is evident through four 'global sentient states': a sense of personal worth, a sense of agency (of self-determination), social confidence and hope. Erickson (1986) writes of the developmental task of individuals in achieving 'ego integrity'; developing a sense of meaning and order in one's life. These criteria are well worth bearing in mind when we evaluate the impact of our current services on people with dementia. Research by Keady (1997) and Robinson et al (1997) indicates that one of the initial strategies used in managing cognitive loss is to hide the symptoms. It is a very private stage of the process of having dementia. Exposure through assessment strategies may therefore be to the detriment of the individual's sense of wellbeing.

The therapeutic pessimism of people with dementia hangs like a pall over their medical treatment. In Chapter 14, Trevor Adams describes how the person with dementia was not even regarded as a legitimate target for therapeutic intervention, health care being diverted into supporting the family carer. However, there is no need for such pessimism if the goal of care is the wellbeing of the individual and the interrelationships within a family.

CONCLUSION

To achieve a partnership between people with dementia, their family carers, and health and social care professionals is not, in my opinion, an impossible dream, but I do think that many things make it difficult to attain. However, these difficulties should not be insurmountable; rather, they require a refocusing of the purposes of professional practice. Through identifying the practices that obstruct partnership we can start to move towards removing them, basing our future care on practices that are non-discriminatory and non-reductionalist.

As I write this, the world is mourning the death of Diana, Princess of Wales. Repeatedly, the word 'humanity' is being used. Perhaps it is this quality that we need to take dementia care forward. Humanity is defined in the *Collins English Dictionary* (1994) as: '1. the human race. 2. the quality of being human. 3. kindness or mercy'; perhaps, then, to base dementia care on practices that are discriminatory and reductionalist does not display the qualities of a humanitarian society. Indeed, to disallow people with dementia a sense of being human is also to deny ourselves our own humanity. It takes no great philosopher, no expert practitioner, no outstanding researcher, to work alongside people in a way that values them as an individual. There is no need to let factors of age, gender, mental health status, culture, knowledge or dependency act as filters to our appreciation of other people. Instead, value them in the context of their life history, their part in a family and in society. Realise and value the impact that all health and social care professionals can have in return on people with dementia and their families. The rest, the development of partnerships in practice, will, I think, follow as surely as day follows night.

REFERENCES

Anderton, J.M., Elfert, H. & Lai, M. (1989) Ideology in the clinical context: chronic illness, ethnicity and the discourse on normalisation. *Sociology of Health and Illness* **11**, 253–275.

Arber, S. & Ginn, J. (1990) The meaning of informal care: gender and the contribution of elderly people. *Ageing and Society* **10**, 429–454.

Arber, S. & Ginn, J. (1997) Class, caring and the life course. In: Arber, S. & Evandrou, M. (eds) *Ageing, Independence and the Life Course*, 2nd edn. London: Jessica Kingsley.

Archibald, C. (1995) Sexuality and sexual needs of the person with dementia. In: Kitwood T. & Benson S. (eds) *The New Culture of Dementia Care*. London: Hawker.

Archibald, C. (1997) Sexuality and dementia? In: Marshall, M. (ed.) *The State of the Art in Dementia Care*. London: Centre for Policy on Ageing.

Askham J., Henshaw, L. & Tarpey, M. (1997) Policies and perceptions of identity: service needs of elderly people from black and minority ethnic backgrounds. In: Arber S. & Evandrou M. (eds) *Ageing, Independence and the Life Course*, 2nd edn. London: Jessica Kingsley.

Barnett, E. (1995) Broadening our approach to spirituality. In: Kitwood T. & Benson S. (eds) *The New Culture of Dementia Care*. London: Hawker.

Barnett, E. (1997) Collaboration and interdependence: care as a two-way street. In: Marshall M. (ed.) *The State of the Art in Dementia Care*. London: Centre for Policy on Ageing.

Clarke, C.L. (1997) In sickness and in health: remembering the relationship in family caregiving for people with dementia. In: Marshall, M. (ed.) *The State of the Art in Dementia Care*. London: Centre for Policy on Ageing.

Clarke, C.L. & Heyman, B. (1998) Risk management for people with dementia. In: Heyman, B. (ed.) *Risk, Health and Health Care: A Qualitative Approach*. London: Chapman & Hall.

Clarke, C. & Watson, D. (1991) Informal carers of the dementing elderly: a study of relationships. *Nursing Practice* **4**, 17–21.

Collins English Dictionary (1994) Glasgow: HarperCollins.

Crisp, J. (1995) Making sense of the stories that people with Alzheimer's tell: a journey with my mother. *Nursing Inquiry* **2**, 133–140.

Cummings, E. & Henry W. (1961) *Growing Old: The Process of Disengagement*. New York: Basic Books.

Dalley, G. (1993) The ideological foundations of informal care. In: Kitson, A. (ed.) *Nursing: Art and Science*. London: Chapman & Hall.

Engel, G.L. (1977) The need for a new medical model: a challenge for biomedicine. *Science* **196**, 129.

Erickson, E. (1986) *Vital Involvement in Old Age*. New York: Norton.

Frank, B.A. (1995) People with dementia can communicate – if we are able to hear In: Kitwood, T. & Benson, S. (eds) *The New Culture of Dementia Care*. London: Hawker

Friedmann, M. (1993) The concept of family nursing. In: Wenger, G.D. & Alexander, R. J. (eds) *Readings in Family Nursing*. Philadelphia: Lippincott.

Froggatt, A. & Moffitt, L. (1997) Spiritual needs and religious practice in dementia care. In: Marshall, M. (ed.) *The State of the Art in Dementia Care*. London: Centre for Policy on Ageing.

Hargrave, T.D. (1994) Using video life reviews with older adults. *Journal of Family Therapy* **16**, 259–267.

Keady, J. (1997) Maintaining involvement: a meta concept to describe the dynamics of dementia. In: Marshall, M. (ed.) *The State of the Art in Dementia Care*. London: Centre for Policy on Ageing.

Keady, J. & Nolan, M. (1994) The Carer-Led Assessment Process (CLASP): a framework for the assessment of need in dementia caregivers. *Journal of Clinical Nursing* **3**, 103–108.

Killick, J. (1997) Confidences: the experience of writing with people with dementia. In: Marshall, M. (ed.) *The State of the Art in Dementia Care*. London: Centre for Policy on Ageing.

King's Fund Centre (1986) *Living Well Into Old Age*. Project Paper No. 23. London: King's Fund.

Kitson, A.L. (1987) A comparative analysis of lay-caring and professional (nursing) caring relationships. *International Journal of Nursing Studies* **24**, 155–165.

Kitwood, T. (1997) The experience of dementia. *Aging and Mental Health* **1**, 13–22.

Kitwood, T. & Benson, S., (eds) (1995) *The New Culture of Dementia Care*. London: Hawker.

Kitwood, T. & Bredin, K. (1992) Towards a theory of dementia care: personhood and well-being. *Ageing and Society* **12**, 269–287.

Langan, J., Means, R. & Rolfe, S. (1996) *Maintaining Independence in Later Life: Older People Speaking*. Oxford: Anchor Trust.

Macintyre, S. (1977) Old age as a social problem: historical notes on an English experience. In: Dingwall, R., Heath, C., Reid, M. & Stacey, M. (eds) *Health Care and Health Knowledge*. London: Croom Helm.

Malmberg, B. (1997) Group homes: an alternative for older people with dementia. In: Marshall, M. (ed.) *The State of the Art in Dementia Care*. London: Centre for Policy on Ageing.

Murphy, C. & Moyes, M. (1997) Life history work. In: Marshall, M. (ed.) *The State of the Art in Dementia Care*. London: Centre for Policy on Ageing.

Murphy, J.W. & Longino, C.F. (1992) What is the justification for a qualitative approach to ageing studies? *Ageing and Society* **12**, 143–156.

Norman, A. (1985) *Triple Jeopardy: Growing Old in a Second Homeland*. Policy Studies on Aging No. 3. London: Centre for Policy on Ageing.

Orona, C.J. (1990) Temporality and identity loss due to Alzheimer's disease. *Social Sciences Medicine* **30**, 1247–1256.

Parker, G. (1993) *With This Body: Caring and Disability in Marriage*. Buckingham: Open University Press.

Perry, J. & Olshansky, E.F. (1996) A family coming to terms with Alzheimer's disease. *Western Journal of Nursing Research* **18**, 12–28.

Phair, L. & Good, V. (1995) *Dementia – A Positive Approach*. Harrow: Scutari.

Reed, J. & Payton, V.R. (1996) Constructing familiarity and managing the self: ways of adapting to life in nursing and residential homes for older people. *Ageing and Society* **16**, 543–560.

Richardson, C.A., Gilleard, C.J., Lieberman, S. & Peeler, R. (1994) Working with older adults and their families – a review. *Journal of Family Therapy* **16**, 225–240.

Robinson, P., Ekman, S.-L., Meleis, A.I., Winbald, B. & Wahlund, L.-O. (1997) Suffering in silence: the experience of early memory loss. *Health Care in Later Life* **2**, 107–120.

Rogers, W.S. (1991) *Explaining Health and Illness: An Exploration of Diversity*. New York: Harvester Wheatsheaf.

Sabat, S.R. & Harré, R. (1992) The construction and deconstruction of self in Alzheimer's disease. *Ageing and Society* **12**, 443–461.

Stevenson, C. (1996) Taking the pith out of reality: a reflexive methodology for psychiatric nursing practice. *Journal of Psychiatric and Mental Health Nursing* **3**, 103–110.

Sweeting, H. & Gilhooly, M. (1997) Dementia and the phenomenon of social death. *Sociology of Health and Illness* **19**, 93–117.

Townsend, P. (1981) The structured dependency of the elderly: a creation of social policy in the twentieth century. *Ageing and Society* **1**, 5–28.

Ungerson, C. (1987) The life course and informal caring: towards a typology. In: Cohen, G. (ed.) *Social Change and the Life Course*. London: Tavistock

Wilson, H.S. (1989) Family caregivers: the experience of Alzheimer's disease. *Applied Nursing Research* **2**, 40–45.

Wuest, J., Ericson, P.K. & Stern, P.N. (1994) Becoming strangers: the changing family caregiving relationship in Alzheimer's disease. *Journal of Advanced Nursing* **20**, 437–443.

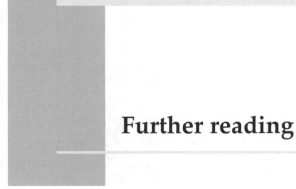

Further reading

Bayles, K. & Kaszniak, A. (1987) *Communication and Cognition in Normal Aging and Dementia*. Boston: College-Hill Press.

This book provides an accessible and comprehensive review of the breakdown of language and other aspects of cognition in different forms of dementia.

Brown, H. & Smith, H., eds (1992) *Normalisation – A Reader for the Nineties*. London: Routledge.

This book acts as a landmark for theories of normalisation up to the 1990s. It is a compilation of a number of informative papers which focus on mental health and learning disability concerns.

Cheston, R. (1996) Stories and metaphors: talking about the past in a psychotherapy group for people with dementia. *Ageing and Society* **16**, 579–602.

A paper that allows the voice of the person with dementia full expression, and uses the data generated to make cogent arguments about the nature of the lived experience of the person with dementia.

Coen, R., O'Mahony, D., O'Boyle, C. et al (1993) Measuring the quality of life of dementia patients using the schedule for the evaluation of individual quality of life. *Irish Journal of Psychology* **14**, 154–163.

A description of a traditional approach to assessing quality issues in people with dementia which differs from Gilloran et al (1993).

Crisp, J. (1995) Making sense of the stories that people with Alzheimer's tell: a journey with my mother. *Nursing Inquiry* **2**, 133–140.
Crisp, J. (1995) Dementia and communication. In: Garrett, S. & Hamilton-Smith, E. (eds) *Rethinking Dementia – An Australian Approach*. Melbourne: Ausmed.

These two items provide a fuller account of strategies for making sense of what people with dementia say, based on Jane Crisp's exploration of the language of people with dementia.

Garrett, S. & Hamilton-Smith, E., eds (1995) *Rethinking Dementia – An Australian Approach*. Melbourne: Ausmed.

This book provides an example of a positive approach to care for people with dementia, founded on a belief in the survival of personhood and in 'enhancing life through optimal stimulus'.

Gilleard, C.J. (1984) *Living with Dementia*. London: Croom Helm.

A seminal work that virtually created the research paradigm of the family carer.

Gilloran, A.J., McGlew, T., McKee, K. et al (1993) Measuring the quality of care in psychogeriatric wards. *Journal of Advanced Nursing* **18**, 269–275.

Goffman, E. (1961) *Asylums*. New York: Doubleday.

A classic analysis of life within total institutions.

Goldsmith, M. (1996) *Hearing the Voice of People with Dementia: Opportunities and Obstacles*. London: Jessica Kingsley.

This book encompasses views both from people with dementia, and from care workers from the whole arena of dementia care. It offers an insight into the problems experienced so far, and thoughts and suggestions about how best to take dementia care forward.

Goldsmith, M. (1997) Hearing their voice. In: Hunter, S. (ed.) *Dementia: Challenges and New Directions*, pp. 107–120. London: Jessica Kingsley.

A well-referenced chapter that provides a useful summary of Goldsmith's study on hearing the voice of people with dementia. In this work, Goldsmith challenges practitioners to understand the art of communication with people with dementia and views time as the most important commodity in this process.

Hamilton, H.E. (1994) *Conversations with an Alzheimer's Patient*. Cambridge: CUP.

This book provides a fascinating case study from a conversation analysis perspective of the changes in conversational participation for one woman with dementia over a 4 year period.

Hansson, R.O. & Carpenter, B.N. (1994) *Relationships in Old Age*. New York: Guilford Press.

A book that shows the similar emotional issues facing individuals at different phases of the lifespan, and which also explores the challenges particular to later life.

Harding, N. & Palfrey, C. (1997) *The Social Construction of Dementia: Confused Professionals?* London: Jessica Kingsley.

An important text which examines the construction of dementia in Western society. Basing their work on an evaluation of community care services for people with dementia, the authors provide a critique of biomedical perspectives and apply social science theories to dementia and dementia care.

Henderson, J.N. & Vesperi, M.D., eds (1995) *The Culture of Long Term Care.* Westport: Bergin & Garvey.

An excellent compendium of ethnographic research that attempts to map the intricacies and intimacies of life for older people in nursing homes.

Jacques, A. (1997) Ethical dilemmas in care and research for people with dementia. In: Hunter, S. (ed.) *Dementia: Challenges and New Directions.* London: Jessica Kingsley.

Jones, J. & Miesen, B.M.L., eds (1992) *Care Giving in Dementia: Research and Applications.* London: Routledge.

This is a standard reference text which brings research into practice, in an accessible manner. Chapters 8–13 (Part II) are particularly relevant to institutionalised care, and offer useful, practical information for care workers trying to grasp an understanding of suitable care strategies in their everyday work.

Jones, R.G. (1993) Ethical and legal issues in the care of demented people. *Reviews in Clinical Gerontology* **3**, 55–68.

Jurnaid, O. & Bruce, J. (1994) Providing a community psychogeriatric service: models of community psychiatric nursing provision in a single health district. *International Journal of Geriatric Psychiatry* **9**, 715–720.

King's Fund (1996) *Living Well into Old Age: Applying Principles of Good Practice to Services for Elderly People with Severe Mental Disabilities.* London: King's Fund.

Kitwood, T. (1990) The dialectics of dementia: with particular reference to Alzheimer's disease. *Ageing and Society* **10**, 177–196.

A discussion of the effects of our attitudes and behaviour on the condition of people with dementia, including a useful list of the types of behaviour through which carers unwittingly diminish the personhood of their charges.

Kitwood, T. & Bredin, K. (1992) Towards a theory of dementia care: personhood and well-being. *Ageing and Society* **12**, 269–287.

A paper that describes new methodologies and new research agendas within dementia care.

Kitwood, T. (1995) Exploring the ethics of dementia research: a response to a response to Berghmans and Ter Meulen: a psycho-social perspective. *International Journal of Geriatric Psychiatry* **10**, 655–657.

Kitwood, T. & Benson, S., eds (1995) *The New Culture of Dementia Care.* Bradford: Hawker/Bradford Dementia Group.

This book attempts to challenge the stereotypes and misconceptions held by care workers, both inside and outside the field. It provides food for thought across a diverse arena, but the underpinning philosophy of maintaining the uniqueness of an individual is a common theme throughout. The content provides ideal material for stimulating lively debate, and if sensitively handled can facilitate a safe medium with which to express deeply held fears and reservations.

Kitwood, T. (1997) The experience of dementia. In: Kitwood, T. (ed.) *Dementia Reconsidered: The Person Comes First*, pp. 70–85. Buckingham: Open University Press.

The chapter provides an interesting overview of the literature on the subjective experience of dementia and suggests that people with dementia require comfort, attachment, inclusion, occupation and identity underpinned by expressions of love. The chapter will be of particular relevance to practitioners working with people with dementia within the context of a continuing relationship.

Lesser, R. & Milroy, L. (1993) *Linguistics and Aphasia: Psycholinguistic and Pragmatic Aspects of Intervention*. London: Longman.

Although this book is written about aphasia, it provides a useful introduction to conversation analysis and its application to disordered communication.

Lubinski, R., ed. (1991) *Dementia and Communication*. Philadelphia: BC Decker.

This book contains several chapters that address communication changes from the family perspective and explore the impact of the environment on those changes.

Mace, N., Rabins, P., Castleton, B., McEwen, E. & Meredith, B. (1992) *The 36 Hour Day: A Guide to Caring at Home for People with Alzheimer's Disease and Other Confusional Illnesses*, 2nd edn. London: Age Concern/Hodder & Stoughton.

This book provides practical advice but also gives health professionals a useful insight into the everyday experiences of caring for a person with dementia. Chapter 12 covers the emotional and physical aspects of caring, and case histories are usefully provided throughout the book.

Orbach, A. (1996) Remembering and forgetting. In: Orbach, A. (ed.) *Not Too late: Psychopathy and Ageing*, pp. 77–86. London: Jessica Kingsley.

This chapter provides an illuminating account of the value of psychoanalysis in working with older people with memory impairment. Discursive commentary on the meaning of language in 'senility' is also included in this chapter.

Procter, A. (1995) Ethical Issues in research with dementia patients: a neuroscience perspective – a response to Berghmans and Ter Meulen. *International Journal of Geriatric Psychiatry* **10**, 653–654.

Reed, J. & MacMillan, J. (1995) Friendship – the proper focus of care? *Reviews in Clincal Gerontology* **5**, 229–237.

A paper that describes new methodologies and new research agendas within dementia care.

Richardson, C.A., Gilleard, C.J., Lieberman, S. & Peeler, R. (1994) Working with older adults and their families – a review. *Journal of Family Therapy* **16**, 225–240.

This paper provides a much-needed review of family work with older people with mental health problems.

Rolfe, G. & Phillips, L.M. (1997) The development and role of an Advanced Nurse Practitioner in dementia – an action research project. *International Journal of Nursing Studies* **34**, 119–127.

Sabat, S.R. & Harré, R. (1992) The construction and deconstruction of self in Alzheimer's disease. *Ageing and Society* **12**, 443–461.

Like the Kitwood papers, this is an important discussion of the effects of our attitudes on people with dementia, and is especially relevant to this book because of its constructivist view of the self and its account of the importance of our recognising and responding to the attempts of someone with dementia to construct a social identity.

Seymour, J., Saunders, P., Wattis, J.P. & Daly, L. (1994) Evaluation of early dementia by a trained nurse. *International Journal of Geriatric Psychiatry* **9**, 37–42.

Spear, J. & Hertzberg, J. (1995) The community psychiatric nurse in the dementia service. *Current Opinion in Psychiatry* **8**, 237–239.

Tarman, V. (1988) Autobiography: the negotiation of a lifetime. *International Journal of Aging and Human Development* **27**, 171–191.

This studies the stories told by older people from a constructivist perspective, and stresses the use of such stories to counteract the stigma associated with old age.

Tennstedt, S., Crawford, S. & McKinlay, J. (1993) Determining the pattern of community care; is co-residence more important than the care giving relationship? *Journal of Gerontology* **48**, S74–S83.

This article provides some useful reading on the theme of partnership and the nature of the caregiving relationship. It raises some interesting points about the importance of co-residence, which contribute to the debate surrounding community care.

Terry, P. (1995) *Counselling the Elderly and Their Carers*. London: Macmillan.

Despite its title, this book is not about techniques but is an interesting account of the author's work as a clinical psychologist, working with older people and their carers. Aspects covered include ageing, loss and change and allow health professionals to reflect on their own work with older people.

Twigg, J. & Atkin, K. (1994) *Carers Perceived: Policy and Practice in Informal Care*. Buckingham: Open University Press.

An invaluable book which landmarks contemporary thinking about family caregiving. In this time of rapid change in conceptualisation of family caregiving, this book provides a very useful reference point.

Index